made INCREDIBLY

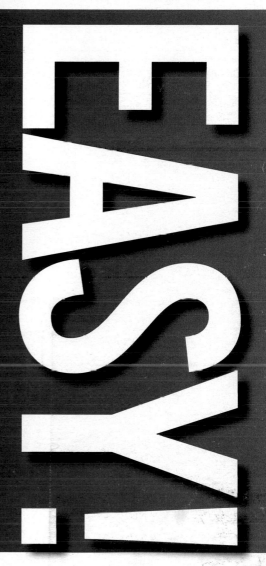

Dosage Calculations

Adapted for the UK by

William N Scott, BSc, MPhil, PhD
Lecturer in Biomedicine, School of
Nursing and Midwifery, Queen's
University Belfast

and

Deirdre McGrath, RN, BSc, MSc
Lecturer in Nursing, School of Nursing
and Midwifery, Queen's University
Belfast

First UK Edition

 Wolters Kluwer | Lippincott Williams & Wilkins
Health

Philadelphia · Baltimore · New York · London
Buenos Aires · Hong Kong · Sydney · Tokyo

Staff

Director, Global Publishing
Cathy Peck

Production Director
Chris Curtis

Senior Production Manager
Richard Owen

Production Editor
Amy Smith

Academic Marketing Executive
Alison Major

Copy Editor
Nik Prowse

Proofreader
Christine Whittle

Illustrator
Bot Roda

Printed in the UK by Stephens & George Ltd, Merthyr Tydfil, Wales. Typeset by Macmillan Publishing Solutions, New Delhi, India.

For information, write to Lippincott Williams & Wilkins, 250 Waterloo Road, London SE1 8RD.

British Library Cataloguing in Publication Data. A catalogue record for this book is available from the British Library.

ISBN13 978-1-901831-03-0
ISBN10 1-901831-03-5

Contents

Acknowledgements

Reviewers of the UK edition

Simone Bedford RN, Dip HE, BSc, PG Dip (Education)
Adult Branch Co-ordinator, School of Health Science, Swansea University

Margaret Buckley, RGN, MSc, RNT
Formerly Lecturer in Nursing, Swansea University

Jane Depledge RGN, MSc, PGDipEd, DipCPC, RNT, FHEA
Senior Lecturer, Buckinghamshire New University

Mrs Fiona Paul, MPhil, BN, RN, EN
Lecturer, School of Nursing and Midwifery, University of Dundee

Heulwen Morgan-Samuel, MSc, BSc, Dip Nursing, RGN
Nurse Tutor, Swansea University

Foreword

As a result of the ever-changing structure of UK healthcare, the role of the nurse has undergone considerable change over the last decade. Rapidly emerging technologies, and a clearer understanding of health and disease, have increased the demands placed on nursing staff. In many cases, nurses' remit now extends to the administration and prescription of medication – and with this additional responsibility comes a legal requirement for competency in dosage calculations.

The nurse is the last link in the chain to protect the patient from medication administration errors. Nurses are responsible for every dose that they administer and are held to the five 'rights' of medication administration: right medication, right dose, right route, right patient, and right time. It may seem daunting and confusing at times, but, with effort, practice and diligence – and *Dosage Calculations Made Incredibly Easy*, First UK Edition – you can be confident in your medication administration every time!

Adapted specifically for the UK healthcare system, this book is the perfect resource to be used in a class or by a self-directed learner who wants to improve their dosage calculations knowledge and skills. It tackles complex dosage calculations in an easy-to-understand manner. However, the text goes beyond being solely a calculations resource – it also incorporates many aspects of current UK practice.

Dosage Calculations Made Incredibly Easy, First UK Edition, starts with the basics. Part I presents fractions, decimals, percentages, ratios and proportions. Part II introduces the metric system, and also discusses unit and millimole systems. Part III looks at what constitutes a legal prescription, looks at the abbreviations that are used and presents the essentials of documentation. This section also includes a chapter devoted to preventing errors and promoting patient safety. Part IV covers oral, topical and rectal drugs. Part V focuses on parenteral administration. Part VI deals with special considerations for paediatric, obstetric and critical care patients.

Entertaining and amusing sketches lighten the tone, making the topics less threatening and more inviting. Objectives at the beginning of each chapter tell you what you'll learn, the body of the chapter teaches crucial information and 'That's a wrap!' summaries provide a review at the end of each chapter. 'Quick quiz' lets you validate that learning has occurred. A recurring section called 'Real-world problems' provides opportunities to perform calculation and conversion using real-life situations.

Icons interspersed throughout the book highlight important information and key concepts:

'Before you give that drug!' contains urgent advice on how to avoid dangerous drug errors.

'Advice from the experts' provides pointers on how to maintain dosage accuracy.

'For maths phobics only' directs you to helpful hints, tips and illustrations to help you get over the 'I hate maths' hurdles.

'Memory jogger' offers mnemonics and other aids to help you understand and remember difficult concepts.

The appendices are also invaluable. In addition to the glossary, a table of conversions and a summary of dosage calculation formulas have been added to this edition. Additional multiple-choice questions are included in the 'Practice makes perfect' section.

You can be a safe, competent nurse, protecting your patient from medication errors. *Dosage Calculations Made Incredibly Easy*, First UK Edition, is a great tool that can help you achieve that crucial goal!

William N Scott, BSc, MPhil, PhD
Lecturer in Biomedicine
School of Nursing and Midwifery
Faculty of Medicine, Health and
Life Sciences
Queen's University, Belfast

Contributors and consultants to the US edition

Melody C Antoon, RN, MSN
Instructor of Nursing
Lamar State College
Port Arthur, Tex.

Christine Frazer, RN, MSN, CNS
Nursing Instructor
Pennsylvania State University
Hershey

Julia A Greenawalt, RNC, MA, MSN
Adjunct Faculty
University of Pittsburgh
School Nurse
Seneca Valley School District
Harmony, Pa.

Nancy Haynes, RN, MN, CCRN
Assistant Professor of Nursing
Saint Luke's College
Kansas City, Mo.

Patricia Lange-Otsuka, APRN, BC, EdD, MSN
Associate Professor of Nursing
Hawaii Pacific University
Kaneohe

Kathy Latch Johnson, RN, MSN
Assistant Professor of Nursing
Baptist College of Health Sciences
Memphis

Linda May-Ludwig, RN, BS, MEd
Practical Nursing Instructor
Canadian Valley Technology Center
El Reno, Okla.

Catherine Todd Magel, RN, BC, EdD
Assistant Professor
Villanova (Pa.) University College of Nursing

Patricia O'Brien, RN, BS, MSN, APRN
Family Nurse Practitioner
Associate Professor, Graduate Nursing
Winona State University
Rochester, Minn.

Terri M Perkins, RN, MN
Instructor, Associate Degree Nursing Program
Bellevue (Wash.) Community College

Dana Reeves, RN, MSN
Assistant Professor
University of Arkansas
Fort Smith

Allison Jones Terry, RN, MSN
Director of Community Certification
State of Alabama Department
   of Mental Health and Mental
   Retardation
Montgomery

Karen Wilkinson, ARNP, MN
Nurse Practitioner, Pain
   Management Program
Children's Hospital and Regional
   Medical Center
Seattle

Sharon Wing, RN, MSN
Assistant Professor
Cleveland State University

Part I

Basic calculations

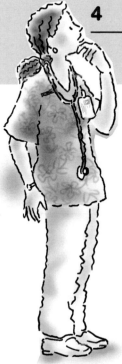

1 Fractions

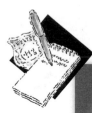

Just the facts

In this chapter, you'll learn:

♦ what a fraction is

♦ about different types of fractions you may use

♦ how to convert fractions, reduce them to their lowest terms and find the lowest common denominator

♦ how to add, subtract, multiply and divide fractions.

A look at fractions

A fraction represents the division of one number by another number. It's a mathematical expression for parts of a whole. (See *Parts of a whole.*)

Parts of a whole

In any fraction, the numerator (top number) and the denominator (bottom number) represent the parts of a whole. The denominator describes the total number of equal parts in the whole; the numerator describes the number of parts being considered.

> The numerator 5 over the denominator 16 shows that we're considering 5 parts out of 16.

> The numerator is on the top.

> The denominator is on the bottom.

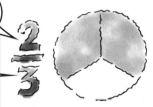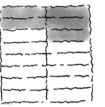

Getting to the bottom of it

The bottom number, or *denominator*, represents the total number of equal parts in the whole. The larger the denominator, the greater the number of equal parts. For example, in the fraction ⅗, the denominator 5 indicates that the whole has been divided into five equal parts. In the fraction ⁷⁄₁₂, the denominator 12 indicates that the whole has been divided into 12 equal parts. So, as the denominator becomes larger, the size of the parts becomes smaller.

Staying on top of it

The top number, or *numerator*, signifies the number of parts of the whole being considered. For example, in the fraction ⅗, only 3 of the 5 equal parts are being considered. In the fraction ⁷⁄₁₂, only 7 of the 12 equal parts are being considered.

Types of fractions

There are four types of fraction:
* common
* complex
* proper
* improper.

Common and complex

In a common fraction, such as ⅔, both the numerator and denominator are whole numbers.

In a complex fraction, the numerator and denominator are fractions. For example:

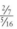

$$\frac{2/7}{5/16}$$

Proper and improper

In a proper fraction, such as ¼, the numerator is smaller than the denominator.

In an improper fraction, such as ⁸⁄₇ or ¹¹⁄₄, the numerator is larger than the denominator. In other words, it's top heavy. An improper fraction represents a number that's greater than 1.

An improper fraction can also be expressed as a mixed number; that is, a whole number and a fraction. Therefore, ⁸⁄₇ can be rewritten as 1⅐ and ¹¹⁄₄ can be rewritten as 2¾.

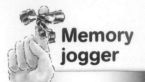

Memory jogger

To remember which number is the numerator and which is the denominator in a fraction, think of:

Nursing

Diagnosis

The **N**umerator is on the top; the **D**enominator is on the bottom.

Working with fractions

You can manipulate fractions in three ways:
- converting mixed numbers to improper fractions and vice versa
- reducing fractions to their lowest terms
- finding a common denominator.

Converting mixed numbers to improper fractions

To convert a mixed number to an improper fraction, follow these steps:

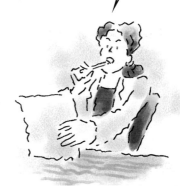

Learning the proper way to make improper fractions takes practice!

☝ Multiply the denominator by the whole number.

✌ Add the product, or resulting number, from the first step to the numerator (this gives you a new numerator).

🖐 Leave the denominator as it is.

Three incredibly easy steps

For example, to convert the mixed number 5⅓ to an improper fraction:

☝ Multiply the denominator 3 by the whole number 5, for a total of 15.

✌ Add 15 to the numerator 1, for a new numerator of 16.

🖐 Leave the denominator as it is. The improper fraction is ¹⁶⁄₃.

$$5\tfrac{1}{3} \text{ is } \frac{16}{3}$$

Encore!

Here's another example! To convert the mixed number 8⅘ to an improper fraction:

☝ Multiply the denominator 5 by the whole number 8, for a total of 40.

✌ Add 40 to the numerator 4, for a new numerator of 44.

🖐 Leave the denominator as it is. The improper fraction is ⁴⁴⁄₅.

$$8\tfrac{4}{5} \text{ is } \frac{44}{5}$$

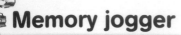

Memory jogger

Here's a way to remember how to convert mixed numbers to improper fractions. Think **MAST**: **M**ultiply, **A**dd and **S**tack on **T**op.

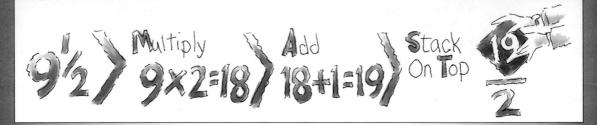

Putting it in reverse

At times, you may want to convert improper fractions back to mixed numbers. To convert the improper fraction $\frac{16}{3}$ back to a mixed number:

Divide the numerator 16 by the denominator 3. When you do this, you get 5 with 1 left over.

The 1 becomes the new numerator, and the denominator stays the same.

The mixed number is $5\frac{1}{3}$.

$$\frac{16}{3} \text{ is } 5\tfrac{1}{3}$$

One more time

To convert the improper fraction $\frac{44}{5}$ back into a mixed number:

Divide the numerator 44 by the denominator 5. The answer is 8 with 4 left over.

Place the 4 over the 5.

The mixed number is $8\frac{4}{5}$.

$$\frac{44}{5} \text{ is } 8\tfrac{4}{5}$$

Reducing fractions to lowest terms

For simplicity's sake, a fraction should usually be reduced to its lowest terms; that is, to the smallest numbers possible in the numerator and denominator. To simplify a fraction, follow these steps:

Determine the largest common divisor of the numerator and the denominator: the largest number by which both can be divided equally.

Divide both the numerator and denominator by that number to reduce the fraction to its lowest terms.

Example numero uno

To reduce the fraction $^8/_{10}$ to its lowest terms:

Determine the largest common divisor of 8 and 10, which is 2.

Divide the numerator and denominator by 2 to reduce the fraction to its lowest terms, or $^4/_5$.

$$\frac{8}{10} \text{ is } \frac{8 \div 2}{10 \div 2} \text{ is } \frac{4}{5}$$

Missed it? Watch again!

To reduce the fraction $^7/_{14}$ to its lowest terms:

Determine that the number 7 is the largest divisor that 7 and 14 have in common.

Divide the numerator and the denominator by 7 to reduce the fraction to its lowest terms, or $^1/_2$. This fraction can't be reduced further.

$$\frac{7}{14} \text{ is } \frac{7 \div 7}{14 \div 7} \text{ is } \frac{1}{2}$$

One more time

To reduce the fraction $^2/_{10}$ to its lowest terms:

Determine that the number 2 is the largest divisor that 2 and 10 have in common.

Divide the numerator and the denominator by 2 to reduce the fraction to its lowest terms, or $^1/_5$.

$$\frac{2}{10} \text{ is } \frac{2 \div 2}{10 \div 2} \text{ is } \frac{1}{5}$$

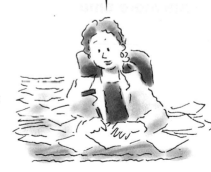

Reducing a fraction to its lowest terms will make my life simpler!

Finding a common denominator

One way to find a common denominator for a set of fractions is to multiply all the denominators. For example, to find a common denominator for the fractions ⅖ and ⁷⁄₁₀, multiply the denominators 5 and 10 to get the multiplied common denominator 50:

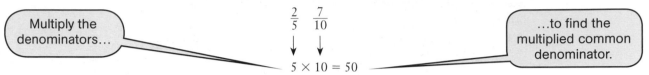

Multiply the denominators...

$$\frac{2}{5} \quad \frac{7}{10}$$

$$5 \times 10 = 50$$

...to find the multiplied common denominator.

To find the multiplied common denominator of the set of fractions ⅛, ¼ and ⅕, simply multiply all the denominators together to find the common denominator 160:

$$8 \times 4 \times 5 = 160$$

Lowest common denominator

Unfortunately, multiplying all the denominators of a set of fractions won't always give you the lowest common denominator. The *lowest common denominator* or *least common multiple* – the smallest number that is a multiple of all the denominators in a set of fractions – is an important tool for working with fractions.

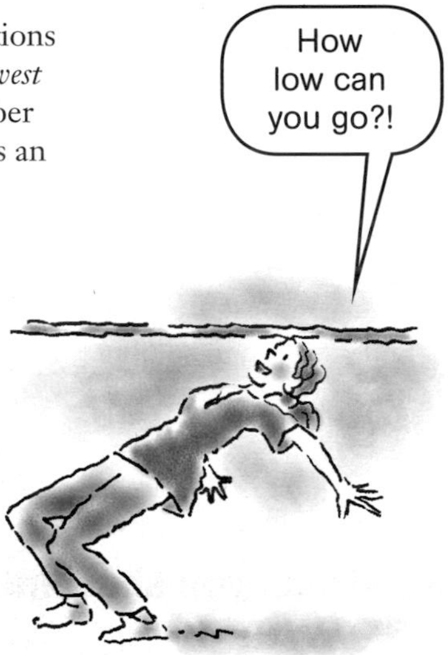

How low can you go?

One way to find the lowest common denominator of a set of fractions is to work with its prime factors. A *prime number* is a number that's evenly divisible only by 1 and itself. Some prime numbers are 2, 3, 5 and 7. *Prime factors* are prime numbers that can be divided into some part of a mathematical expression, in this case, the denominators in a set of fractions.

How low can you go?!

Prime factoring

Let's say you want to find the lowest common denominator for ⅛, ¼ and ⅕. Here's a useful technique, called *prime factoring*:
* Make a table with two headings: 'Prime factors' and 'Denominators'.
* Write the denominators 8, 4 and 5 over the top right-hand columns.

Prime factors	Denominators		
	8	4	5

* Divide the three denominators by the prime factors for each, starting with the smallest prime factor by which one of the denominators can be divided – in this case, 2. Write 2 in the left-hand

column and divide the denominators by it. (Divide the denominator 8 by the prime factor 2 and write the answer, 4, in the column under the 8. Then divide the denominator 4 by the prime factor 2 and write the answer, 2, in the column under the denominator 4.)
• Bring down the numbers in the right-hand columns that aren't evenly divisible by the prime factor in the left-hand column. (In this case, the denominator 5 isn't divisible by the prime factor 2, so just bring the 5 down.)

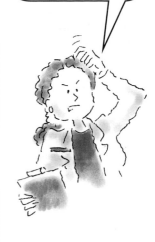

Primarily, I have to remember to divide denominators by the *smallest* prime first!

Prime factors	Denominators		
	8	4	5
2	4	2	5

• Repeat this process until the numbers in the bottom row can't be divided further.

Prime factors	Denominators		
	8	4	5
2	4	2	5
2	2	1	5
2	1	1	5

• Then multiply the prime factors in the left-hand column by the numbers in the bottom row. To say it with numbers:

$$2 \times 2 \times 2 \times 1 \times 1 \times 5 = 40$$

• The lowest common denominator for this set of fractions is 40.

Wow! Can you show me again?

OK. Let's use prime factoring to find the lowest common denominator for ⅛ and ⅚. Create a table that lists the denominators horizontally; then find the prime factors.
• Set up a table like this:

Prime factors	Denominators	
	8	6
2	4	3
2	2	3
2	1	3

- Then multiply the prime factors in the left-hand column by the numbers in the bottom row:

$$2 \times 2 \times 2 \times 1 \times 3 = 24$$

> Lowest common denominator

Once more, please

Now, use prime factoring to find the lowest common denominator for $\frac{1}{3}$, $\frac{1}{4}$ and $\frac{1}{2}$.
- Set up the table:

Prime factors	Denominators		
	3	4	2
2	3	2	1
2	3	1	1

> Yes! I finally get it! I'm Dominator of the denominators now!

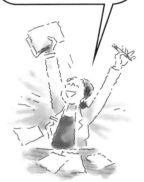

- Then multiply the prime factors in the left-hand column by the numbers in the bottom row:

$$2 \times 2 \times 3 \times 1 \times 1 = 12$$

> Lowest common denominator

Converting fractions

When you know the lowest common denominator of a set of fractions, you can *convert* the fractions so that they all have the same denominator: the *lowest common denominator*.

One way to convert a set of fractions is to multiply each fraction by 1 in the form of a fraction; that is, a fraction with the same number in the numerator and denominator. You can find this fraction by taking the lowest common denominator and dividing it by the original denominator.

Here's what the formula looks like:

$$\frac{\text{original}}{\text{fraction}} \times \frac{\text{lowest common denominator} \div \text{original denominator}}{\text{lowest common denominator} \div \text{original denominator}}$$

> This is how you convert a fraction using 1 in the form of a fraction.

Conversion excursion

Convert the set of fractions $\frac{1}{8}$, $\frac{1}{4}$ and $\frac{1}{5}$ so that each has the lowest common denominator. We already know that the lowest common denominator for this set of fractions is 40.
- Here's the conversion of the first fraction, $\frac{1}{8}$, to $\frac{5}{40}$:

$$\frac{1}{8} = \frac{1}{8} \times \frac{40 \div 8}{40 \div 8} = \frac{1}{8} \times \frac{5}{5} = \frac{1 \times 5}{8 \times 5} = \frac{5}{40}$$

- Convert the next fraction, ¼, to ¹⁰⁄₄₀:

$$\frac{1}{4} = \frac{1}{4} \times \frac{40 \div 4}{40 \div 4} = \frac{1}{4} \times \frac{10}{10} = \frac{1 \times 10}{4 \times 10} = \frac{10}{40}$$

- Convert the last fraction in the set, ⅕, to ⁸⁄₄₀:

$$\frac{1}{5} = \frac{1}{5} \times \frac{40 \div 5}{40 \div 5} = \frac{1}{5} \times \frac{8}{8} = \frac{1 \times 8}{5 \times 8} = \frac{8}{40}$$

Do it again

This is how to convert ⅜ and ⅚ to fractions with the lowest common denominator, which is 24.
- Convert the first fraction, ⅜, to ⁹⁄₂₄:

$$\frac{3}{8} = \frac{3}{8} \times \frac{24 \div 8}{24 \div 8} = \frac{3}{8} \times \frac{3}{3} = \frac{3 \times 3}{8 \times 3} = \frac{9}{24}$$

- Convert the other fraction, ⅚, to ²⁰⁄₂₄:

$$\frac{5}{6} = \frac{5}{8} \times \frac{24 \div 6}{24 \div 6} = \frac{5}{6} \times \frac{4}{4} = \frac{5 \times 4}{6 \times 4} = \frac{20}{24}$$

Once more

OK. Now convert ⅓, ¼ and ½ to fractions with the lowest common denominator, which is 12.
- Convert ⅓ to ⁴⁄₁₂:

$$\frac{1}{3} = \frac{1}{3} \times \frac{12 \div 3}{12 \div 3} = \frac{1}{3} \times \frac{4}{4} = \frac{1 \times 4}{3 \times 4} = \frac{4}{12}$$

- Convert ¼ to ³⁄₁₂:

$$\frac{1}{4} = \frac{1}{4} \times \frac{12 \div 4}{12 \div 4} = \frac{1}{4} \times \frac{3}{3} = \frac{1 \times 3}{4 \times 3} = \frac{3}{12}$$

- Convert the last fraction, ½, to ⁶⁄₁₂:

$$\frac{1}{2} = \frac{1}{2} \times \frac{12 \div 2}{12 \div 2} = \frac{1}{2} \times \frac{6}{6} = \frac{1 \times 6}{2 \times 6} = \frac{6}{12}$$

Divide and conquer

You can also convert a set of fractions by using long division. To convert each fraction, follow these steps:

Divide the lowest common denominator by the original denominator.

Multiply the *quotient*, or resulting number, by the original numerator to determine the new numerator.

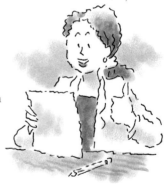

Hey, I'm getting pretty good at this!

Place the new numerator over the lowest common denominator. Here's how to set up the conversion for each fraction:

$$\underset{\substack{\text{original} \\ \text{denominator}}}{} \overline{)\,\underset{\substack{\text{lowest common} \\ \text{denominator}}}{\text{quotient}}} \overset{\substack{\text{original} \\ \text{}}}{\times} \text{numerator} = \frac{\text{new numerator}}{\substack{\text{lowest common} \\ \text{denominator}}}$$

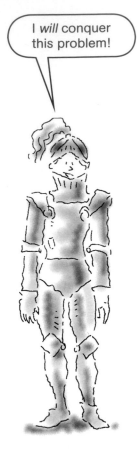

I *will* conquer this problem!

Set 'em up

This is how to convert ⅜, ¼ and ⅖. The lowest common denominator is 40.
*   Convert the first fraction in the set, ⅜, to ¹⁵⁄₄₀:

$$\frac{3}{8} = 8\overline{)40}^{\,5} \times 3 = \frac{15}{40}$$

*   Convert ¼ to ¹⁰⁄₄₀:

$$\frac{1}{4} = 4\overline{)40}^{\,10} \times 1 = \frac{10}{40}$$

*   Convert ⅖ to ¹⁶⁄₄₀:

$$\frac{2}{5} = 5\overline{)40}^{\,8} \times 2 = \frac{16}{40}$$

Amazing! Let's see that again

This is how to convert ⅜ and ⅚. The lowest common denominator is 24.
*   Convert the fraction ⅜ to ⁹⁄₂₄:

$$\frac{3}{8} = 8\overline{)24}^{\,3} \times 3 = \frac{9}{24}$$

*   Convert ⅚ to ²⁰⁄₂₄:

$$\frac{5}{6} = 6\overline{)24}^{\,4} \times 5 = \frac{20}{24}$$

One last time

And this is how to convert ⅓, ¼ and ½. The lowest common denominator is 12.
*   Convert ⅓ to ⁴⁄₁₂:

$$\frac{1}{3} = 3\overline{)12}^{\,4} \times 1 = \frac{4}{12}$$

*   Convert ¼ to ³⁄₁₂:

$$\frac{1}{4} = 4\overline{)12}^{\,3} \times 1 = \frac{3}{12}$$

- Convert ½ to 6/12:

$$\frac{1}{2} = 2\overline{)12}^{\;6} \times 1 = \frac{6}{12}$$

Comparing fraction size

Why are these calculations important? Because finding the lowest common denominator in a set of fractions allows you to compare the *relative size* of the fractions. (See *Denominators can be deceptive*.)

Consider the following set of fractions: 1/100, 1/150 and 1/200. Which of these do you think is largest? Follow these steps:

 Using the prime factor method, first find the lowest common denominator for these three fractions. The table looks like this:

Prime factors	Denominators		
	100	150	200
2	50	75	100
2	25	75	50
5	5	15	10
5	1	3	2

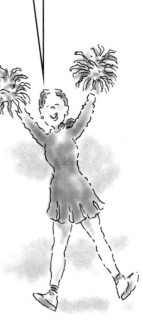

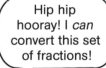
Hip hip hooray! I *can* convert this set of fractions!

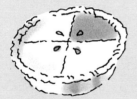

For maths phobics only

Denominators can be deceptive

If you were hungry, would you rather have 1 slice from a pie that was cut into 4 slices, 8 slices, or 16 slices? You'd choose 4, of course, because the slices would be bigger. You can judge the size of fractions the same way. When the fractions all have the same numerators — in this case, ¼, ⅛ and 1/16 — the fraction with the lowest denominator is the biggest one. Don't fall into the trap of thinking that the bigger the denominator, the bigger the fraction. Think in terms of a pie, as shown below.

 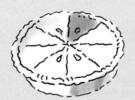 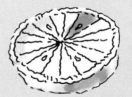

Then multiply the prime factors in the left column and the numbers in the bottom row. In other words:

$$2 \times 2 \times 5 \times 5 \times 1 \times 3 \times 2 = 600$$

> Lowest common denominator

Finding common ground

Next, convert all three fractions – $\frac{1}{100}$, $\frac{1}{150}$ and $\frac{1}{200}$ – to new fractions with the lowest common denominator of 600. To do this, multiply each fraction by 1 in the form of a fraction (create this fraction by dividing the lowest common denominator by the original denominator).

Here's the conversion:

- The fraction $\frac{1}{100}$ is converted to $\frac{6}{600}$:

$$\frac{1}{100} = \frac{1}{100} \times \frac{600 \div 100}{600 \div 100} = \frac{1}{100} \times \frac{6}{6} = \frac{1 \times 6}{100 \times 6} = \frac{6}{600}$$

- $\frac{1}{150}$ is converted to $\frac{4}{600}$:

$$\frac{1}{150} = \frac{1}{150} \times \frac{600 \div 150}{600 \div 150} = \frac{1}{150} \times \frac{4}{4} = \frac{1 \times 4}{150 \times 4} = \frac{4}{600}$$

- $\frac{1}{200}$ is converted to $\frac{3}{600}$:

$$\frac{1}{200} = \frac{1}{200} \times \frac{600 \div 200}{600 \div 200} = \frac{1}{200} \times \frac{3}{3} = \frac{1 \times 3}{200 \times 3} = \frac{3}{600}$$

Comparing the three final fractions, you'll see that $\frac{1}{100}$ is the largest of these: $\frac{6}{600}$.

Same destination, different route

You can arrive at the same conclusion by dividing the lowest common denominator (600) by the denominator, multiplying the numerator by the number obtained and placing the result over the lowest common denominator.

- The fraction $\frac{1}{100}$ is converted to $\frac{6}{600}$ this way:

$$\frac{1}{100} = 100\overline{)600}^{\,6} \times 1 = \frac{6}{600}$$

- $\frac{1}{150}$ is converted to $\frac{4}{600}$:

$$\frac{1}{150} = 150\overline{)600}^{\,4} \times 1 = \frac{4}{600}$$

- $\frac{1}{200}$ is converted to $\frac{3}{600}$:

$$\frac{1}{200} = 200\overline{)600}^{\,3} \times 1 = \frac{3}{600}$$

> Hmm…it appears there are two ways to arrive at the same conclusion.

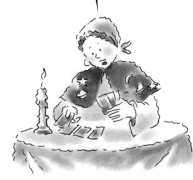

Fraction fact

When comparing fractions that have common denominators, the fraction with the largest numerator is the largest number. In the set of fractions above, $\frac{9}{600}$ is the largest number.

A common hero

The lowest common denominator also enables you to add and subtract fractions. Reducing fractions to their lowest terms and converting improper fractions to mixed numbers let you present the answers to addition, subtraction, multiplication and division problems in a useful way.

Remember: Whenever you perform these functions, always reduce the final answer to its lowest terms and, if it's an improper fraction, convert it to a mixed number.

Adding fractions

To add fractions, first convert them to fractions with common denominators. (See *Comparing apples with apples*.)

It all adds up

Here's an example of adding fractions. Follow the steps below to add the fractions $\frac{1}{2}$ and $\frac{1}{3}$.

Comparing apples with apples

When adding or subtracting fractions, don't forget to convert them to fractions with common denominators. That way, you'll be comparing apples with apples.

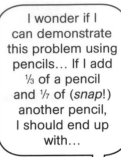

> I wonder if I can demonstrate this problem using pencils… If I add ⅓ of a pencil and ⅐ of (*snap!*) another pencil, I should end up with…

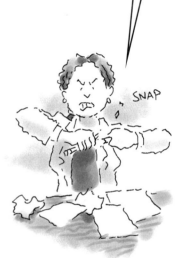

SNAP

Find the lowest common denominator. Because the denominators in ⅐ and ⅓ are both prime numbers, multiply 7 by 3 to find the lowest common denominator, 21.

Then convert the fractions by multiplying each by 1 (in the form of a fraction) to yield fractions with the lowest common denominator.

Start by converting ⅐ to ³⁄₂₁:

$$\frac{1}{7} = \frac{1}{7} \times \frac{21 \div 7}{21 \div 7} = \frac{1}{7} \times \frac{3}{3} = \frac{1 \times 3}{7 \times 3} = \frac{3}{21}$$

Then convert ⅓ to ⁷⁄₂₁:

$$\frac{1}{3} = \frac{1}{3} \times \frac{21 \div 3}{21 \div 3} = \frac{1}{3} \times \frac{7}{7} = \frac{1 \times 3}{3 \times 7} = \frac{7}{21}$$

Now, add the new fractions. To add fractions with a common denominator, add the numerators and place the result over the common denominator. The resulting fraction is your answer. (Reduce it to its lowest terms, if possible.)

$$\frac{3}{21} + \frac{7}{21} = \frac{3 + 7}{21} = \frac{10}{21}$$

Additional addition

To add ½ and ⅕, follow these steps:

Find the lowest common denominator. In this case, because the denominators 2 and 5 are both prime numbers, multiply 2 by 5 to find the lowest common denominator, 10.

Convert the fractions by multiplying each by 1 (in the form of a fraction) to yield fractions with the lowest common denominator.

Convert the fraction ½ to ⁵⁄₁₀:

$$\frac{1}{2} = \frac{1}{2} \times \frac{10 \div 2}{10 \div 2} = \frac{1}{2} \times \frac{5}{5} = \frac{1 \times 5}{2 \times 5} = \frac{5}{10}$$

Then convert ⅕ to ²⁄₁₀:

$$\frac{1}{5} = \frac{1}{5} \times \frac{10 \div 5}{10 \div 5} = \frac{1}{5} \times \frac{2}{2} = \frac{1 \times 2}{5 \times 2} = \frac{2}{10}$$

Now, add the converted fractions. To do this, add the numerators and place the result over the common denominator:

$$\frac{5}{10} + \frac{2}{10} = \frac{5+2}{10} = \frac{7}{10}$$

Another additional addition

To add ⅗ and ⅔, follow these steps:

Find the lowest common denominator – in this case, 15.

Convert the fractions by multiplying each by 1 (in the form of a fraction) to yield fractions with the lowest common denominator.

Convert ⅗ to %₁₅:

$$\frac{3}{5} = \frac{3}{5} \times \frac{15 \div 5}{15 \div 5} = \frac{3}{5} \times \frac{3}{3} = \frac{3 \times 3}{5 \times 3} = \frac{9}{15}$$

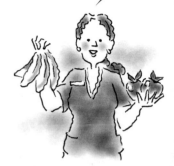

Apples with apples? Why do I end up with apples and bananas?

Then convert ⅔ to ¹⁰⁄₁₅:

$$\frac{2}{3} = \frac{2}{3} \times \frac{15 \div 3}{15 \div 3} = \frac{2}{3} \times \frac{5}{5} = \frac{2 \times 5}{3 \times 5} = \frac{10}{15}$$

To add the converted fractions, add the new numerators and place the result over the common denominator:

$$\frac{9}{15} + \frac{10}{15} = \frac{9 + 10}{15} = \frac{19}{15}$$

It all adds up!

Reduce the fraction to its lowest terms:

$$\frac{19}{15} = 1\frac{4}{15}$$

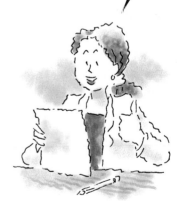

Subtracting fractions

Like addition, subtraction requires converting fractions to terms with common denominators.

Fraction subtraction

Here's an example of how to subtract one fraction from another. Follow the steps below to subtract ⅙ from ⁵⁄₁₂.

Find the lowest common denominator in this case, 12. The fraction ⁵⁄₁₂ already has the lowest common denominator.

Convert the fraction ⅙ to a fraction with the lowest common denominator. To do this, multiply the fraction by the number 1 (in the form of a fraction):

$$\frac{1}{6} = \frac{1}{6} \times \frac{12 \div 6}{12 \div 6} = \frac{1}{6} \times \frac{2}{2} = \frac{1 \times 2}{6 \times 2} = \frac{2}{12}$$

Now, subtract the numerators and place the result over the common denominator:

$$\frac{5}{12} - \frac{2}{12} = \frac{5 - 2}{12} = \frac{3}{12}$$

Reduce the fraction to its lowest terms, if possible. The resulting fraction is your answer:

$$\frac{3}{12} = \frac{1}{4}$$

A second subtraction

To subtract ⅑ from ⅚, follow these steps:

Find the lowest common denominator – in this case, 18. (To find the lowest common denominator in this case, try prime factoring on your own.)

Convert the fractions to those with the lowest common denominator by multiplying each fraction by the number 1 (in the form of a fraction).

Convert ⅚ to ¹⁵⁄₁₈:

$$\frac{5}{6} = \frac{5}{6} \times \frac{18 \div 6}{18 \div 6} = \frac{5}{6} \times \frac{3}{3} = \frac{5 \times 3}{6 \times 3} = \frac{15}{18}$$

Then convert ⅑ to ²⁄₁₈:

$$\frac{1}{9} = \frac{1}{9} \times \frac{18 \div 9}{18 \div 9} = \frac{1}{9} \times \frac{2}{2} = \frac{1 \times 2}{9 \times 2} = \frac{2}{18}$$

Then subtract the numerators and place the result over the common denominator. Reduce the fraction to its lowest terms, if possible. In this case, the fraction can't be reduced:

$$\frac{15}{18} - \frac{2}{18} = \frac{15 - 2}{18} = \frac{13}{18}$$

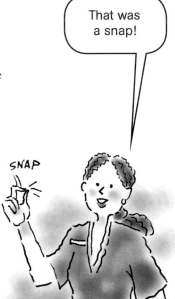

That was a snap!

SNAP

More subtraction action

To subtract ¼ from ⅔, follow these steps:

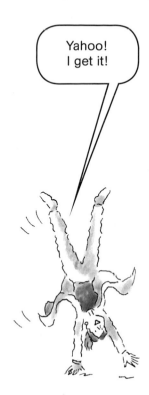

Yahoo!
I get it!

Find the lowest common denominator – in this case, 12.

Convert the fractions to those with the lowest common denominator by multiplying each fraction by the number 1 (in the form of a fraction).

Convert ⅔ to ⁸⁄₁₂:

$$\frac{2}{3} = \frac{2}{3} \times \frac{12 \div 3}{12 \div 3} = \frac{2}{3} \times \frac{4}{4} = \frac{2 \times 4}{3 \times 4} = \frac{8}{12}$$

Convert ¼ to ³⁄₁₂:

$$\frac{1}{4} = \frac{1}{4} \times \frac{12 \div 4}{12 \div 4} = \frac{1}{4} \times \frac{3}{3} = \frac{1 \times 3}{4 \times 3} = \frac{3}{12}$$

Subtract the numerators and place the result over the common denominator:

$$\frac{8}{12} - \frac{3}{12} = \frac{8-3}{12} = \frac{5}{12}$$

Multiplying fractions

Good news! There's no need to convert to common denominators when multiplying fractions. Simply multiply the numerators and denominators in turn to find the product.

For example, to multiply ⁴⁄₇ by ⅝, multiply the numerators 4 and 5 and the denominators 7 and 8 to get a new fraction. Here's the calculation:

• Set up the equation:

$$\frac{4}{7} \times \frac{5}{8}$$

• Multiply the numerators and multiply the denominators:

$$\frac{4 \times 5}{7 \times 8} = \frac{20}{56}$$

• Reduce the answer to its lowest terms:

$$\frac{5}{14}$$

Let's see it again!

To multiply ⅚ by ⅓, multiply the numerators 5 and 1 and the denominators 6 and 3 to get the answer:

$$\frac{5}{6} \times \frac{1}{3} = \frac{5 \times 1}{6 \times 3} = \frac{5}{18}$$

A whole other matter

To multiply a fraction by a whole number, for example ⅑ by 4, follow these simple steps:
* First, convert the whole number 4 to the fraction ⁴⁄₁.
* Then multiply the numerators and denominators. The complete calculation looks like this:

$$\frac{1}{9} \times 4 = \frac{1}{9} \times \frac{4}{1} = \frac{1 \times 4}{9 \times 1} = \frac{4}{9}$$

Dividing fractions

In division (as in multiplication), you don't need to convert the fractions but you do need to invert the divisor. Division problems are usually written as two fractions separated by a division sign. The first fraction is the number to be divided (the *dividend*), and the second fraction is the number doing the dividing (the *divisor*); the answer is the *quotient*. (See *Divvying up the problem* for a quick review.)
To divide ⁵⁄₇ by ⅔, first set up the problem:

> This fraction is the dividend.

$$\frac{5}{7} \div \frac{2}{3}$$

> This fraction is the divisor.

To divide fractions, multiply the dividend by the divisor's *reciprocal*, or the inverted divisor.
* To divide ⁵⁄₇ by ⅔ (the divisor), first multiply ⁵⁄₇ (the dividend) by ³⁄₂ (the divisor's reciprocal):

$$\frac{5}{7} \div \frac{2}{3} = \frac{5}{7} \times \frac{3}{2}$$

> Here's the divisor's reciprocal.

* Then complete the calculation and reduce the answer (the quotient) to its lowest terms:

$$\frac{5 \times 3}{7 \times 2} = \frac{15}{14} = 1\frac{1}{14}$$

A part divided by a whole

To divide a fraction by a whole number, use the same principle.

Divvying up the problem

Before you can divide numbers, you need to know what each part of a division problem is called. The division problem below can be written two different ways, but the terms remain the same.

> Divisor

> Dividend

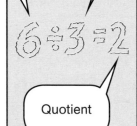

> Quotient

> Quotient

> Divisor

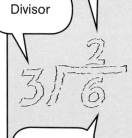

> Dividend

- To divide ⅗ by 2, first convert the whole number 2 to the fraction 2/1:

$$\frac{3}{5} \div 2 = \frac{3}{5} \div \frac{2}{1}$$

- Then multiply the dividend (⅗) by the reciprocal of the divisor (½). Reduce the answer to its lowest terms:

$$\frac{3}{5} \times \frac{1}{2} = \frac{3 \times 1}{5 \times 2} = \frac{3}{10}$$

In this case, the answer can't be further reduced.

Making things less complex

In complex fractions, the numerators and denominators are fractions themselves. Complex fractions can be simplified by following the rules for division of fractions. Think of the line separating the two fractions as a division sign. For example, follow the simple steps below to simplify the complex fraction:

$$\frac{\tfrac{1}{3}}{\tfrac{5}{8}}$$

First, rewrite the complex fraction as a division problem:

$$\frac{\tfrac{1}{3}}{\tfrac{5}{8}} = \frac{1}{3} \div \frac{5}{8}$$

Multiply the dividend (⅓) by the reciprocal of the divisor (⅝):

$$\frac{1}{3} \times \frac{8}{5}$$

Lastly, complete the calculation:

$$\frac{1 \times 8}{3 \times 5} = \frac{8}{15}$$

Real-world problem

A nurse is calculating a patient's recent fluid intake. In the past 8 hours, the patient drank ½ of a cup of milk, ⅔ of a cup of orange juice and ¾ of a cup of water. How many cups of liquid has the patient had to drink?

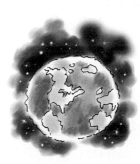

Adding for a liquid solution

To solve this problem, you need to add fractions.

- First, find the lowest common denominator for ½, ⅔ and ¾ – in this case, 12.
- Next, convert each fraction by multiplying each by 1 (in the form of a fraction) to yield fractions with the lowest common denominator:

$$\frac{1}{2} = \frac{1}{2} \times \frac{12 \div 2}{12 \div 2} = \frac{1}{2} \times \frac{6}{6} = \frac{1 \times 6}{2 \times 6} = \frac{6}{12}$$

$$\frac{2}{3} = \frac{2}{3} \times \frac{12 \div 3}{12 \div 3} = \frac{2}{3} \times \frac{4}{4} = \frac{2 \times 4}{3 \times 4} = \frac{8}{12}$$

$$\frac{3}{4} = \frac{3}{4} \times \frac{12 \div 4}{12 \div 4} = \frac{3}{4} \times \frac{3}{3} = \frac{3 \times 3}{4 \times 3} = \frac{9}{12}$$

- Lastly, add the converted fractions, and reduce to the lowest terms:

$$\frac{6}{12} + \frac{8}{12} + \frac{9}{12} = \frac{6 + 8 + 9}{12} = \frac{23}{12} = 1^{11}/_{12}$$

- The patient has had $1^{11}/_{12}$ cups of liquid to drink in the past 8 hours.

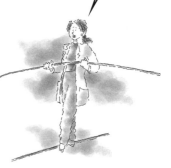

In the real world, you don't get three tries to get it right. So now is the time to practise, practise, practise!

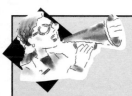

That's a wrap!

Fractions review

Here are some important facts about fractions you'll need to remember.

Fraction basics

- A fraction is a mathematical expression for parts of a whole.
- The denominator (bottom number) represents the total number of equal parts in the whole.
- The numerator (top number) represents the number of parts of the whole being considered.

Types of fraction

- Common fraction: both the numerator and denominator are whole numbers (such as ⅔).

- Complex fraction: the numerator and denominator are fractions (such as $\frac{2/7}{5/16}$).
- Proper fraction: the numerator is smaller than the denominator (such as ¼).
- Improper fraction: the numerator is larger than the denominator (such as ⅔).

Converting to improper fractions

- Multiply the denominator by the whole number.
- Add the product to the numerator.
- The resulting sum is the new numerator.
- Leave the denominator as it is.

(continued)

Fractions review *(continued)*

Reducing fractions

- Determine the largest common divisor.
- Divide the numerator and denominator by that number.

Common denominators

- Multiply all the denominators in a set of fractions to find the common denominator.
- The smallest multiple of the denominators is the lowest common denominator.
- Use prime factoring to determine the lowest common denominator.

Adding and subtracting fractions

- Always convert to fractions with common denominators first, then add or subtract the numerators and keep the denominator as it is.

Multiplying fractions

- Don't convert fractions to common denominators.
- Multiply the numerators and denominators in turn.

Dividing fractions

- Don't convert fractions to common denominators.
- Write them as two fractions separated by a division sign.
- Invert the divisor.
- Multiply the dividend by the inverted divisor (reciprocal).

Don't forget!

- Always reduce the final answer to its lowest terms.
- If the fraction is improper, convert to a mixed number.

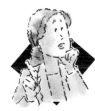

Quick quiz

1. The product of $\frac{2}{3} \times \frac{5}{7}$ is:
   A. $\frac{14}{15}$
   B. $\frac{10}{21}$
   C. $\frac{7}{5}$
   D. $\frac{1}{21}$

   Answer: B. To multiply two common fractions, multiply the numerators and then the denominators. The calculation looks like this:

   $$\frac{2}{3} \times \frac{5}{7} = \frac{2 \times 5}{3 \times 7} = \frac{10}{21}$$

2. In the fraction $\frac{4}{5}$, the denominator is:
   A. $\frac{5}{4}$
   B. $1\frac{1}{5}$
   C. 4
   D. 5

   Answer: D. The denominator is the bottom number of a fraction. The numerator is the top number.

3. When you reduce the fraction ⁸⁄₂₄ to its lowest terms, you get:
    A. ²⁄₆
    B. ¾
    C. ⅓
    D. ⅛

Answer: C. Both the numerator and the denominator are divisible by 8, leaving the reduced fraction ⅓.

4. Which of the following is an improper fraction?
    A. ⁹⁄₁₇
    B. ¹¹⁄₂
    C. ⅓
    D. ¾

Answer: B. An improper fraction has a numerator that's larger than the denominator.

5. When adding the fractions ⅓ and ½, you get:
    A. ²⁄₅
    B. ⅚
    C. ³⁄₆
    D. ⁵⁄₂₀

Answer: B. To add ½ and ⅓, first find the common denominator, which is 6. Convert the fractions to ³⁄₆ and ²⁄₆. Then add the numerators and place the result over the common denominator. The calculation looks like this:

$$\frac{1}{2} + \frac{1}{3} = \frac{3}{6} + \frac{2}{6} = \frac{3+2}{6} = \frac{5}{6}$$

6. Which of the following is a prime number?
    A. 4
    B. 5
    C. 6
    D. 8

Answer: B. The number 5 is a prime number because it can be divided only by itself and 1.

Scoring

⭐⭐⭐ If you answered all six items correctly, wow! You're a number 1 maths whiz (which is the same as a ²⁄₂, a ³⁄₃ or a ⁶⁄₆ maths whiz).

⭐⭐ If you answered four or five items correctly, fantastic! You're a freewheeling fraction fiend.

⭐ If you answered fewer than four items correctly, stick with it! You've shown great derring-do in dealing with dividends and divisors.

2 Decimals and percentages

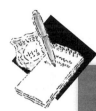

Just the facts

In this chapter, you'll learn:

♦ what decimals and percentages are

♦ how to add, subtract, multiply, divide and round off decimal fractions

♦ how to convert common fractions to decimal fractions and vice versa

♦ how to convert percentages to decimal fractions and common fractions and vice versa

♦ how to solve percentage problems.

A look at decimals and percentages

For most people, decimals and percentages are a part of everyday life. Calculating a tip at a restaurant, balancing a cheque book and interpreting the results of an election or a survey are just three ways in which people use decimals and percentages.

As a nurse, you also encounter decimals and percentages every day at work. The metric system – the most common worldwide system for measuring medications – is based on decimal numbers. You also use decimals and percentages when administering solutions such as 0.9% sodium chloride solution and drugs such as a 2.5% cream.

In the know

To administer medications accurately and efficiently, you must understand what decimals and percentages are and how to work with them in common calculations. You also need to know how to convert from percentages to decimal fractions and common

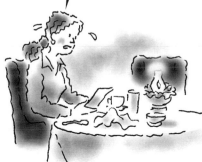

…all these decimals and percentages. I just want to figure out the tip!

fractions and then back to percentages. This chapter will sharpen your calculation skills and help you build confidence.

Deciphering decimals

A *decimal fraction* is a proper fraction in which the denominator is a power of 10, signified by a decimal point placed at the left of the numerator. An example of a decimal fraction is 0.2, which is the same as ²⁄₁₀.

In a *decimal number* – for example, 2.25 – the decimal point separates the whole number from the decimal fraction.

Look to the left...

Each number or place to the left of the decimal point represents a whole number that's a power of 10, starting with ones and working up to tens, hundreds, thousands, ten thousands and so on.

...and then to the right

Each place to the right of the decimal point signifies a fraction whose denominator is a power of 10, starting with tenths and working up to hundredths, thousandths, ten thousandths and so on. When working as a nurse, you'll rarely encounter decimal fractions beyond the thousandths. (See *Know your places*.)

Know your places

Based on its position relative to the decimal point, each decimal place represents a power of 10 or a fraction with a denominator that's a power of 10, as shown below.

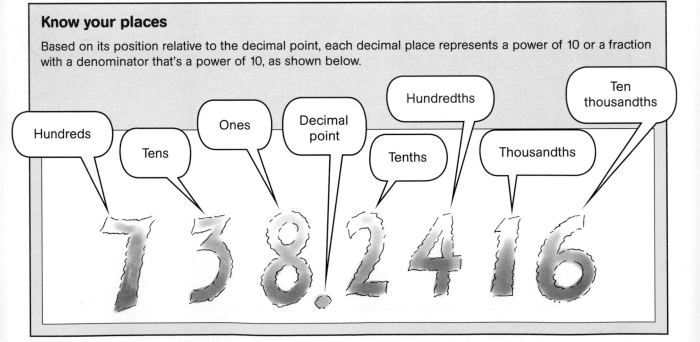

Getting to the point

When discussing money, people use the word *and* to signify the decimal point, for example, saying £5.20 as '5 pounds and 20 pence'. However, when discussing decimal numbers in dosage calculations, use the word *point* to signify the decimal point. For example, say the number 5.2 as '5 point 2'.

Zeroing in on zeros

Now that you've learned the basic terms used with decimal fractions, you're ready to review the decimal calculations most often performed by nurses. But first, review these two important rules:

• After performing mathematical functions with decimal numbers, you may eliminate zeros to the right of the decimal point that don't appear before other numbers (See *Zap those zeros.*) In other cases, you may wish to *add* zeros at the end of fractions (for example, as place holders). Deleting or adding zeros at the end of a decimal fraction doesn't change the value of the number.

• When writing answers to mathematical calculations and specifying drug dosages, always put a zero to the left of the decimal point if no other number appears there. This helps prevent errors. (See *Disappearing decimal alert.*)

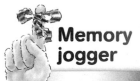

Memory jogger

To remember which zeros you can safely eliminate in a decimal number, think of the letters 'l' and 'r' in the words 'left' and 'right':

• **Leave** a zero to the **left** of the decimal point if no other number appears there and you need a place holder (as in 0.5 ml).

• **Remove** any trailing zeros to the **right** of the decimal point if no other number follows and you don't need a place holder (as in 7.50 mg).

Zap those zeros

Are you solving a problem with decimal numbers? In most cases, you can delete all zeros to the right of the decimal point that don't appear before other numbers.

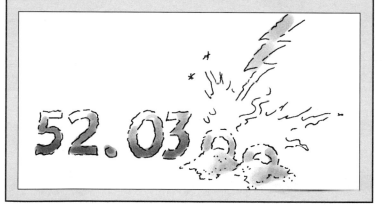

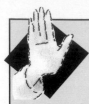

Before you give that drug!

Disappearing decimal alert

Decimal points and zeros may be small items, but they're big deals on prescription sheets and administration records. When you get a prescription, study it closely. If a dose doesn't sound right, maybe a decimal point was left out or incorrectly placed.

For instance, a prescription that calls for '*.5 mg lorazepam intravenous*' may be mistaken for '*5 mg lorazepam intravenous*.' The correct way to write this prescription is to use a zero as a place holder before the decimal point. The prescription would then become '*0.5 mg lorazepam intravenous*'.

Adding and subtracting decimal fractions

Before adding and subtracting decimal fractions, align the decimal points vertically to help you keep track of the decimal positions.

Place holders, take your place

To maintain column alignment, add zeros as place holders in decimal fractions.

Here's how to use zeros to align the decimal fractions 2.61, 0.315 and 4.8 before adding:

$$
\begin{array}{r}
2.610 \\
0.315 \\
+\ 4.800 \\
\hline
7.725
\end{array}
$$

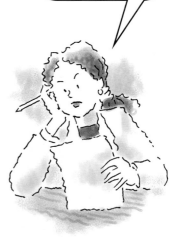

One sneaky decimal point can make a good dosage go bad!

Working it out

Here are two more examples of adding and subtracting decimal fractions. First, add 0.017, 4.8 and 1.22:

$$
\begin{array}{r}
0.017 \\
4.800 \\
+\ 1.220 \\
\hline
6.037
\end{array}
$$

Next, subtract 0.05 from 4.726:

$$
\begin{array}{r}
4.726 \\
-\ 0.050 \\
\hline
4.676
\end{array}
$$

Multiplying decimal fractions

Aligning the decimal points isn't necessary before doing a multiplication problem with decimal fractions. Just leave the decimal points in their original positions and multiply the factors to find the product.

To determine where to place the decimal point in the final product, first add together the number of decimal places in both factors being multiplied. Then count out the same total number of places in the answer, starting from the right and moving to the left, and place the decimal point just to the left of the last place counted. Here's how you would multiply 2.7 and 0.81:

$$
\begin{array}{r}
2.70 \\
\times\ 0.81 \\
\hline
2.1870
\end{array}
$$

> The decimal point goes here because there are four decimal places in the factors.

Multiple multiplication

Here are two more examples of multiplying decimal fractions. First, multiply 1.423 and 8.59:

$$
\begin{array}{r}
1.423 \\
\times\ 8.59 \\
\hline
12.22357
\end{array}
$$

Next, multiply 42.1 and 0.376:

$$
\begin{array}{r}
42.1 \\
\times\ 0.376 \\
\hline
15.8296
\end{array}
$$

Dividing decimal fractions

When dividing decimal fractions, align the decimal points but don't add zeros as place holders. *Remember:* the number to be divided is the *dividend*, the number that does the dividing is the *divisor* and the answer is the *quotient*.

> All decimal points, please report to your proper places... All decimal points, please report...

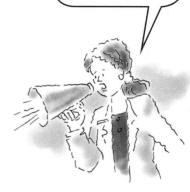

Whole-number divisors

Decimal point placement is easiest when the divisor is a whole number. Just place the decimal point in the quotient directly above the decimal point in the dividend and then work the problem. For example, here's how to divide 4.68 by 2:

$$2)\overline{4.68} = 2.34$$

> Align decimal points.

Revisiting decimal division

Here are two more examples of decimal point placement when the divisor is a whole number. First, divide 44.02 by 10:

$$10)\overline{44.020} = 4.402$$

Next, divide 9.093 by 3:

$$3)\overline{9.093} = 3.031$$

> Align decimal points.

Decimal-fraction divisors

Of course, not every divisor is a whole number – some are decimal fractions. Dividing one decimal fraction into another requires moving the decimal points in both the divisor and the dividend. (See *Dividing decimal fractions*.)

Rounding off decimal fractions

Most of the instruments and measuring devices a nurse uses measure accurately only to a tenth or, at most, to a hundredth. So you'll need to round off decimal fractions – that is, convert long fractions to those with fewer decimal places. (See *Remember rounding*.)

Whittling decimals down

To round off a decimal fraction, follow these steps:

Suppose you want to round off the decimal fraction 0.4293. First, decide how many places to the right of the decimal point you want to keep. If you decide to round the number off to hundredths, you'll keep two places to the right of the decimal point and delete the rest (the 9 and the 3).

Now, look at the first number that you've deleted. Is this number 5 or greater than 5? If so, add 1 to the number in the

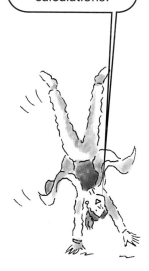

> Rounding off is part of most dosage calculations!

For maths phobics only

Dividing decimal fractions

When dividing one decimal fraction by another, move the divisor's decimal point all the way to the right to convert it to a whole number. Move the dividend's decimal point the same number of places to the right. After completing the division problem, place the quotient's decimal point directly above the new decimal point in the dividend.

   The example below shows how to divide 10.45 by 2.6. The quotient is rounded to the nearest hundredth.

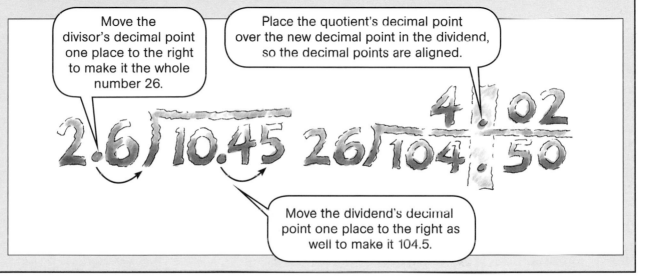

Move the divisor's decimal point one place to the right to make it the whole number 26.

Place the quotient's decimal point over the new decimal point in the dividend, so the decimal points are aligned.

Move the dividend's decimal point one place to the right as well to make it 104.5.

hundredths place – that is, to the number 2. Your rounded-off number is now 0.43.

Suppose the number that you delete is less than 5. Then don't add 1 to the number on the left. For example, to round off 1.9085 to the nearest tenth, identify the number in the tenths position (9) and delete all the numbers to the right of it (0, 8 and 5). Because the number directly to the right of 9 – the 0 – is less than 5, the number 9 stays the same. The number 1.9085 rounded off to the nearest tenth is 1.9.

A practice round

Try rounding off 14.723 to the nearest hundredth:
- First, decide what number is in the hundredths place (2) and delete all the numbers to the right of it (only the number 3).
- Because 3 is lower than 5, you don't add 1 to the 2. Thus, the rounded-off number is 14.72.

Now, round off 0.9875 to the nearest thousandth:
• The number in the thousandth place is 7. All numbers to the right of the 7 – the 5 – will be deleted.
• Because the number to be deleted is a 5, the 7 is rounded up to 8 (7 + 1). The rounded-off number is therefore 0.988.

Converting fractions

Many measuring devices have metric calibrations, so you'll often need to convert common fractions to decimal fractions. At times, you may also need to convert decimal fractions back into common fractions.

Converting common fractions to decimal fractions

Changing a common, proper fraction into a decimal fraction is simple. Just divide the numerator by the denominator. Add a zero as a place holder to the left of the decimal point.

Commence converting

For example, here's how to convert ⁴⁄₁₀ to a decimal fraction:

$$\frac{4}{10} = 4 \div 10 = 10\overline{)4.0}^{\,0.4}$$

Keep on converting

Here are two more examples. First, convert ²⁄₅ to a decimal fraction:

$$\frac{2}{5} = 2 \div 5 = 5\overline{)2.0}^{\,0.4}$$

Next, convert ³⁄₈ to a decimal fraction:

$$\frac{3}{8} = 3 \div 8 = 8\overline{)3.000}^{\,0.375}$$

Converting mixed numbers to decimal fractions

How do you convert a mixed number to a decimal fraction? First, convert it to an improper fraction and then divide the numerator by the denominator, as shown above.

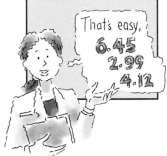

That's easy,
6.45
2.99
4.12

Mixing it up

Here's an example. To convert $4\frac{3}{4}$ to a decimal fraction, first convert the mixed number $4\frac{3}{4}$ to the improper fraction $\frac{19}{4}$. Then divide 19 by 4 to find the decimal fraction:

$$4\frac{3}{4} = \frac{19}{4} = 19 \div 4 = 4\overline{)19.00}^{\,4.75}$$

Let's see that again

Here are two more calculations to try. First, convert $10\frac{7}{8}$ to a decimal fraction:

$$10\frac{7}{8} = \frac{87}{8} = 87 \div 8 = 8\overline{)87.00}^{\,10.88}$$

Note that the quotient above has been rounded off to the nearest hundredth.

Next, convert $1\frac{2}{9}$ to a decimal fraction:

$$1\frac{2}{9} = \frac{11}{9} = 11 \div 9 = 9\overline{)11.00}^{\,1.22}$$

Converting decimal fractions to common fractions

To convert a decimal fraction to a common fraction, count the number of decimal places in the decimal fraction. This number reflects the number of zeros in the denominator of the common fraction.

For example, to convert the decimal fraction 0.33 into a common fraction, follow these steps:

Count the number of decimal places in 0.33. There are two decimal places, so the denominator of its common fraction is 100 because 100 has two zeros.

Remove the decimal point from 0.33 and use this number as the numerator. Reduce the fraction, if possible.

The calculation looks like this:

$$0.33 = \frac{33}{100}$$

This fraction can't be reduced further.

Practise, practise, practise

Try two more calculations. First, convert 0.413 to a common fraction. Here, the denominator is 1000 because the decimal fraction (0.413) has three places after the decimal point.

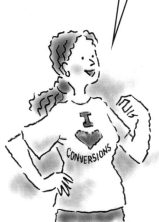

You needn't have an aversion to conversion. It can be incredibly easy!

The calculation looks like this:

$$0.413 = \frac{413}{1000}$$

This fraction can't be reduced further.

Now convert 0.65 to a common fraction. The denominator is 100 because this decimal fraction has two places after the decimal point.

The calculation looks like this:

$$0.65 = \frac{65}{100} = \frac{13}{20}$$

Note that this fraction has been reduced to its lowest terms.

Converting decimal fractions to mixed numbers

Use the same method as described previously to convert a decimal fraction to a mixed number (or to an improper fraction).

Mixed up but methodical

For example, to convert 5.75 to a fraction, use 100 as the denominator because 5.75 has two decimal places. Then convert the fraction to a mixed number.

The calculation looks like this:

$$5.75 = \frac{575}{100} = 5^{75}/_{100} = 5\tfrac{3}{4}$$

Note that this mixed number has been reduced to its lowest terms.

That was brilliant! Do it again!

Below are two more sample calculations. First, convert 3.25 to a fraction. Use 100 as the denominator because 3.25 has two decimal places. Then convert the fraction to a mixed number.

The calculation looks like this:

$$3.25 = \frac{325}{100} = 3^{25}/_{100} = 3\tfrac{1}{4}$$

Note that this mixed number has been reduced.

Once more and you got it!

Convert 1.9 to a fraction. Use 10 as the denominator because 1.9 has one decimal place. Then convert the fraction to a mixed number.

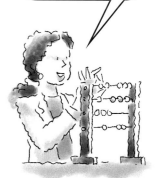

You mean figuring out the denominator is just a matter of counting decimal places?

The calculation looks like this:

$$1.9 = \frac{19}{10} = 1\%_{10}$$

Note that this mixed number can't be reduced further.

Understanding percentages

Percentages are another way to express fractions and numerical relationships. The per cent symbol may be used with a whole number such as 21%, or a decimal number such as 0.9% (See *A point about percentages*.)

From discounts to drug doses

You use percentages in everyday life when working out shopping discounts or tips in restaurants. You also use them in nursing when calculating solutions and drug doses. Because percentages are such an important part of your work, you must know how to convert easily from percentages to decimal fractions and common fractions and vice versa.

Converting percentages to decimals

To change a percentage to a decimal fraction, remove the % sign and multiply the number in the percentage by $\frac{1}{100}$, or 0.01. For example, you would convert 84% and 35% to decimal fractions in this way:

$$84 \times 0.01 = 0.84$$

$$35 \times 0.01 = 0.35$$

Watch that decimal point!

Make sure that you shift the decimal point in the right direction (to the left, when converting a percentage to a decimal), otherwise you could calculate a drug dose incorrectly. (See *From percentages to decimals (and back again)*.)

Converting percentages to common fractions

Suppose you want to convert 50% to a common fraction. To convert a percentage to a common fraction, follow these steps:

A point about percentages

When you see %, the per cent sign, think 'for every hundred'. Why? Because percentage means any quantity stated as parts per hundred. In other words, 75% is actually $\frac{75}{100}$ because the per cent sign takes the place of the denominator 100.

Watch the direction in which you shift that decimal point!

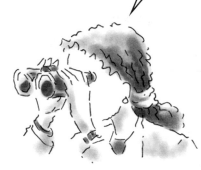

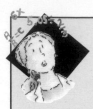

For maths phobics only

From percentages to decimals (and back again)

Although it seems like a harmless dot, a misplaced decimal point can lead to a serious drug error. Study the examples below to see how to perform conversions quickly and accurately.

Jump to the left

To convert from a percentage to a decimal, remove the per cent sign and move the decimal point two places to the left. Here's how:

$$97\% = 0.97$$

> Remove the per cent sign and move the decimal point two places to the left.

Jump to the right

To convert a decimal to a percentage, reverse the process. Move the decimal point two places to the right; add a zero as a place holder, if necessary; and then add a per cent sign. If the resulting percentage is a whole number, remove the decimal because it's understood. Here's what the calculation looks like:

$$0.20 = 20\%$$

> Move the decimal point two places to the right and add a per cent sign.

First, remove the per cent sign and put the decimal point two places to the left, creating the decimal fraction 0.50:

$$50\% = 0.50$$

Next, convert 0.50 to a common fraction with a denominator that's a factor of 10. The result is $\frac{50}{100}$ because 0.50 has two decimal places:

$$0.50 = \frac{50}{100}$$

Lastly, reduce the fraction to its lowest terms, which is ½:

$$\frac{50}{100} = \frac{1}{2}$$

so,

$$50\% = \frac{1}{2}$$

Incredible! Do it again!

Here's another example. To convert 32.7% to a common fraction, remove the per cent sign and put the decimal point two places to the left, creating the decimal fraction 0.327. Convert 0.327 to a common fraction using 1000 as the denominator because 0.327 has three decimal places:

$$32.7\% = 0.327 = \frac{327}{1000}$$

The result is $^{327}/_{1000}$ – a fraction that's already reduced to its lowest terms.

Again?

All right, here's one last example: to convert 20.05% to a common fraction, remove the per cent sign and put the decimal point two places to the left, creating the decimal fraction 0.2005. Use 10 000 as the denominator because 0.2005 has four decimal places:

$$20.05\% = 0.2005 = \frac{2005}{10\,000} = \frac{401}{2000}$$

The result is $^{2005}/_{10\,000}$, which becomes $^{401}/_{2000}$ when reduced.

Converting common fractions to percentages

Converting a common fraction to a percentage involves two simple steps. Suppose you want to convert ⅖ to a percentage. First, create a decimal fraction by dividing the numerator, 2, by the denominator, 5. You can do this by hand or with a calculator. (See *Thank heaven for calculators*.)

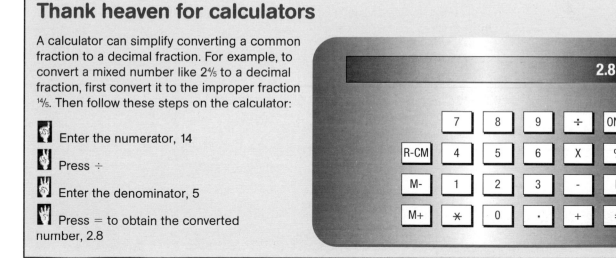

Thank heaven for calculators

A calculator can simplify converting a common fraction to a decimal fraction. For example, to convert a mixed number like 2⅘ to a decimal fraction, first convert it to the improper fraction ¹⁴⁄₅. Then follow these steps on the calculator:

Enter the numerator, 14

Press ÷

Enter the denominator, 5

Press = to obtain the converted number, 2.8

The calculation looks like this:

$$\frac{2}{5} = 2 \div 5 = 5\overline{)2.0}^{\,0.4}$$

Next, convert the decimal fraction to a percentage by moving the decimal point two places to the right (you'll need to add a 0 as a place holder) and then adding the per cent sign.
Here's what the calculation looks like:

$$0.40 = 40\%$$

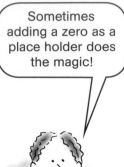

Sometimes adding a zero as a place holder does the magic!

More practice to make you perfect

Here's a second example. To convert ⅓ to a percentage, create a decimal fraction by dividing 1 by 3. Round off the quotient to two decimal places:

$$\frac{1}{3} = 1 \div 3 = 0.333 = 0.33$$

Then convert the decimal fraction to a percentage by moving the decimal point two places to the right and adding the per cent sign:

$$0.33 = 33\%$$

Once more to make sure

Here's a third example. To convert ⅜ to a percentage, create a decimal fraction by dividing 3 by 8:

$$\frac{3}{8} = 3 \div 8 = 0.375$$

Then convert the decimal fraction to a percentage by moving the decimal point two places to the right and adding the per cent sign.
The result is:

$$0.375 = 37.5\%$$

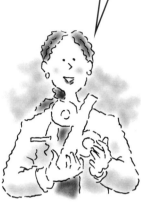

Solving percentage problems

Solving percentage problems involves three types of calculations.
They are:
• finding a percentage of a number
• finding what percentage one number is of another

- finding a number when a percentage of it is known. (See *Percentage problems: watch the wording*.)

You'll have an easier time solving these calculations if you follow a few simple guidelines.

Finding a percentage of a number

The question 'what is 40% of 200?' is an example of the first type of calculation. To solve it, change the word *of* to a multiplication sign. This gives you:

$$40\% \times 200 = ?$$

Next, convert 40% to a decimal fraction by removing the per cent sign and moving the decimal point two places to the left. This gives you:

$$40\% = 0.40$$

Then multiply the two numbers to get the answer, 80:

$$0.40 \times 200 = 80$$

> 40% of 200 is 80.

Practice time (again)

Now, try solving the problem, 'what is 5% of 150?' First, restate it as a multiplication problem:

$$5\% \times 150 = ?$$

Next, convert 5% to the decimal fraction 0.05:

$$5\% = 0.05$$

Then multiply the two numbers to get the answer, 7.5:

$$0.05 \times 150 = 7.5$$

> 5% of 150 is 7.5.

Therefore, 7.5 is 5% of 150.

Percentage problems: watch the wording

When a percentage problem is worded this way: 'What is 25% of 80?' mentally change the *of* to a multiplication sign so the problem becomes 'What is 25% (or, using a decimal fraction, 0.25) × 80?' Then continue with the calculation. (The answer is 20.)

If a problem is worded as '25 is what percentage of 80?' treat the *what* as a division sign so the problem becomes $^{25}/_{80}$. Then continue with the calculation. (The answer is 0.3125, or 31.25%.)

More practice (and you thought the piano was rough)

Here's one more example: 'what is 7% of 300?' First, restate the question as a multiplication problem:

$$7\% \times 300 = ?$$

Convert 7% to the decimal fraction 0.07:

$$7\% = 0.07$$

Then multiply the two numbers to get the answer, 21:

$$0.07 \times 300 = 21$$

> 21 is 7% of 300.

Finding what percentage one number is of another

The question '10 is what percentage of 200?' is an example of this type of calculation. To solve it, restate the question as a division problem, with the number 10 as the dividend and the number 200 as the divisor. Here's how the calculation looks so far:

$$200\overline{)10.00}^{0.05}$$

Now, move the decimal point in the quotient two places to the right and add a per cent sign:

$$0.05 = 5\%$$

> 10 is 5% of 200.

Again (with a twist)

This type of problem can also be expressed in this way: 'what percentage of 28 is 14?' To solve it, restate the question as a division problem by making 28 the divisor and 14 the dividend:

$$28\overline{)14.00}^{0.50}$$

Then move the decimal point two places to the right and add a per cent sign:

$$0.50 = 50\%$$

> 14 is 50% of 28.

One more time

Here's one last problem: 'what percentage of 30 is 6?' First, restate the question as a division problem by making 30 the divisor and 6 the dividend:

$$\begin{array}{r} 0.20 \\ 30\overline{)6.00} \end{array}$$

Move the decimal point two places to the right and add a per cent sign:

$$0.20 = 20\%$$

> 6 is 20% of 30.

Finding a number when you know a percentage of it

The third type of problem – finding a number when you know a percentage of it – also requires division. For example, consider the following question: '70% of what number is 7?' Here's how to do this calculation.

First, convert 70% into a decimal fraction by removing the per cent sign and moving the decimal point two places to the left:

$$70\% = 0.70$$

Next, divide 7 by 0.70. Move the decimal point two places to the right in both the divisor (to make it a whole number) and the dividend. The quotient is 10:

$$\begin{array}{r} 10.0 \\ 0.70\overline{)7.00\ 0} \end{array}$$

> 70% of 10 is 7.

Do you feel perfect yet?

Now try the problem '30% of what number is 90?' To solve it, convert 30% to a decimal fraction by removing the per cent sign and moving the decimal point two places to the left:

$$30\% = 0.30$$

Then divide 90 by 0.30. Move the decimal point two places to the right in both the divisor (to make it a whole number) and the dividend. The quotient is 300:

$$
\begin{array}{r}
300.0 \\
0.30\overline{)90.000}
\end{array}
$$

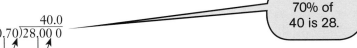

30% of 300 is 90.

Now you're getting the hang of it!

Here's a third example: '70% of what number is 28?' To solve this problem, convert 70% to a decimal fraction by removing the per cent sign and moving the decimal point two places to the left:

$$70\% = 0.70$$

Then divide 28 by 0.70. Move the decimal point two places to the right in both the divisor (to make it a whole number) and the dividend. The quotient is 40:

$$
\begin{array}{r}
40.0 \\
0.70\overline{)28.00\,0}
\end{array}
$$

70% of 40 is 28.

Real-world problem

A patient received 600 ml of I.V. fluid out of 1000 ml that was prescribed. What percentage of I.V. fluid did the patient receive?

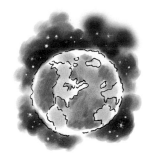

Devising the division

What you really want to find out in this problem is '600 is what percentage of 1000?'
• First, restate it as a division problem, with 600 as the dividend and 1000 as the divisor:

$$
\begin{array}{r}
0.60 \\
1000\overline{)600.00} \\
\underline{6000} \\
00
\end{array}
$$

• Next, move the decimal point in the quotient two places to the right and add a per cent sign:

$$0.60 = 60\%$$

So, 600 is 60% of 1000.

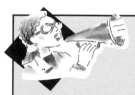

That's a wrap!

Decimals and percentages review

Keep in mind these important facts when working with decimals and percentages.

Decimals and percentages

- A decimal fraction is a proper fraction in which the denominator is a power of 10, signified by a decimal point placed at the left of the numerator.
- Each number or place to the left of the decimal point represents a whole number that's a power of 10.
- Each place to the right of the decimal point represents a fraction whose denominator is a power of 10.
- A percentage is any quantity stated as parts per hundred (the per cent sign takes the place of the denominator 100).

Writing decimals

- Eliminate zeros to the right of the decimal point that don't appear before other numbers.
- Always place a zero to the left of the decimal point if no other number appears there.

Adding and subtracting decimals

- Align the decimal points vertically.
- Use zeros to maintain column alignment.

Multiplying decimals

- Don't move decimal points.
- The number of decimal places in the product equals the sum of the decimal places in the numbers multiplied.

Dividing decimals

- When a whole number is the divisor, place the quotient's decimal point directly above the dividend's decimal point.
- When a decimal fraction is the divisor, move the divisor's decimal point to the right to convert to a whole number, then move the dividend's decimal point the same number of places to the right and, lastly, place the quotient's decimal point directly above the dividend's decimal point.

Rounding off decimals

- Check the number to the right of the decimal place that will be rounded off.
- If that number is less than 5, leave the number in the decimal place alone and delete the number less than 5.
- If that number is 5 or greater, add 1 to the decimal place and delete the number greater than 5.

Converting percentages to decimals

- Multiply the percentage number by $\frac{1}{100}$ (or 0.01).
- Or, shift the decimal point two places to the left.

Converting decimals to percentages

- Divide the decimal fraction by $\frac{1}{100}$ (or 0.01).

(continued)

Decimals and percentages review *(continued)*

- Or, shift the decimal point two places to the right.

Converting percentages to common fractions

- Remove the per cent sign.
- Move the decimal point two places to the left.
- Convert to a common fraction with a denominator that's a factor of 10.

Converting common fractions to percentages

- Divide the numerator by the denominator.
- Convert to a percentage by moving the decimal point two places to the right.

Finding a percentage of a number

- Restate as a multiplication problem by changing the word *of* to a multiplication sign.
- Convert the percentage to a decimal fraction.
- Multiply the two numbers.

Finding what percentage one number is of another

- Restate as a division problem.
- Convert the quotient to a percentage.

Finding a number when you know a percentage of it

- Convert the percentage to a decimal fraction.
- Divide the number by the decimal fraction.

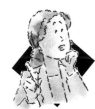

Quick quiz

1. What number is 16% of 79?
    A. 0.20
    B. 4.16
    C. 4.93
    D. 12.64

Answer: D. To solve this, restate the question as a multiplication problem. Convert 16% to a decimal fraction by removing the per cent sign and moving the decimal point two places to the left. The decimal fraction is 0.16. Then multiply 0.16 by 79.

2. In the decimal fraction 1.2058, the tenths place is represented by what number?
    A. 2
    B. 0
    C. 1
    D. 5

Answer: A. The tenths place is to the immediate right of the decimal point.

3. When 3% is converted to a decimal fraction, it becomes what number?

    A.   3.0
    B.   0.30
    C.   0.03
    D.   0.33

Answer: C. Remove the per cent sign and move the decimal point two places to the left.

4. Converting the common fraction ⅛ to a percentage yields which of the following?

    A.   12.5%
    B.   8%
    C.   1.25%
    D.   0.125%

Answer: A. To obtain 12.5, divide 1 by 8; then convert the answer to a percentage by moving the decimal point two places to the right and adding the per cent sign.

5. The decimal fraction 1.8 divided by 2.4 yields what number?

    A.   1.5
    B.   0.75
    C.   6.08
    D.   10.55

Answer: B. To solve this, move the decimal points of both the divisor and the dividend one place to the right before dividing. Place the quotient's decimal point over the new decimal point in the dividend.

6. Multiplying 4.9 by 10.203 yields which product?

    A.   49.9947
    B.   49994.7
    C.   0.499947
    D.   499.947

Answer: A. When multiplying, the number of decimal places in the final product equals the sum of the decimal places in the numbers being multiplied. Count the decimal places starting from the right and place the decimal point there.

Scoring

☆☆☆   If you answered all six items correctly, that's 100% (or %, or, if you prefer decimal fractions, 1.00).

☆☆   If you answered four or five items correctly, excellent! As they say, ⅘ to ⅚ isn't bad.

☆   If you answered fewer than four items correctly, here's what to do: subtract the number you got right from 6 and add the result back to your score. Now you've got 100%. Reward yourself with a new calculator!

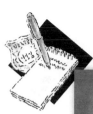

Just the facts

In this chapter, you'll learn:

♦ definitions of ratios and proportions

♦ how to set up proportions using ratios and fractions

♦ how to solve for *X* in an equation

♦ how ratios, proportions and solving for *X* relate to dosage calculations.

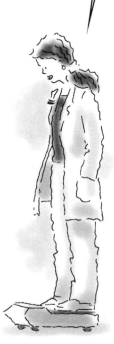

You can convert weights easily! Wait, that number can't be right, can it?

A look at numerical relationships

Ratios, fractions and proportions describe relationships between numbers. Ratios use a colon between the numbers in the relationship, as in 4 : 9. Fractions use a slash between numbers in the relationship, as in ⅘.

Proportions are statements of equality between two ratios. For example, to show that 4 : 9 is equal to 8 : 18, you would write:

$$4 : 9 :: 8 : 18$$

or

$$\frac{4}{9} = \frac{8}{18}$$

Three major problem-solvers

When calculating dosages, you'll use ratios, fractions and proportions frequently. You'll also use them to perform many other related tasks, such as calculating intravenous (I.V.) infusion rates, converting weights between systems of measurement and, in speciality settings, performing oxygenation and haemodynamic calculations. However, before you can use ratios, fractions and proportions, you need to know how to develop and express them appropriately.

Ratios and fractions

Ratios and fractions are numerical ways to compare items.

Dare to compare

If 100 syringes come in 1 box, then the number of syringes compared to the number of boxes is 100 to 1. This can be written as the ratio 100 : 1 or as the fraction $^{100}/_{1}$.

Conversely, the number of boxes to syringes would be 1 : 100 or the fraction $^{1}/_{100}$, so pay attention to which item is mentioned first.

Twice more, with feeling

Here are two more examples.

If a hospital's intensive care area requires 1 registered nurse for every 2 patients, then the relationship of registered nurses to patients is 1 to 2. You can express this with the ratio 1 : 2 or with the fraction ½.

Suppose a vial has 8 mg of a drug in 1 ml of solution. By using a ratio, you can express this as 8 mg : 1 ml. By using a fraction, you can describe it as $^{8\,mg}/_{1\,ml}$.

Proportions

Any proportion that's expressed as two ratios also can be expressed as two fractions.

Using ratios in proportions

When using ratios in a proportion, separate them with double colons. Double colons represent equality between the two ratios.

For example, if the ratio of syringes to boxes is 100 : 1, then 200 syringes are provided in 2 boxes. This proportion can be written as:

100 syringes : 1 box : : 200 syringes : 2 boxes

or

100 : 1 : : 200 : 2

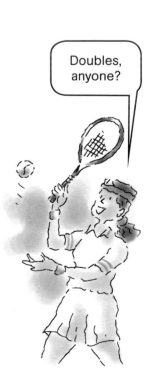

Doubles, anyone?

Proportion practice

Here's another example. If the intensive care area has 1 nurse for every 2 patients, you can express this as the ratio 1 : 2. You can also say that this equals a ratio of 3 nurses for every 6 patients. In a proportion, you can express this relationship with the ratios:

1 nurse : 2 patients : : 3 nurses : 6 patients

or

1 : 2 : : 3 : 6

Another portion of proportions

Now, suppose you have a vial that contains 8 mg of a drug in 1 ml of a solution. You can state this as the ratio 8 mg : 1 ml, which equals 16 mg : 2 ml. This proportion can be expressed with ratios as follows:

8 mg : 1 ml : : 16 mg : 2 ml

or

8 : 1 : : 16 : 2

Using fractions in proportions

Any proportion that can be expressed with ratios can also be expressed with fractions. Here's how to do this using the previous examples.

If 100 syringes come in 1 box, this means that 200 syringes come in 2 boxes. Using fractions, you can write this proportion as:

$$\frac{100 \text{ syringes}}{1 \text{ box}} = \frac{200 \text{ syringes}}{2 \text{ boxes}}$$

or

$$\frac{100}{1} = \frac{200}{2}$$

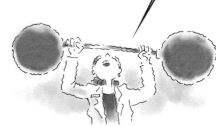

Working out ratios, fractions and proportions puts you in good shape for dosage calculations.

Fraction action

If the intensive care area has 1 nurse for every 2 patients, this means that it has 3 nurses for every 6 patients. Using fractions, you can express this relationship as:

$$\frac{1 \text{ nurse}}{2 \text{ patients}} = \frac{3 \text{ nurses}}{6 \text{ patients}}$$

or

$$\frac{1}{2} = \frac{3}{6}$$

Vial trial run

If there are 8 mg of a drug in 1 ml, this means there are 16 mg in 2 ml. This proportion can be expressed with fractions as:

$$\frac{8 \text{ mg}}{1 \text{ ml}} = \frac{16 \text{ mg}}{2 \text{ ml}}$$

or

$$\frac{8}{1} = \frac{16}{2}$$

Solving for *X*

We know that a proportion is a set of two equal ratios or fractions, but what if one ratio or fraction is incomplete? In this case, the unknown part of the ratio or fraction is represented by X. You can solve for X to determine the value of the unknown quantity. (See *An explanation of* X.)

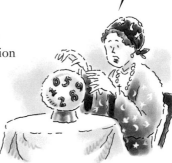

You don't need supernatural powers to solve for *X*. Just use your brain power and follow these steps!

Solving common-fraction equations

The method used to solve common-fraction equations forms the basis for solving other types of simple equations to find the value of X. For example, here's how to solve the common-fraction equation:

$$X = \frac{1}{5} \times \frac{3}{9}$$

Multiply the numerators:

$$1 \times 3 = 3$$

Multiply the denominators:

$$5 \times 9 = 45$$

Restate the equation with this new information:

$$X = \frac{1 \times 3}{5 \times 9} = \frac{3}{45}$$

Advice from the experts

An explanation of X

Being able to find the value of X is vital in making dosage calculations. For example, suppose a drug is prescribed for your patient, but the drug isn't available in the prescribed strength. How do you decide on the right amount of drug to administer?

Here's how

Suppose you receive a prescription to administer 0.1 mg of adrenaline (epinephrine) subcutaneously, but the only adrenaline on hand is a 1-ml ampoule that contains 1 mg of adrenaline. To calculate the volume for injection, state the problem in a proportion:

$$1\,mg : 1\,ml :: 0.1\,mg : X\,ml$$

Rewrite the problem as an equation by applying the principle that the product of the means (the numbers in the middle of the proportion) equals the product of the extremes (the numbers at either end of the proportion).

$$1\,ml \times 0.1\,mg = 1\,mg \times X\,ml$$

Solve for X by dividing both sides of the equation by the known value that appears on the same side of the equation as the unknown value X. Then cancel out units that appear in the numerator and denominator. (This isolates X on one side of the equation.)

$$\frac{1\,ml \times 0.1\,\cancel{mg}}{1\,\cancel{mg}} = \frac{1\,\cancel{mg} \times X\,ml}{1\,\cancel{mg}}$$

$$X = 0.1\,ml$$

Reduce the fraction by dividing the numerator and denominator by the lowest common denominator (3), to find that $X = \frac{1}{15}$:

$$X = \frac{3 \div 3}{45 \div 3} = \frac{1}{15}$$

Most dosage calculations require your answer to be in decimal form, so convert $\frac{1}{15}$ to a decimal fraction by dividing the numerator by the denominator. Round the answer off to the nearest hundredth. The final result is $X = 0.07$:

$$X = \frac{1}{15} = 1 \div 15 = 0.07$$

Try this X-ample

Now, solve for X in the equation:

$$X = \frac{2}{3} \times \frac{5}{8}$$

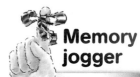

Memory jogger

The term X factor is commonly used to describe a person or event that could cause unexpected, or unknown, outcomes. Keep this in mind and you'll remember that X represents the unknown part of a ratio or fraction.

Multiply the numerators:

$$2 \times 5 = 10$$

Multiply the denominators:

$$3 \times 8 = 24$$

Restate the equation with this new information:

$$X = \frac{2 \times 5}{3 \times 8} = \frac{10}{24}$$

Reduce the fraction by dividing the numerator and denominator by the lowest common denominator (2), to find that $X = \frac{5}{12}$:

$$X = \frac{10 \div 2}{24 \div 2} = \frac{5}{12}$$

Convert $\frac{5}{12}$ to a decimal fraction by dividing the numerator by the denominator and then rounding it off. The final result is $X = 0.42$.

$$\frac{5}{12} = 5 \div 12 = 0.42$$

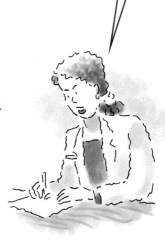

Multiply, multiply, restate, reduce, convert...

Here comes a twist

In this example, the whole number 3 is involved. (See *Making whole numbers fractions*.)

Here's how to solve for X in an equation with a whole number:

$$X = \frac{125}{500} \times 3$$

Convert the whole number 3 into the fraction $\frac{3}{1}$. The equation becomes:

$$X = \frac{125}{500} \times \frac{3}{1}$$

Next, reduce $\frac{125}{500}$ by dividing the numerator and denominator by the lowest common denominator (125) to get $\frac{1}{4}$. The equation becomes:

$$X = \frac{125 \div 125}{500 \div 125} \times \frac{3}{1}$$

or

$$X = \frac{1}{4} \times \frac{3}{1}$$

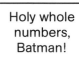

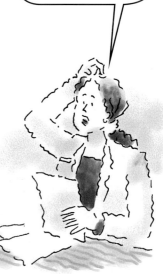

Holy whole numbers, Batman!

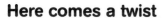

Then proceed as usual.

 Multiply the numerators:

$$1 \times 3 = 3$$

 Multiply the denominators:

$$4 \times 1 = 4$$

 Restate the equation with this new information:

$$X = \frac{1 \times 3}{4 \times 1} = \frac{3}{4}$$

 The fraction ¾ can't be reduced. Convert it to a decimal fraction by dividing the numerator by the denominator. The final result is $X = 0.75$:

$$X = \frac{3}{4} = 3 \div 4 = 0.75$$

For maths phobics only

Making whole numbers fractions

You can change any whole number into a fraction by making the whole number the numerator and placing it over a 1, which is the denominator. The value of the number doesn't change.

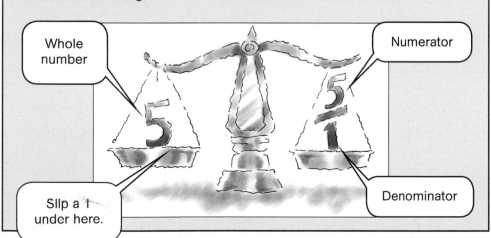

Whole number

Numerator

Denominator

Slip a 1 under here.

Solving decimal-fraction equations

To solve for X in equations with decimal fractions, use a method similar to that used in the previous examples. Here's how to solve for X in the equation:

$$X = \frac{0.05}{0.02} \times 3$$

Remove the decimal points from the fraction by moving them two spaces to the right. Then remove the zeros. The equation becomes:

$$X = \frac{5}{2} \times 3$$

Next, convert the whole number 3 to the fraction ³⁄₁. The equation becomes:

$$X = \frac{5}{2} \times \frac{3}{1}$$

Then multiply the numerators:

$$5 \times 3 = 15$$

Multiply the denominators:

$$2 \times 1 = 2$$

Restate the equation with this new information:

$$X = \frac{5 \times 3}{2 \times 1} = \frac{15}{2}$$

Convert the answer to decimal form by dividing 15 by 2. The final result is $X = 7.5$.

$$X = \frac{15}{2} = 15 \div 2 = 7.5$$

X-tra credit

Here's another practice problem:

$$X = \frac{0.33}{0.11} \times 0.6$$

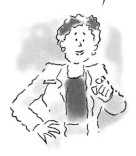

You won't be decimated by decimal-fraction equations!

Remove the decimal points from the fraction by moving them two spaces to the right. Then remove the zeros. The equation becomes:

$$X = \frac{33}{11} \times 0.6$$

Convert the number 0.6 into the fraction $^{0.6}\!/_1$. The equation becomes:

$$X = \frac{33}{11} \times \frac{0.6}{1}$$

Multiply the numerators:

$$33 \times 0.6 = 19.8$$

Multiply the denominators:

$$11 \times 1 = 11$$

Restate the equation with this new information:

$$X = \frac{33 \times 0.6}{11 \times 1} = \frac{19.8}{11}$$

Convert the answer to decimal form by dividing 19.8 by 11. The final result is $X = 1.8$:

$$X = \frac{19.8}{11} = 19.8 \div 11 = 1.8$$

Now we're heading into the home stretch of practice problems!

X-tra, *X*-tra credit

Here's the last problem:

$$X = \frac{0.04}{0.05} \times 4$$

Remove the decimal points from the fraction by moving them two places to the right. Then delete the zeros. The equation becomes:

$$X = \frac{4}{5} \times 4$$

Turn 4 into the fraction ⁴⁄₁. The equation becomes:

$$X = \frac{4}{5} \times \frac{4}{1}$$

Multiply the numerators:

$$4 \times 4 = 16$$

Multiply the denominators:

$$5 \times 1 = 5$$

Restate the equation with this new information:

$$X = \frac{4 \times 4}{5 \times 1} = \frac{16}{5}$$

Convert the answer to decimal form by dividing 16 by 5. The final answer is $X = 3.2$:

$$X = \frac{16}{5} = 16 \div 5 = 3.2$$

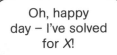

Oh, happy day – I've solved for X!

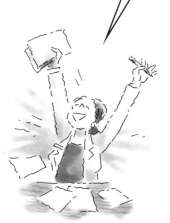

Solving proportion problems with ratios

A proportion can be written with ratios, as in:

Extreme

Extreme

Mean

Mean

$$4 : 1 :: 20 : 5$$

The outer or end numbers are called the *extremes*, and the inner or middle numbers are called the *means*. In such a proportion, the product of the means equals the product of the extremes. In this case,

The product of the means…

$$1 \times 20 = 4 \times 5$$

…equals the product of the extremes.

This principle lets you solve for any of four unknown parts in a proportion.

X marks another spot

Here's an example. Solve for X in the proportion:

$$4 : 8 :: 8 : X$$

Follow these steps:

 Rewrite the problem so that the means and the extremes are multiplied:

$$8 \times 8 = 4 \times X$$

Obtain the products of the means and extremes and put them into an equation:

$$64 = 4X$$

Solve for *X* by dividing both sides by 4. Cancel the number (4) that appears in both the numerator and denominator. This isolates *X* on one side of the equation:

$$\frac{64}{4} = \frac{\cancel{4}X}{\cancel{4}}$$

Find *X*:

$$64 \div 4 = X$$

or

$$X = 16$$

Replace *X* with 16 and restate the proportion in ratios:

$$4 : 8 :: 8 : 16$$

X moves back to the front

Solve for *X* in the proportion:

$$X : 12 :: 6 : 24$$

Follow these steps:

Rewrite the problem so that the means and the extremes are multiplied:

$$12 \times 6 - X \times 24$$

Obtain the products of the means and extremes and put them into an equation:

$$72 = 24X$$

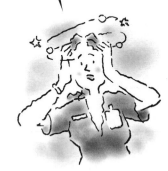

Arrrgh! That *X* keeps moving around!

Solve for X by dividing both sides by 24. Cancel the number (24) that appears in both the numerator and denominator. This isolates X on one side of the equation:

$$\frac{72}{24} = \frac{24X}{24}$$

 Find X:

$$72 \div 24 = X$$

or

$$X = 3$$

 Replace X with 24 and restate the proportion in ratios:

$$3 : 12 :: 6 : 24$$

Another *X*-treme shift

Try one last problem, using this proportion:

$$10 : 20 :: X : 40$$

 Rewrite the problem so that the means and the extremes are multiplied:

$$20 \times X = 10 \times 40$$

 Obtain the products of the means and extremes and put them into an equation:

$$20X = 400$$

 Solve for X by dividing both sides by 20. Cancel the number (20) that appears in both the numerator and denominator. This isolates X on one side of the equation:

$$\frac{20X}{20} = \frac{400}{20}$$

 Find X:

$$X = \frac{400}{20}$$

or

$$X = 20$$

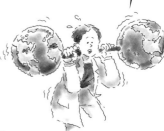

Practising solving for *X* helps limber up your mathematical muscles for the real world of dosage calculations.

Replace *X* with 20 and restate the original proportion in ratios:

$$10 : 20 : : 20 : 40$$

Solving proportion problems with fractions

Proportion problems may also be set up with fractions. In a proportion expressed as a fraction, cross products are equal – just as the means and extremes are equal in a proportion with ratios. (See *Cross product principle*.)

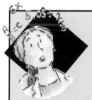

For maths phobics only

Cross product principle

In a proportion expressed as fractions, cross products are equal. In other words, the numerator on the equation's left-hand side multiplied by the denominator on the right-hand side equals the denominator on the equation's left-hand side multiplied by the numerator on the right-hand side.

The above statement has a lot of words. The same meaning is communicated more simply in the illustration below.

The principle applies to ratios as well

Note that the same principle applies to ratios. In a proportion expressed as ratios, the product of the **m**eans (numbers in the **m**iddle) equals the product of the **e**xtremes (numbers on the **e**nds). Consider the illustration to the right.

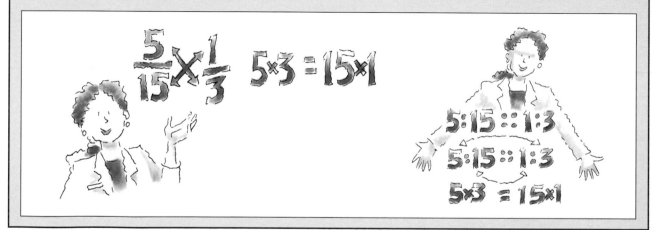

Using the cross products of a proportion, you can solve for any of four unknown parts. Once again, the position of the X doesn't matter because the cross products of a proportion are always equal. (See *Cross products to the rescue*.)

Keeping things in proportion

After studying the example in *Cross products to the rescue*, practise solving for X using this proportion:

$$\frac{3}{4} = \frac{9}{X}$$

Follow these steps:

 Rewrite the problem so the cross products are multiplied:

$$3 \times X = 4 \times 9$$

 Obtain the cross products and put them into an equation:

$$3X = 36$$

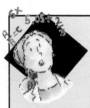

For maths phobics only

Cross products to the rescue

Fractions can be used to describe the relative proportion of ingredients, such as the amount of a drug relative to its solution.

Suppose you have a vial containing 10 mg/ml of morphine. You can write this fraction to describe it:

Amount of drug

$$\frac{10 \text{ mg}}{1 \text{ ml}}$$

Amount of solution

The plot thickens

Now, suppose you need to administer 8 mg of morphine to your patient. How much of the solution should you use?

1. Write a second fraction to represent the amount of solution:

An unknown quantity

$$\frac{8 \text{ mg}}{X \text{ ml}}$$

2. Set up the equation. Keep the fractions in the same relative proportion of drug to solution.

3. Rewrite the problem so cross products are multiplied:

Cross-multiply

$$\frac{10 \text{ mg}}{1 \text{ ml}} \bowtie \frac{8 \text{ mg}}{X \text{ ml}}$$

4. This gives you:

$$10X = 8$$

5. Solve for X by dividing both sides by 10, and you're left with:

$$X = \frac{8}{10}$$

6. Convert this to a decimal fraction because you'll be drawing up medication and need to work with a decimal:

$$X = 0.8 \text{ ml}$$

The answer!

This is how much morphine you should use.

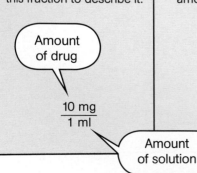

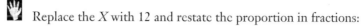 Solve for *X* by dividing both sides by 3. Cancel the number (3) that appears in both the numerator and denominator. This isolates *X* on one side of the equation:

$$\frac{\cancel{3}X}{\cancel{3}} = \frac{36}{3}$$

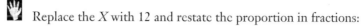 Find *X*:

$$X = \frac{36}{3}$$

or

$$X = 12$$

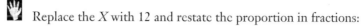 Replace the *X* with 12 and restate the proportion in fractions:

$$\frac{3}{4} = \frac{9}{12}$$

Final practice problem (Yippee!)

Solve one more problem:

$$\frac{12}{25} = \frac{X}{50}$$

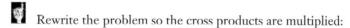 Rewrite the problem so the cross products are multiplied:

$$12 \times 50 = 25 \times X$$

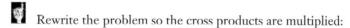 Obtain the cross products and put them into an equation:

$$600 = 25X$$

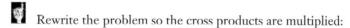 Solve for *X* by dividing both sides by 25:

$$\frac{600}{25} = \frac{\cancel{25}X}{\cancel{25}}$$

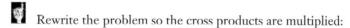 Find *X*:

$$X = 24$$

 Replace *X* with 24 and restate the proportion in fractions:

$$\frac{12}{25} = \frac{24}{50}$$

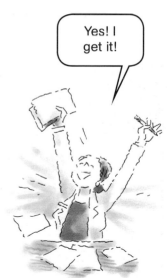

Yes! I get it!

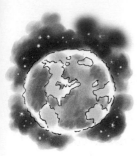

Real-world problems

Next, you'll find three practical examples of proportions in everyday nursing practice.

How do you set up a proportion to solve a real-world problem? Just place the known ratio on one side of the double colon and the unknown ratio on the other side. Make sure that the units of measure in each ratio are in the same positions on both sides of the proportion. (See *Write it down*.)

How much hydrogen peroxide?

Set up a proportion to find out how much hydrogen peroxide (H_2O_2) you should add to 1000 ml of water (H_2O) to make a solution that contains 50 ml of H_2O_2 for every 100 ml of H_2O.

The ratio approach

To solve this problem using ratios, follow these steps:

 Decide what part of the ratio is X. In this case, it's the amount of H_2O_2 in 1000 ml of H_2O.

Set up the proportion so that similar parts of each ratio are in the same position:

$$X : 1000 \text{ ml } H_2O :: 50 \text{ ml } H_2O_2 : 100 \text{ ml } H_2O$$

Multiply the means and the extremes and restate the problem as an equation:

$$1000 \text{ ml } H_2O \times 50 \text{ ml } H_2O_2 = X \text{ ml } H_2O_2 \times 100 \text{ ml } H_2O$$

Solve for X by dividing both sides of the equation by 100 ml H_2O and cancelling units that appear in both the numerator and denominator:

$$\frac{1000 \text{ ml } H_2O \times 50 \text{ ml } H_2O_2}{100 \text{ ml } H_2O} = \frac{X \text{ ml } H_2O_2 \times 100 \text{ ml } H_2O}{100 \text{ ml } H_2O}$$

Find X:

$$\frac{50\,000 \text{ ml } H_2O_2}{100} = X$$

or

$$X = 500 \text{ ml } H_2O_2$$

Advice from the experts

Write it down

When calculating dosages, you may be able to figure out some problems in your head. For instance, 4 mg in 2 ml is the same as 2 mg in 1 ml. If you're stumped, don't be shy about writing the proportion down on paper. Taking the time to see the numbers will help you avoid confusion and solve for X more quickly and accurately.

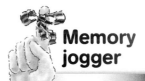

Memory jogger

When working with ratios, the product of the **means** always equals the product of the **extremes**. To differentiate these terms, remember:

means (**m**iddle numbers)

extremes (**e**nd numbers)

The fraction approach

If you set up a proportion with fractions, place similar units of measure for each fraction in the same position. Here's what the previous example looks like in fraction form:

$$\frac{X}{1000 \text{ ml } H_2O} = \frac{50 \text{ ml } H_2O_2}{100 \text{ ml } H_2O}$$

Rewrite the equation by cross-multiplying the fractions:

$$X \times 100 \text{ ml } H_2O_2 = 1000 \text{ ml } H_2O \times 50 \text{ ml } H_2O_2$$

Solve for X by dividing both sides of the equation by 100 ml H_2O and cancelling units that appear in both the numerator and denominator:

$$\frac{X \times \cancel{100 \text{ ml } H_2O}}{\cancel{100 \text{ ml } H_2O}} = \frac{1000 \cancel{\text{ ml } H_2O} \times 50 \text{ ml } H_2O_2}{100 \cancel{\text{ ml } H_2O}}$$

Find X:

$$X = \frac{50\,000 \text{ ml } H_2O_2}{100}$$

$$X = 500 \text{ ml } H_2O_2$$

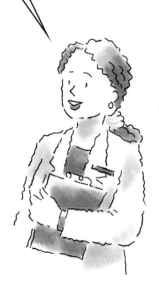

Now do you see all that fractions and ratios can do?

How many clinical demonstrators?

Set up another proportion problem with both ratios and fractions. If a school of nursing requires 1 clinical demonstrator for every 8 students, how many demonstrators are needed for a class of 24 students?

Resolving it with ratios

Use ratios first. Follow these steps:

Decide what part of the proportion is X. In this case, it's the number of demonstrators for 24 students.

Set up the proportion so that the units of measure (demonstrators and students) in each ratio are in the same position:

1 demonstrator : 8 students : : X : 24 students

Multiply the means and the extremes and set up the equation:

8 students $\times X$ = 1 demonstrator $\times$ 24 students

Solve for X by dividing both sides of the equation by 8 students and cancelling units that appear in both the numerator and denominator:

$$\frac{8 \text{ students} \times X}{8 \text{ students}} = \frac{1 \text{ demonstrator} \times 24 \text{ students}}{8 \text{ students}}$$

$$X = \frac{24}{8}$$

Find X:

$$X = 3 \text{ demonstrators}$$

Figuring it out with fractions

If you prefer to solve the previous problem using fractions, follow these steps:

Set up the proportion so that the units of measure are in the same position in each fraction. Here's what the problem looks like in fraction form:

$$\frac{1 \text{ demonstrator}}{8 \text{ students}} = \frac{X}{24 \text{ students}}$$

Rewrite the equation by cross-multiplying the fractions:

$$1 \text{ demonstrator} \times 24 \text{ students} = X \text{ demonstrators} \times 8 \text{ students}$$

Solve for X by dividing both sides of the equation by 8 students and cancelling units that appear in both the numerator and denominator:

$$\frac{1 \text{ demonstrator} \times 24 \text{ students}}{8 \text{ students}} = \frac{X \times 8 \text{ students}}{8 \text{ students}}$$

or

$$24 \div 8 = X \text{ demonstrators}$$

Find X:

$$X = 3 \text{ demonstrators}$$

OK… time to break into smaller, equal groups. We have 3 demonstrators and 24 students. Let's figure out the equation together.

How many bags of I.V. fluid?

Here's one more problem. One case of I.V. fluid holds 20 bags. If your community practice receives 6 cases, how many bags of I.V. fluid does it have?

The ratio rally

Solve this problem using ratios first. Follow these steps:

 Decide what part of the ratio is X. In this case, it's the number of bags of I.V. fluid in 6 cases.

Set up the proportion so that the units of measure in each ratio are in the same position:

$$1 \text{ case} : 20 \text{ bags} : : 6 \text{ cases} : X$$

Multiply the means and the extremes and set up the equation:

$$20 \text{ bags} \times 6 \text{ cases} = X \text{ bags} \times 1 \text{ case}$$

Solve for X by dividing both sides of the equation by 1 case and cancelling units that appear in both the numerator and denominator:

$$\frac{20 \text{ bags} \times 6 \text{ cases}}{1 \text{ case}} = \frac{X \times 1 \text{ case}}{1 \text{ case}}$$

Find X:

$$120 \text{ bags} = X$$

The fraction finale

Now, use fractions to solve the problem. Here's what the equation looks like in fraction form:

$$\frac{1 \text{ case}}{20 \text{ bags}} = \frac{6 \text{ cases}}{X}$$

Rewrite the equation by cross-multiplying the fractions. Then solve for X by dividing each side of the equation by 1 case and cancelling units that appear in both the numerator and denominator:

$$\frac{1 \text{ case} \times X}{1 \text{ case}} = \frac{6 \text{ cases} \times 20 \text{ bags}}{1 \text{ case}}$$

$$X = \frac{120}{1}$$

$$X = 120 \text{ bags}$$

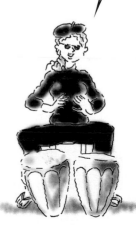

Now that's what I call a big finish. Groovy!

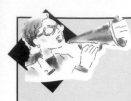

That's a wrap!

Ratios, fractions, proportions and solving for *X* review

Some important facts about ratios, fractions, proportions and solving for *X* are outlined below.

Numerical relationship basics

- Ratio: a ratio uses a colon between the numbers in a numerical relationship.
- Fraction: a fraction uses a slash between numbers in a numerical relationship.
- Proportion: a proportion is a statement of equality between two ratios or two fractions.

Solving common-fraction equations

- Multiply numerators.
- Multiply denominators.
- Restate the equation.
- Reduce the fraction.
- Convert the fraction to decimal form by dividing the numerator by the denominator.

Solving decimal-fraction equations

- Move the decimal points two spaces to the right.

- Remove the zeros.
- Convert the whole number to a fraction.
- Multiply the numerators.
- Multiply the denominators.
- Restate the equation.
- Convert the answer to decimal form by dividing the numerator by the denominator.

Solving proportions with ratios

- Means—middle numbers
- Extremes—end numbers
- Product of the means = product of the extremes
- Isolate *X* on one side of the equation.
- Solve for *X*.

Solving proportions with fractions

- Cross products of a proportion are always equal.
- Multiply the cross products.
- Put the cross products into the equation, and isolate *X* on one side of the equation.
- Solve for *X*.

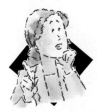

Quick quiz

1. Which is an example of a proportion?
   A. 4 : 5 :: 8 : 12
   B. 6 : 1 :: 18 : 3
   C. 7 : 1 :: 14 : 7
   D. 3 : 8 :: 2 : 6

   Answer: B. In a proportion, the ratios are equal.

2. The proportion 1 : 5 :: 2 : 10 can be restated in fraction form as which of the following?

    A. $\frac{1}{5} = \frac{2}{10}$

    B. $\frac{5}{1} = \frac{2}{10}$

    C. $\frac{2}{5} = \frac{1}{10}$

    D. $\frac{5}{2} = \frac{10}{1}$

Answer: A. Make the ratios on both sides into fractions by substituting slashes for colons.

3. If there are 50 mg of a drug in 5 ml of solution, the amount of drug in 15 ml of solution is:

    A. 10 mg

    B. 150 mg

    C. 75 mg

    D. 100 mg

Answer: B. Substitute X for the amount of drug in 15 ml of solution and then set up a proportion with ratios or fractions.

4. The amount of salt you should add to 200 ml of water to make a solution with 0.5 g of salt for every 50 ml of water is:

    A. 2 g

    B. 1 g

    C. 0.5 g

    D. 0.25 g

Answer: A. Substitute X for the amount of salt in 200 ml of water and then set up a proportion with ratios or fractions.

5. A patient is prescribed 0.125 mg of a drug. The vial you have from the pharmacy contains 0.25 mg per ml of solution. How many millilitres of the solution should you administer?

    A. 1 ml

    B. 2 ml

    C. 0.5 ml

    D. 1.5 ml

Answer: C. Substitute X for the amount of solution needed to administer 0.125 mg of the drug and then set up a proportion with ratios or fractions.

Scoring

☆☆☆ If you answered all five items correctly, wow! You're a whiz at relationships (numerical relationships, that is).

☆☆ If you answered four items correctly, all right! You have everything in proportion.

☆ If you answered fewer than four items correctly, a quick review will get your numbers back on track!

Way to go, partner! Now get ready for a whole new dimension!

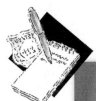
Just the facts

In this chapter, you'll learn:

♦ what dimensional analysis is

♦ how to set up an equation using dimensional analysis

♦ how to identify conversion factors

♦ how to solve dosage calculations using dimensional analysis.

A look at dimensional analysis

Dimensional analysis, also known as *factor analysis* or *factor labelling*, is an alternative way of solving mathematical problems. It's a basic and easy approach to calculating drug dosages because it eliminates the need to memorise formulas. Only one equation is required to determine each answer.

Factors are the main actors

When using dimensional analysis, a series of ratios, called factors, are arranged in a fractional equation. Each factor, written as a fraction, consists of two quantities of measurement that are related to each other in a given problem. Dimensional analysis uses the same terms as fractions, specifically the terms *numerator* and *denominator*.

Setting the stage

Let's say you want to change 200 centimetres (cm) to metres (m). (You can see that the abbreviations for centimetres and metres are 'cm' and 'm', respectively.) The problem is written as follows:

$$200\,cm = X\,m$$

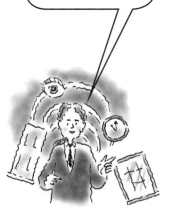

Some people think dimensional analysis is like the Twilight Zone... a whole new dimension.

Some problems contain all of the information needed to identify the factors, set up the equation and find the solution. Other problems, such as this one, require a conversion factor.

Conversion factors

Conversion factors are equivalents between two measurement systems or units of measurement. For example, 1 day equals 24 hours. In this case, day and hour are units of measurement and, when stated as 1 day = 24 hours, they're equivalent. This conversion factor can be used to solve problems involving the measure of time. There are many commonly used conversion factors. (See *Common conversion factors*.)

Putting it into practice

In the previous problem of how many metres are in 200 cm, use the conversion factor 100 cm equals 1 m.

Because the quantities and units of measurement are equivalent, they can serve as the numerator or denominator. The conversion can be written as:

$$\frac{100}{1}$$

or

$$\frac{1}{100}$$

Setting up the equation

Solving a problem using dimensional analysis is like climbing a staircase: it requires steps. Six simple steps need to be followed to solve any problem. (See *Following the steps*.)

Stepping up to the problem

Let's take it one step at a time:

Given quantity – this is the beginning point of the problem. Identify the given quantity in the problem. In this case, it's:

$$200\,cm$$

Wanted quantity – this is the answer to the problem. Identify the wanted quantity in the problem as an unknown unit. In this problem, it's:

$$X\,m$$

Advice from the experts

Common conversion factors

Keep this chart handy for quick reference to breeze through problems that call for these common conversions.

1 kg	=	2.2 lb
1 lb	=	16 oz
1 m	=	100 cm
1 L	=	1000 ml
1′	=	12″
1 yd	=	3′

Advice from the experts

Following the steps

Remember these steps when calculating an equation using dimensional analysis, and you'll soon be standing on top of a solution.

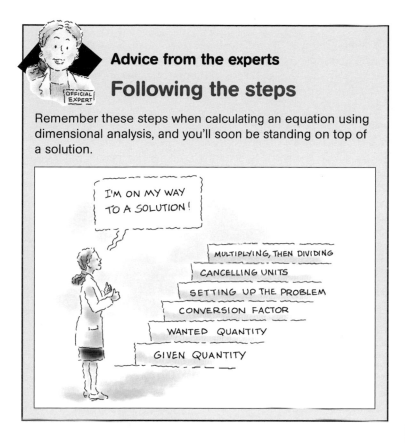

I'M ON MY WAY TO A SOLUTION!

MULTIPLYING, THEN DIVIDING

CANCELLING UNITS

SETTING UP THE PROBLEM

CONVERSION FACTOR

WANTED QUANTITY

GIVEN QUANTITY

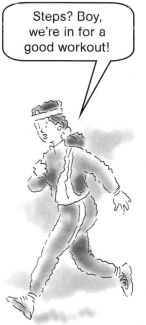

Steps? Boy, we're in for a good workout!

Conversion factors–again, these are the equivalents that are necessary to convert between systems. The conversion factor for this problem is:

$$100\,cm = 1\,m$$

Set up the problem using necessary equivalents as conversion factors. When setting up equations, make sure that units you want cancelled out appear in both a numerator and a denominator. If an unwanted unit appears in two numerators, for example, you won't be able to cancel it. In this example, you want to cancel the centimetres and get the answer in metres. To do this, you must multiply 200 cm by a fraction that has centimetres in the denominator and metres in the numerator. The problem should be set up as:

$$\frac{200\,cm}{1} \times \frac{1\,m}{100\,cm}$$

Just as with any type of mathematical problem, you'll cancel units that appear in both the numerator and denominator to isolate the unit you're seeking. In this case, you'll cancel centimetres, thereby isolating metres, which is the desired measurement. The step will look like this:

$$\frac{200 \; \cancel{cm}}{1} \times \frac{1 \; m}{100 \; \cancel{cm}}$$

Multiply the numerators, multiply the denominators and divide the product of the numerators by the product of the denominators to reach the wanted quantity:

$$\frac{200}{1} \times \frac{1 \; m}{100} = \frac{200 \times 1 \; m}{1 \times 100} = \frac{200 \; m}{100} = 2 \; m$$

There are 2 m in 200 cm.

Let's step to it again!

Now try to solve another problem using dimensional analysis. A package weighs 38 ounces (oz). How many pounds (or lb) does it weigh?

- Identify the given:

$$38 \; oz$$

- Identify the wanted:

$$X \; pounds$$

- Identify the conversion factor:

$$1 \; lb = 16 \; oz$$

- Set up the equation:

$$\frac{38 \; oz}{1} \times \frac{1 \; lb}{16 \; oz}$$

- Cancel units that appear in both the numerator and denominator:

$$\frac{38 \; \cancel{oz}}{1} \times \frac{1 \; lb}{16 \; \cancel{oz}}$$

- Multiply the numerators and denominators and divide the products:

$$\frac{38 \times 1 \; lb}{1 \times 16} = \frac{38 \; lb}{16} = 2.4 \; lb$$

There are 2.4 lb in 38 oz.

I wonder if converting this to kilograms will help make it feel any lighter?

Feel the conversion burn!

Now see how we can use dimensional analysis to take this same example a little further. If the same package weighs 38 oz, what does it weigh in kilograms? (Kilograms can be abbreviated to 'kg'.)
- Identify the given:

$$38\,oz$$

- Identify the wanted:

$$X\,kilograms$$

- Identify the conversion factors (in this case, there are two):

$$1\,lb = 16\,oz$$

$$1\,kg = 2.2\,lb$$

- Set up the equation:

$$\frac{38\,oz}{1} \times \frac{1\,lb}{16\,oz} \times \frac{1\,kg}{2.2\,lb}$$

- Cancel units that appear in both the numerator and denominator:

$$\frac{38\,\cancel{oz}}{1} \times \frac{1\,\cancel{lb}}{16\,\cancel{oz}} \times \frac{1\,kg}{2.2\,\cancel{lb}}$$

- Multiply the numerators and denominators and divide the products:

$$\frac{38 \times 1 \times 1\,kg}{1 \times 16 \times 2.2} = \frac{38\,kg}{35.2} = 1.08\,kg$$

There are 1.08 kg in 38 oz.

Take a breath and let's review

Now that you've made it through the steps again, let's pause to study some key ideas. Dimensional analysis is a method of problem-solving that can be used whenever two quantities are directly proportional to each other. One of the quantities can be converted to another unit of measurement by using common equivalents or conversion factors. The problem is treated as an equation using fractions. (See *Quick guide to dimensional analysis*.)

Now on your feet and do it again!

Apply the concepts you just reviewed above. Tom is recovering from orthopaedic surgery. As part of his rehabilitation, he walks

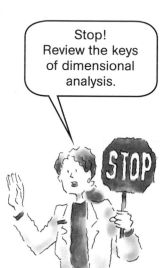

Stop! Review the keys of dimensional analysis.

Advice from the experts

Quick guide to dimensional analysis

Need to calculate a dosage? Need to figure out a drip rate? Don't panic! Just follow this step-by-step guide to dimensional analysis to come up with the number you need quickly and accurately.

Step 1: Given

Identify the given quantity in the problem.

Step 2: Wanted

Identify the wanted quantity in the problem (the unknown unit, or the answer to the problem).

Step 3: Conversion factor

Write down the equivalents that are necessary to convert between systems.

Step 4: The problem

Set up the fractions so that the units you need to cancel appear as both a numerator and a denominator. Units can't be cancelled if they appear only as numerators or only as denominators.

Step 5: Unwanted units

Cancel unwanted units that appear in the numerator and denominator to isolate the unit you're seeking for the answer.

Step 6: Multiply, multiply and divide

This is where you use maths to solve the problem. Multiply the numerators, multiply the denominators and divide the products.

Fun with dimensional analysis!

Now try this sample problem using the steps identified above.

A doctor prescribes 75 mg of a drug. The pharmacy stocks a solution containing the drug at a concentration of 100 mg/ml. What dose should you give in millilitres?

- Step 1: Given = 75 mg
- Step 2: Wanted = X ml
- Step 3: Conversion factor: 100 mg = 1 ml
- Step 4: Set up the equation (remember that units you want cancelled should be positioned in both a numerator and a denominator):

$$\frac{75\,mg}{1} \times \frac{1\,ml}{100\,mg}$$

- Step 5: Cancel unwanted units:

$$\frac{75\,\cancel{mg}}{1} \times \frac{1\,ml}{100\,\cancel{mg}}$$

- Step 6: Multiply, multiply and divide:

$$\frac{75 \times 1\,ml}{1 \times 100} = \frac{75}{100} = 0.75\,ml \text{ of the solution}$$

2 kilometres (km) each day. If he usually walks at a pace of 2.5 km per hour, how long will it take Tom to complete his walk?

- Identify the given:

$$2\,km$$

- Identify the wanted:

$$X\,hours$$

- Identify the conversion factor:

$$2.5 \, km = 1 \, hour$$

- Set up the equation:

$$\frac{2 \, km}{1} \times \frac{1 \, hour}{2.5 \, km}$$

- Cancel units that appear in both the numerator and denominator:

$$\frac{2 \, \cancel{km}}{1} \times \frac{1 \, hour}{2.5 \, \cancel{km}}$$

- Multiply the numerators and denominators and divide the products:

$$\frac{2 \times 1 \, hour}{1 \times 2.5} = \frac{2 \, hours}{2.5} = 0.8 \, hours$$

It will take Tom 0.8 hours to complete his walk.

Real-world problems

A patient is prescribed 70 mg of enoxaparin. It's available in vials that contain 40 mg per 0.4 ml. How much should be prepared?

- Begin by identifying the given quantity:

$$70 \, mg$$

- Then isolate what you're looking for:

$$X \, ml$$

- Know your conversion factor:

$$40 \, mg = 0.4 \, ml$$

- Set up the equation:

$$\frac{70 \, mg}{1} \times \frac{0.4 \, ml}{40 \, mg}$$

- Identify and cancel units that appear in both the numerator and denominator:

$$\frac{70 \, \cancel{mg}}{1} \times \frac{0.4 \, ml}{40 \, \cancel{mg}}$$

- Lastly, multiply the numerators and denominators and divide the products:

$$\frac{70 \times 0.4 \, ml}{1 \times 40} = \frac{28}{40} = 0.7 \, ml$$

The patient would receive 0.7 ml of enoxaparin.

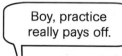

Boy, practice really pays off.

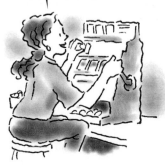

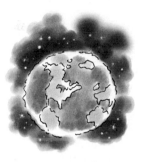

Solve for ibuprofen

A patient is to receive 50 mg of ibuprofen. The drug is available as 100 mg per 5 ml. How many millilitres should the nurse prepare?

- The given quantity:

$$50\,mg$$

- The wanted quantity:

$$X\,ml$$

- The conversion factor:

$$100\,mg = 5\,ml$$

- Set up the equation:

$$\frac{50\ mg}{1} \times \frac{5\ ml}{100\ mg}$$

- Cancel units that appear in both the numerator and denominator:

$$\frac{50\ \cancel{mg}}{1} \times \frac{5\ ml}{100\ \cancel{mg}}$$

- Then multiply the numerators and denominators and divide the products:

$$\frac{50 \times 5\ ml}{1 \times 100} = \frac{250}{100} = 2.5\ ml$$

The nurse should prepare 2.5 ml of ibuprofen.

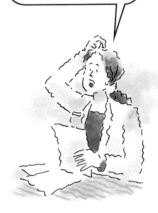

Now where did I see that conversion factor? And did I remember to cancel out the right units? It wouldn't hurt to double-check!

How much heparin?

A patient is prescribed 10 000 units of heparin in 500 ml of 5% glucose in water, at 1200 units/hour. How many drops per minute should you administer if the I.V. tubing delivers 20 drops/ml?

- The given quantities (in this case there are three):

$$\text{1st quantity:} \quad \frac{20\ drops}{1\ ml}$$

$$\text{2nd quantity:} \quad \frac{500\ ml}{10\,000\ units}$$

$$\text{3rd quantity:} \quad \frac{1200\ units}{1\ hour}$$

- The wanted quantity:

$$X\,drops/minute$$

- The conversion factor:

$$\frac{1\ hour}{60\ minutes}$$

- Set up the equation:

$$\frac{20\ \text{drops}}{1\ \text{ml}} \times \frac{500\ \text{ml}}{10\,000\ \text{units}} \times \frac{1200\ \text{units}}{1\ \text{hour}} \times \frac{1\ \text{hour}}{60\ \text{minutes}}$$

- Cancel the units that appear in both the numerator and denominator:

$$\frac{20\ \text{drops}}{1\ \cancel{\text{ml}}} \times \frac{500\ \cancel{\text{ml}}}{10\,000\ \cancel{\text{units}}} \times \frac{1200\ \cancel{\text{units}}}{1\ \cancel{\text{hour}}} \times \frac{1\ \cancel{\text{hour}}}{60\ \text{minutes}}$$

- Then multiply the numerators and denominators and divide the products:

$$\frac{20 \times 500 \times 1200\ \text{drops}}{10\,000 \times 60} = \frac{12\,000\,000}{600\,000\ \text{minutes}} = 20\ \text{drops/minute}$$

You should administer the heparin at a rate of 20 drops/minute.

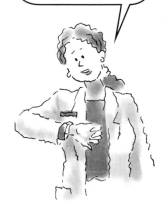

Looks like we have time for one more practice problem.

Featuring furosemide fractions

Let's try one more problem. Your patient is to receive 20 mg of furosemide oral solution. The bottle is labelled 40 mg per 5 ml. How many millilitres will the patient receive?

- The given quantity:

$$20\,\text{mg}$$

- The wanted quantity:

$$X\,\text{ml}$$

- The conversion factor:

$$40\,\text{mg} = 5\,\text{ml}$$

- Set up the equation:

$$\frac{20\ \text{mg}}{1} \times \frac{5\ \text{ml}}{40\ \text{mg}}$$

- Cancel units that appear in both the numerator and denominator:

$$\frac{20\ \cancel{\text{mg}}}{1} \times \frac{5\ \text{ml}}{40\ \cancel{\text{mg}}}$$

- Multiply the numerators and denominators and divide the products:

$$\frac{20 \times 5\ \text{ml}}{1 \times 40} = \frac{100\ \text{ml}}{40} = 2.5\ \text{ml}$$

The patient would receive 2.5 ml of furosemide oral solution.

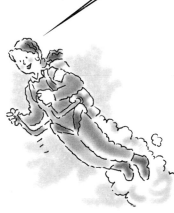

I've just experienced another dimension of the expanding nursing universe!

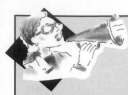

That's a wrap!
Dimensional analysis review

Remember these important facts about dimensional analysis for dosage calculations.

Dimensional analysis basics

- Use whenever two quantities are directly proportional to each other.
- Use common equivalents or conversion factors to convert to the same unit of measurement.
- Set up the problem using fractions.

Performing dimensional analysis: 6 steps

- Determine the given quantity.
- Determine the wanted quantity.
- Select conversion factors.
- Set up the problem.
- Cancel unwanted units.
- Multiply the numerators, multiply the denominators and divide the products.

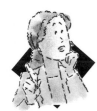

Quick quiz

1. When using dimensional analysis, factors are written as:
   A. fractions.
   B. whole numbers.
   C. percentages.
   D. ratios.

Answer: A. Factors are always written as common fractions. When a problem includes a quantity and its unit of measurement is unrelated to any other factor in the problem, that quantity serves as the numerator of the fraction, and 1 (which is implied) becomes the denominator.

2. Conversion factors in a dimensional analysis equation are:
   A. identified as the given quantity and the wanted quantity.
   B. equivalents necessary to convert between two systems.
   C. always placed as numerators.
   D. always placed as denominators.

Answer: B. Conversion factors involve equivalent measurements that allow for conversion between different systems.

3. Dimensional analysis involves calculations that can be solved:
   A. in three simple steps.
   B. in a single equation.
   C. using formulas that must be memorised.
   D. using common denominators.

Answer: B. Although dimensional analysis uses a step-by-step approach, the problem can be simplified in one single equation.

4. Your patient is 142 cm tall. How much is this in metres?
    A.   0.71 m
    B.   1.42 m
    C.   14.2 m
    D.   142 m

Answer: B. Use the conversion factor 100 cm equals 1 m. Then set up the equation and follow the steps:

$$\frac{142 \ \cancel{cm}}{1} \times \frac{1 \ m}{100 \ \cancel{cm}}$$

$$\frac{142 \times 1 \ m}{1 \times 100} = \frac{142 \ m}{100} = 1.42 \ m$$

5. How many pounds are in 48 oz?
    A.   4 lb
    B.   6 lb
    C.   5 lb
    D.   3 lb

Answer: D. Use the conversion factor 16 oz equals 1 lb to solve:

$$\frac{48 \ \cancel{oz}}{1} \times \frac{1 \ lb}{16 \ \cancel{oz}}$$

$$\frac{48 \times 1 \ lb}{1 \times 16} = \frac{48 \ lb}{16} = 3 \ lb$$

6. A container weighs 11 lb. How much is this in kilograms?
    A.   6 kg
    B.   7 kg
    C.   8 kg
    D.   9 kg

Answer: C. Use the conversion factor 2.2 lb equals 1 kg to solve:

$$\frac{11 \ \cancel{lb}}{1} \times \frac{1 \ kg}{2.2 \ \cancel{lb}}$$

$$\frac{11 \times 1 \ kg}{1 \times 2.2} = \frac{11 \ lb}{2.2} = 5 \ kg$$

Scoring

☆☆☆ If you answered all six items correctly, congratulations! You've added an impressive dimension to your intellect!

☆☆ If you answered four or five items correctly, label yourself a factor to be reckoned with. Don't convert to lazy ways; keep up the good work!

☆ If you answered fewer than three items correctly, please retrace your steps to discover where you went wrong. You'll soon be the equivalent of an expert!

Part II

Measurement systems

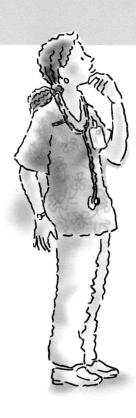

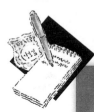

Just the facts

In this chapter, you'll learn:

♦ metric units of measure

♦ how to convert measurements from one metric unit to another

♦ how to solve basic arithmetic problems in metric units

♦ how to calculate drug dosages using the metric system.

A look at the metric system

Today, most nations of the world rely on the metric system of measurement. It's also the most widely used system for measuring amounts of drugs.

The metric system is a *decimal* system. That means it's based on the number 10 and multiples and subdivisions of 10. The metric system offers three advantages over other systems:
• It eliminates common fractions.
• It simplifies the calculation of large and small units.
• It simplifies the calculation of drug doses. (See *Tips for going metric.*)

Beginning with the basics

The three basic units of measurement in the metric system (along with the abbreviation for each) are the metre (m), litre (L) and gram (g):
• The metre is the basic unit of length.
• The litre is the basic unit of volume – it's equivalent to 1 cubic decimetre.
• The gram is the basic unit of weight – it represents the weight of 1 cubic centimetre (cm³ or cc) of water at 4°C.

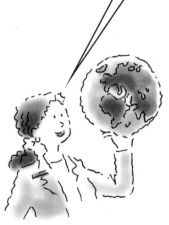

The metric system makes my world a lot easier to handle!

What's in a name?

All other units of measure are based on these three major units. When you see the root word *metre*, *litre* or *gram* within a measurement, you can easily tell if you're measuring length, volume or weight.

For example, centi*metre* (cm) and milli*metre* (mm) are units of length, centi*litre* (cl) and milli*litre* (ml) are units of volume, and kilo*gram* (kg) and milli*gram* (mg) are units of weight.

Measure for measure

Three devices – the metric ruler, the metric graduate and metric weights – are used to measure metres, litres and grams.

Building on the basics

Multiples and subdivisions of metres, litres and grams are indicated by using a prefix before the basic unit. Each prefix that's used in the metric system represents a multiple or subdivision of 10.

Consider the gram. The most common multiple of a gram is the *kilo*gram, which is 1000 times greater than the gram. The most common subdivision of a gram is the *milli*gram, which represents $\frac{1}{1000}$ of a gram, or 0.001 g.

Keeping it brief

Any metric measurement can be represented by a number and an abbreviation that represents the unit of measure. The abbreviation

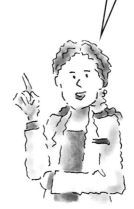

Metres, litres and grams. I can build on that foundation!

Advice from the experts

Tips for going metric

Remember these tips when using the metric system.

Tip	Example
Use the correct abbreviation for each unit of measurement. The abbreviation always follows a number that represents a quantity.	Five kilograms is abbreviated as 5 kg. Five and a half milligrams is abbreviated as 5.5 mg.
Use decimal fractions to represent a part of a whole.	2.5 mg represents 2 milligrams plus five out of ten parts of 1 milligram.
Place a zero before the decimal point for amounts that are less than 1.	0.5 mg, 0.2 ml and 0.65 mcg are less than 1.
Eliminate extra zeros so they aren't misread.	Use 5 mg (not 5.0 mg) and 0.5 ml (not 0.500 ml).

What a little prefix can do

In the metric system, the addition of a prefix to one of the basic units of measure indicates a multiple or subdivision of that unit. Here's a list of prefixes, abbreviations, and multiples and subdivisions of each unit.

Prefix	Abbreviation	Multiples and subdivisions
kilo	k	1000
hecto	h	100
deca	da	10
deci	d	0.1 ($\frac{1}{10}$)
centi	c	0.01 ($\frac{1}{100}$)
milli	m	0.001 ($\frac{1}{1000}$)
micro	mc	0.000001 ($\frac{1}{1000\,000}$)
nano	n	0.000000001 ($\frac{1}{1000\,000\,000}$)
pico	p	0.000000000001 ($\frac{1}{1000\,000\,000\,000}$)

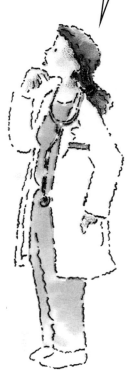

Knowing these prefixes can help me fix almost any dosage muddle.

stands for the basic unit of measure – gram (g), metre (m), litre (L) – and the prefix, such as kilo (k), centi (c) or milli (m). For example, *kg* stands for kilogram, *cm* for centimetre and *ml* for millilitre. (See *What a little prefix can do*.)

A cubic curiosity

The metric system also includes one unusual unit of volume – the cubic centimetre (cc). Because a cubic centimetre occupies the same space as 1 ml of liquid, the two units of volume are considered equal and may be used interchangeably. However, cubic centimetres usually refer to gas volumes, and millilitres usually describe liquid volumes.

Failing to meet standards

The International System of Units (abbreviated to **SI** from the French *Système International d'Unités*) is the modern form of the metric system. It is the world's most widely used system of units, in both science and medicine. The International Bureau of Weights and Measures adopted the International System of Units in 1960 to promote the standard use of metric abbreviations and prevent errors in drug transcriptions. Although alternative measurement systems are sometimes used (particularly in the USA), these systems should be avoided in favour of the standard metric system.

Metric conversions

Because the metric system is decimal-based, converting from one metric unit to another is easy. To convert a smaller unit to a larger unit, move the decimal point to the left. To convert a larger unit to a smaller unit, move the decimal point to the right.

Because all metric units are multiples or subdivisions of the major units, you can also convert a smaller unit to a larger unit by dividing by the appropriate multiple or multiplying by the appropriate subdivision. To convert a larger unit to a smaller unit, multiply by the appropriate multiple or divide by the appropriate subdivision.

Turning the tables on measurements

Luckily, there are tables you can turn to for help in quickly converting measurements. (See *Insta-metric conversion table* and *Amazing metric decimal place finder*.)

Converting metres to kilometres

Suppose you want to convert 15 metres (m) to kilometres (km). There are two ways to get this done.

Dancing decimal

Using the *Amazing metric decimal place finder*, you can follow these steps:

Count the number of places to the right or left of *metres* it takes to reach *kilo*. You'll see that *kilo* is *three* places to the left, indicating

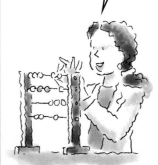

Boy, that table will sure fit more easily in my pocket than this old thing!

Insta-metric conversion table

Want a quick and easy way to jump back and forth between different metric measures? Just use the fantastic 'insta-metric' table below. Make a copy of it to post in a conspicuous spot on your unit. Always remember, a millilitre is to a litre as a microgram is to a milligram.

Liquids	Solids
1 ml = 1 cm³ (or cc)	1000 ng = 1 mcg
1000 ml = 1 L	1000 mcg = 1 mg
100 cl = 1 L	1000 mg = 1 g
10 dl = 1 L	1000 g = 1 kg

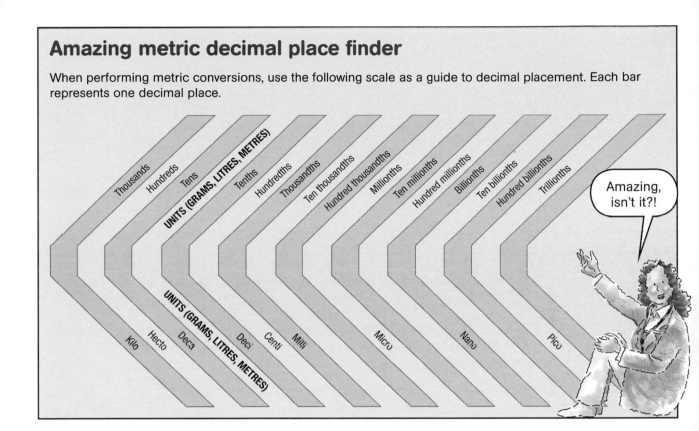

Amazing metric decimal place finder

When performing metric conversions, use the following scale as a guide to decimal placement. Each bar represents one decimal place.

that a kilometre is 1000 times larger than a metre (note the three zeros in 1000).

Move the decimal point in 15.0 three places to the *left*, creating the number 0.015. So, 15 m = 0.015 km. Remember to place a zero in front of the decimal point to draw attention to the decimal point's presence.

On another road to conversion

Another way to complete this conversion is to use the chart in *What a little prefix can do*. First, find *kilo*. You'll see that it indicates a multiple of 1000. When using this chart to go from smaller units to larger units (as you're doing with metres to kilometres), you divide by the multiple.

Here's why: 1 m multiplied by 1000 equals 1 km. Think of driving in Europe, where road distance is measured in kilometres; if you drive 1 m of a 1-km road, you're 1/1000 of the way there. Therefore, 1 m equals 1/1000 km.

To convert 15 m to kilometres, divide by 1000. You might want to set up a simple equation:

$$X = \frac{15 \text{ m}}{1000}$$

$$X = 0.015 \text{ km}$$

So, 15 m = 0.015 km, or 15 thousandths of a kilometre.

Converting grams to milligrams

Now let's say that you want to convert 5 g to milligrams. Again, you can use one of two methods.

Decimal dances again

Using the *Amazing metric decimal place finder*, follow these steps:

Count the number of places to the right or left of *grams* it takes to reach *milli*. You'll see that *milli* is three places to the right, indicating that a milligram is 1000 times smaller than a gram (note the three zeros in 1000).

Move the decimal point in 5.0 three places to the right, creating the number 5000. So 5 g = 5000 mg.

The multiplying subdivision

Or, as before, the chart in *What a little prefix can do* can help you complete your conversion. This time, find *milli*. You'll see that its subdivision is 0.001, or ¹⁄₁₀₀₀. When using this table to go from a larger unit to a smaller unit (such as grams to milligrams), divide by the subdivision.

Here's why: 1 mg is ¹⁄₁₀₀₀ of a gram. Therefore, 1 g equals 1000 mg. If you divide 1 g by the subdivision (¹⁄₁₀₀₀), you get 1000 mg (dividing by ¹⁄₁₀₀₀ is the same as multiplying by 1000). So to convert 5 g to milligrams, divide 5 g by ¹⁄₁₀₀₀ (or multiply it by 1000):

$$X = \frac{5 \text{ g}}{\frac{1}{1\,000}}$$

As you can see, 5 g = 5000 mg.

Converting centilitres to litres

How do you convert 350 cl to litres? Here's how using both charts.

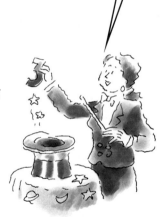

You don't need hocus pocus when you have the one... the only... *Amazing Metric Decimal Place Finder*!

Dancing decimal never rests

Using the *Amazing metric decimal place finder*, follow these steps:

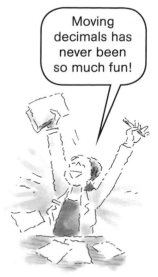

Count the number of places to the right or left of *centi* it takes to reach *litres*. You'll see that *litres* is two places to the left, indicating that a litre is 100 times larger than a centilitre.

To show this, move the decimal point in 350.0 two places to the left, creating the number 3.5. So, 350 cl = 3.5 L.

Another vision of subdivision

Now refer to the chart in *What a little prefix can do*. First, find *centi*. You'll see that its subdivision is 0.01 or ¹⁄₁₀₀. When using this chart to go from a smaller unit to a larger one (centilitres to litres), you multiply by the subdivision.

Here's why: 1 L equals 100 cl. Therefore, 1 cl is ¹⁄₁₀₀ L (or 1 L divided by 100). To convert 350 cl to litres, multiply 350 cl by ¹⁄₁₀₀ (which is the same as dividing by 100) to get 3.5 L:

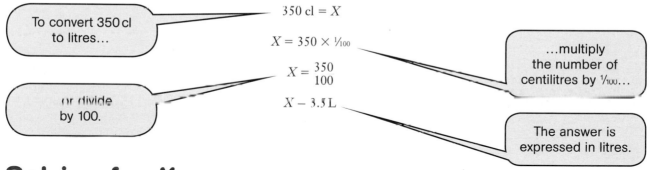

Moving decimals has never been so much fun!

To convert 350 cl to litres...

or divide by 100.

$$350 \text{ cl} = X$$

$$X = 350 \times \tfrac{1}{100}$$

$$X = \frac{350}{100}$$

$$X = 3.5 \text{ L}$$

...multiply the number of centilitres by ¹⁄₁₀₀...

The answer is expressed in litres.

Solving for X

Another way to convert between metric units is by solving for X. The following examples show how to solve for X in three clinical situations. If you don't like fractions, see *Overcoming fear of fractions*.

How much does that baby weigh?

An infant weighs 6.5 kg. How much does he weigh in grams? To solve the problem, follow these steps:

First, refer to the *Insta-metric conversion table*. You'll see that 1000 g equals 1 kg.

For maths phobics only

Overcoming fear of fractions

If you don't like working with fractions, here's an alternative to solving for *X* in problems. In this example about determining an infant's weight in grams, the equation that's expressed in fractions can also be set up as a ratio and proportion:

$$1000\,g : 1\,kg :: X : 6.5\,kg$$

- Multiply the means and extremes:

$$X \times 1\,kg = 1000\,g \times 6.5\,kg$$

- Divide both sides of the equation by 1 kg to isolate *X*.
- Cancel units that appear in both the numerator and denominator:

$$X = 6500\,g$$

The infant weighs 6500 g.

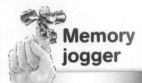

Memory jogger

To remember the difference between **means** and **extremes** in a ratio, think of:

Means = **m**iddle numbers

Extremes = **e**nd numbers

Now set up the following equation, substituting X for the unknown weight in grams:

$$\frac{1000\,g}{1\,kg} = \frac{X}{6.5\,kg}$$

Cross-multiply the fractions:

$$\frac{1000\,g}{1\,kg} \bowtie \frac{X}{6.5\,kg}$$

$$X \times 1\,kg = 6.5\,kg \times 1000\,g$$

Divide both sides of the equation by 1 kg to isolate X. Cancel units that appear in both the numerator and denominator:

$$\frac{X \times 1\,kg}{1\,kg} = \frac{6.5\,kg \times 1000\,g}{1\,kg}$$

$$X = 6500\,g$$

The infant weighs 6500 g.

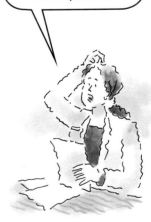

Oh, I remember. *X* stands for the unknown quantity in the equation.

How much I.V. fluid?

If a patient received 0.375 L of Ringer-lactate solution, how many millilitres did he receive?
- Refer to the *Insta-metric conversion table*. You'll see that 1 L is equal to 1000 ml.
- Now set up the following equation, substituting X for the unknown amount of I.V. solution in millilitres:

$$\frac{1\,L}{1000\,ml} = \frac{0.375\,L}{X}$$

- Cross-multiply the fractions:

$$\frac{1\,L}{1000\,ml} \diagdown\!\!\!\!\diagup \frac{0.375\,L}{X}$$

$$X \times 1\,L = 0.375\,L \times 1000\,ml$$

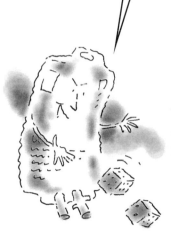

No need to gamble on this dosage. Just convert, cross-multiply, divide and cancel!

- Divide both sides of the equation by 1 L to isolate X. Cancel units that appear in both the numerator and denominator:

$$\frac{X \times \cancel{1\,L}}{\cancel{1\,L}} = \frac{0.375\,\cancel{L} \times 1000\,ml}{1\,\cancel{L}}$$

$$X = 375\,ml$$

The patient received 375 ml of I.V. fluid.

How much medication?

A nurse administered 2 g of ceftriaxone. How many milligrams of this medication did the patient receive?
- Refer to the *Insta-metric conversion table*. You'll see that 1 g is equal to 1000 mg.
- Now set up the following equation, substituting X for the unknown amount of medication in milligrams:

$$\frac{1\,g}{1000\,mg} = \frac{2\,g}{X}$$

- Cross-multiply the fractions:

$$\frac{1\,g}{1000\,mg} \diagdown\!\!\!\!\diagup \frac{2\,g}{X}$$

$$X \times 1\,g = 2\,g \times 1000\,mg$$

- Divide each side of the equation by 1 g, to isolate X. Cancel units that appear in both the numerator and denominator:

$$\frac{X \times \cancel{1\,g}}{\cancel{1\,g}} = \frac{2\,\cancel{g} \times 1000\,mg}{1\,\cancel{g}}$$

$$X = 2000\,mg$$

The patient received 2000 mg of ceftriaxone.

Metric mathematics

To add, subtract, multiply or divide different metric units, first convert all quantities to the same unit. Unless the problem calls for an answer in a specific unit, use the common unit that's easiest for you to work with and then perform the arithmetic.

For example, suppose you want to add 2 kg, 202 mg and 222 g, expressing the total in grams. Here's how to do this:

First, convert all the measurements to grams. (Refer to the *Insta-metric conversion table.*)

1 kg equals 1000 g. Therefore, you can multiply 2 kg by 1000 to get 2000 g.

1000 mg equals 1 g and 1 mg equals $\frac{1}{1000}$ g. Therefore, you can divide 202 mg by 1000 to get 0.202 g.

Now do the addition:

$$2000 + 0.202 + 222 = 2222.202 \text{ g}$$

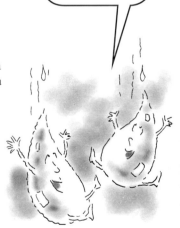

How many of us are left? Just add, convert and subtract. Wheeee!

Real-world problems

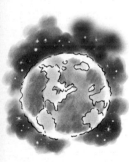

A patient with a 1-L bag of I.V. fluid received 500 ml of fluid over an initial 8-hour period, 225 ml over a second 8 hours and 150 ml over a third 8 hours. How many millilitres of fluid remain in the I.V. bag at the end of 24 hours?
• First, determine how much fluid the patient received. To do this, add:

$$500 + 225 + 150 = 875 \text{ ml}$$

• Because you're trying to determine the number of millilitres remaining, you need to convert only 1 L to millilitres. Refer to the *Insta-metric conversion table*, where you'll see that 1 L = 1000 ml.
• Lastly, compute the amount of fluid remaining in the I.V. bag by subtracting 875 ml from 1000 ml. The answer is 125 ml.

A tantalizing tablet tabulation!

A patient is to receive 5 g of erythromycin before intestinal surgery. If erythromycin is available in 500-mg tablets, how many tablets should be administered?
• First, convert all the measures to the same units. Because you're trying to determine the number of 500-mg tablets to administer,

convert 5 g to milligrams. Refer to the *Insta-metric conversion table,* where you'll see that 1 g is equal to 1000 mg.

• To find how many milligrams are in 5 g, set up this proportion using fractions:

$$\frac{1000 \text{ mg}}{1 \text{ g}} = \frac{X}{5 \text{ g}}$$

• Then cross-multiply the fractions and divide each side of the resulting equation by 1 g to solve for X:

$$\frac{1000 \text{ mg}}{1 \text{ g}} \diagup\!\!\!\!\diagdown \frac{X}{5 \text{ g}}$$

$$X \times 1 \text{ g} = 1000 \text{ mg} \times 5 \text{ g}$$

$$\frac{X \times \cancel{1 \text{ g}}}{\cancel{1 \text{ g}}} = \frac{1000 \text{ mg} \times 5 \, \cancel{g}}{1 \, \cancel{g}}$$

$$X = 5000 \text{ mg}$$

• You find that X is 5000 mg.
• To determine the number of 500-mg tablets that need to be administered to provide 5000 mg, set up another proportion using fractions:

$$\frac{500 \text{ mg}}{1 \text{ tablet}} = \frac{5000 \text{ mg}}{X}$$

• Cross-multiply the fractions and divide each side of the resulting equation by 500 mg to solve for X:

$$\frac{500 \text{ mg}}{1 \text{ tablet}} \diagup\!\!\!\!\diagdown \frac{5000 \text{ mg}}{X}$$

$$X \times 500 \text{ mg} = 5000 \text{ mg} \times 1 \text{ tablet}$$

$$\frac{X \times \cancel{500 \text{ mg}}}{\cancel{500 \text{ mg}}} = \frac{1 \text{ tablet} \times 5000 \, \cancel{mg}}{500 \, \cancel{mg}}$$

• You find that X is 10 tablets.
  You should administer 10 tablets of erythromycin. (See *Did I get it right?*)

Yes! I've mastered metric maths and measurements!

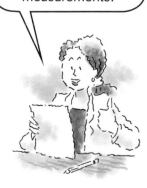

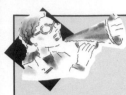

That's a wrap!

Metric system review

Knowing these important facts about the metric system will make your calculations incredibly easy!

Metric basics

- It's the most widely used system for measuring amounts of drugs.
- It's a decimal system (based on the number 10 and its multiples and subdivisions).
- Three basic units of measurement are used in the metric system:
  - *metre*, basic unit of length
  - *litre*, basic unit of volume
  - *gram*, basic unit of weight.
- Multiples and subdivisions of metres, litres and grams are indicated by using a prefix before the basic unit, such as *kilo*, *centi* or *milli*.

Metric conversions

- To convert a smaller unit to a larger unit:
  - move the decimal point to the left
  - OR divide by the appropriate multiple
  - OR multiply by the appropriate subdivision.

- To convert a larger unit to a smaller unit:
  - move the decimal point to the right
  - OR multiply by the appropriate multiple
  - OR divide by the appropriate subdivision.

Solving for *X*

- Set up an equation, substituting *X* for the unknown you're trying to determine.
- Cross-multiply the fractions.
- Divide both sides to isolate *X* on one side.
- Cancel units that appear in both the numerator and denominator.
- Do the maths!

Metric maths

- First, convert all quantities to the same unit.
- Use the common unit that's easiest (unless the problem calls for a specific unit).
- Do the maths!

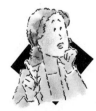

Quick quiz

1. According to the International System of Units (the SI system), the correct abbreviation for gram is:

   A. gm
   B. g
   C. Gm
   D. GM

Answer: B. The standard abbreviation for gram is g.

2. The number of milligrams in 3120 mcg is:
  A. 3 120 000 mg
  B. 0.312 mg
  C. 31.2 mg
  D. 3.12 mg

Answer: D. Locate *milli* and *micro* on the *Amazing metric decimal place finder*, count the number of places *milli* is to the left of *micro*, then move the decimal point three places to the left.

3. The total volume in millilitres of 312 ml, 3.12 L and 312 L is:
  A. 327.12 ml
  B. 315 432 ml
  C. 31 543.2 L
  D. 3154 ml

Answer: B. Convert all the measures to millilitres and then add all three numbers.

4. The measure that's equivalent to a millilitre (ml) is:
  A. cubic centimetre
  B. kilolitre
  C. hectolitre
  D. centimetre

Answer: A. A millilitre of liquid occupies a cubic centimetre of space.

5. The weight in grams of a baby who weighs 5.2 kg is:
  A. 5.2 g
  B. 5.02 g
  C. 50.2 g
  D. 5200 g

Answer: D. Knowing that 1 kg is equal to 1000 g, set up an equation with X grams as the unknown quantity and multiply 5.2 kg by 1000 g/kg.

6. The number of millilitres left in a 4-L bag of normal saline solution after you remove 50 ml, 250 ml, 2.5 L and 750 ml is:
  A. 3550 ml
  B. 450 ml
  C. 50 ml
  D. 40 ml

Answer: B. Convert all the measurements to millilitres, add the last four numbers to find out how many millilitres were removed from the bag, then subtract this number from the amount of fluid in the bag.

Scoring

☆☆☆ If you answered all six items correctly, give yourself 6 points! If each point equalled a gram, you would have 6 grams, or 60 decigrams or 600 centigrams…

☆☆ If you answered five items correctly, dig those decimals! You're a metric master.

☆ If you answered fewer than five items correctly, leapin' millilitres! Review the chapter and you'll soon be doing a hecto of a good job.

6 Alternative measurement systems

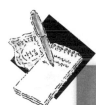

Just the facts

In this chapter, you'll learn:
♦ what the unit system is and how it works
♦ what the millimole system is and how it works
♦ how to perform common conversions.

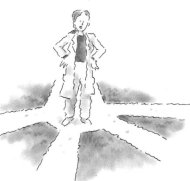

Choosing an alternative measurement system could make all the difference!

A look at alternative measurement systems

Although the metric system is most commonly used in clinical settings, you'll work with other systems from time to time. These include the unit and millimole systems.

Unit system

Some drugs are measured in International Units (IU). The measurement of the unit is unique to each drug that's expressed using this type of measurment.

U-niquely insulin

The most common drug that's measured in units is insulin, which comes in such measurements as U-100 strength.

With insulin, the U refers to the number of units per millilitre. For example, 1 ml of U-100 insulin contains 100 units. The U-100 strength, which is based on metric measurements, makes measurement in a standard syringe easy.

More units singled out

Some other drugs are also measured in units, such as the anticoagulant heparin, and penicillin antibiotics. The hormone calcitonin and the fat-soluble vitamins A, D and E are measured in IU.

All out of proportion

To calculate the dose to be administered when the medication is available in units, use this proportion:

$$\frac{\text{amount of drug in ml or other measure}}{\text{dose required in units}} = \frac{\text{1 ml or other measure}}{\text{drug available in units}}$$

Unit system conversions

The examples in this section show how to perform conversions in the unit system.

Drip…drip…drip…

A standard heparin drip of 25 000 units in 500 ml of half-normal saline solution is prescribed for your patient. The heparin vial that's available has 5000 units/ml. How many millilitres of heparin should you add to the I.V. fluid? This is how to solve this problem:

• Set up a proportion using X as the unknown quantity:

$$\frac{X}{25\,000\ \text{units}} = \frac{1\ \text{ml}}{5000\ \text{units}}$$

• Cross-multiply the fractions:

$$X \times 5000\ \text{units} = 1\ \text{ml} \times 25\,000\ \text{units}$$

• Find X by dividing both sides of the equation by 5000 units and cancelling units that appear in both the numerator and denominator:

$$\frac{X \times 5000\ \cancel{\text{units}}}{5000\ \cancel{\text{units}}} = \frac{1\ \text{ml} \times 25\,000\ \cancel{\text{units}}}{5000\ \cancel{\text{units}}}$$

$$X = 5\ \text{ml}$$

You should add 5 ml of heparin to the I.V. fluid.

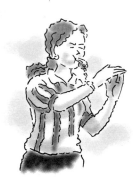

To calculate the perfect dosage, try a unit conversion!

Penicillin problem

Your patient needs 500 000 units of penicillin by intramuscular (I.M.) injection. The vial of penicillin that's available contains 1 000 000 units/ml. How much of the drug should you draw up? This is how to solve this problem:

- Set up a proportion using X as the unknown quantity:

$$\frac{X}{500\ 000\ \text{units}} = \frac{1\ \text{ml}}{1\ 000\ 000\ \text{units}}$$

- Cross-multiply the fractions:

$$X \times 1\ 000\ 000\ \text{units} = 1\ \text{ml} \times 500\ 000\ \text{units}$$

- Find X by dividing each side of the equation by 1 000 000 units and cancelling units that appear in both the numerator and denominator:

$$\frac{X \times 1\ 000\ 000\ \cancel{\text{units}}}{1\ 000\ 000\ \cancel{\text{units}}} = \frac{1\ \text{ml} \times 500\ 000\ \cancel{\text{units}}}{1\ 000\ 000\ \cancel{\text{units}}}$$

$$X = 0.5\ \text{ml}$$

You should inject 0.5 ml of penicillin.

Millilitre mystery

Your patient has been prescribed a bolus of 3000 units of heparin. The heparin vial that's available contains 1000 units/ml. How many millilitres should you administer?

- Set up a proportion using X as the unknown quantity of heparin:

$$\frac{X}{3000\ \text{units}} = \frac{1\ \text{ml}}{1000\ \text{units}}$$

- Cross-multiply the fractions:

$$X \times 1000\ \text{units} = 1\ \text{ml} \times 3000\ \text{units}$$

- Find X by dividing both sides of the equation by 1000 units and cancelling units that appear in both the numerator and denominator:

$$\frac{X \times 1000\ \cancel{\text{units}}}{1000\ \cancel{\text{units}}} = \frac{1\ \text{ml} \times 3000\ \cancel{\text{units}}}{1000\ \cancel{\text{units}}}$$

$$X = 3\ \text{ml}$$

You should administer a 3-ml bolus of heparin.

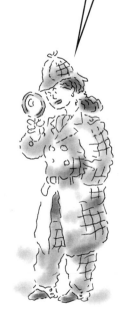

Ah, yes, the Great Millilitre Mystery – I remember it well. Unit conversions made it elementary.

Millimole system

Some electrolytes, such as potassium and sodium, are measured in millimoles (mmol). Drug manufacturers dispense information about the number of metric units required to provide the prescribed number of millimoles. For example, the manufacturer's instructions may indicate that 1 ml equals 4 mmol.

Electrolyte example

The electrolyte potassium chloride is usually prescribed in millimoles. Potassium preparations are available for use in I.V. fluids, as oral suspensions or elixirs, and in solid tablet or powder form. Potassium is also available in the combination drug potassium phosphate. The phosphate in this drug is also measured in millimoles.

A promising proportion

To calculate the dose to be administered when the medication is available in millimoles, use this proportion:

$$\frac{\text{amount of drug in ml or other measure}}{\text{dose required in mmol}} = \frac{\text{1 ml or other measure}}{\text{drug available in mmol}}$$

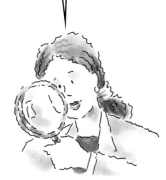

Millimoles sound small but they can be a big dosage problem without the right calculation tools!

Millimole system conversions

The problems below show how to do conversions using the millimole system.

Finding the solution solution

Your patient has been prescribed an I.V. infusion of 40 mmol of potassium chloride in 100 ml of normal saline solution. The potassium vial that's available contains 10 mmol/ml. How many millilitres of potassium chloride should you add to the normal saline solution? This is how to solve this problem:

• Set up a proportion using X as the unknown quantity:

$$\frac{X}{40 \text{ mmol}} = \frac{1 \text{ ml}}{10 \text{ mmol}}$$

• Cross-multiply the fractions:

$$X \times 10 \text{ mmol} = 1 \text{ ml} \times 40 \text{ mmol}$$

- Find X by dividing each side of the equation by 10 mmol and cancelling units that appear in both the numerator and denominator:

$$\frac{X \times 10 \text{ mmol}}{10 \text{ mmol}} = \frac{1 \text{ ml} \times 40 \text{ mmol}}{10 \text{ mmol}}$$

$$X = 4 \text{ ml}$$

You should dilute 4 ml of potassium chloride in 100 ml of normal saline solution.

Calculate that sodium bicarbonate!

Your patient needs 25 mmol of sodium bicarbonate. The vial from the pharmacy contains 50 mmol in 50 ml. How many millilitres of the solution should you administer? Here's how to solve this problem:

- Set up a proportion using X as the unknown quantity:

$$\frac{X}{25 \text{ mmol}} = \frac{50 \text{ ml}}{50 \text{ mmol}}$$

- Cross-multiply the fractions:

$$X \times 50 \text{ mmol} = 50 \text{ ml} \times 25 \text{ mmol}$$

- Find X by dividing both sides of the equation by 50 mmol and cancelling units that appear in both the numerator and denominator:

$$\frac{X \times 50 \text{ mmol}}{50 \text{ mmol}} = \frac{50 \text{ ml} \times 25 \text{ mmol}}{50 \text{ mmol}}$$

$$X = 25 \text{ ml}$$

You should administer 25 ml of sodium bicarbonate solution.

Potassium puzzle

Your patient has been prescribed 30 mmol of potassium chloride oral solution. The solution contains 60 mmol in every 15 ml. How many millilitres of solution should you give the patient? Here's how to solve this problem:

- Set up a proportion using X as the unknown quantity:

$$\frac{X}{30 \text{ mmol}} = \frac{15 \text{ ml}}{60 \text{ mmol}}$$

- Cross-multiply the fractions:

$$X \times 60 \text{ mmol} = 15 \text{ ml} \times 30 \text{ mmol}$$

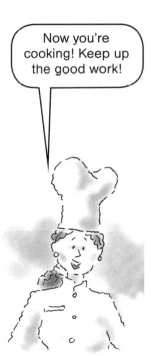

Now you're cooking! Keep up the good work!

- Find X by dividing both sides of the equation by 60 mmol and cancelling units that appear in both the numerator and denominator:

$$\frac{X \times 60 \text{ mmol}}{60 \text{ mmol}} = \frac{15 \text{ ml} \times 30 \text{ mmol}}{60 \text{ mmol}}$$

$$X = 7.5 \text{ ml}$$

You should administer 7.5 ml of oral potassium chloride solution.

Frequently used conversions

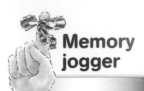

Memory jogger

Remember this jingle when converting inches to centimetres and vice versa: '2.54, that's 1 inch and no more.'

Although use of the metric system is preferred, in clinical practice, it is sometimes necessary to convert between various measurement systems, as some patients may not be familiar with the metric system. This frequently occurs with measurements of weight or height, although it should be avoided whenever possible.

To convert from one system to another, you must know the equivalent measures. If you have trouble remembering the most commonly used equivalents, jot the equivalents on an index card, laminate the card and tuck it into your pocket for easy reference.

A conversion excursion

Two conversions that are commonly used, especially in adult and paediatric intensive care units, are pounds (lb) to kilograms (kg) and inches (″) to centimetres (cm). These conversions are used to determine body weight and body surface.

Making these conversions isn't difficult if you remember the general rules:
- Remember that 1 kg equals 2.2 lb. To convert pounds into kilograms, just divide the number of pounds by 2.2. To convert kilograms to pounds, multiply the number of kilograms by 2.2.
- Remember that 1″ equals 2.54 cm. To convert inches to centimetres, just multiply the number of inches by 2.54. To convert centimetres to inches, divide the number of centimetres by 2.54.

Equivalent-measure conversions

The following examples show how to do equivalent-measure conversions.

You say pounds, I say kilograms

To prepare medications for your hypotensive patient, you must determine her weight in kilograms. You know that she weighs 125 lb, but how much is this in kilograms? Here's how to find out:

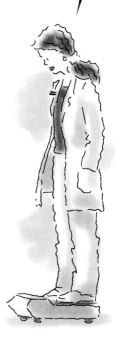

I prefer expressing my weight in kilograms!

- You know that 1 kg equals 2.2 lb. So set up a proportion using X as the unknown weight:

$$\frac{X}{125 \text{ lb}} = \frac{1 \text{ kg}}{2.2 \text{ lb}}$$

- Cross-multiply the fractions:

$$X \times 2.2 \text{ lb} = 1 \text{ kg} \times 125 \text{ lb}$$

- Find X by dividing both sides of the equation by 2.2 lb and cancelling units that appear in both the numerator and denominator:

$$\frac{X \times 2.2 \text{ lb}}{2.2 \text{ lb}} = \frac{1 \text{ kg} \times 125 \text{ lb}}{2.2 \text{ lb}}$$

$$X = 56.8 \text{ kg}$$

Your patient weighs 56.8 kg.

You say inches, I say centimetres

Your patient's height is 58″. How many centimetres is this equivalent to?
- You know that 1″ equals 2.54 cm. So set up a proportion using X as the unknown height:

$$\frac{X}{58''} = \frac{2.54 \text{ cm}}{1''}$$

- Cross-multiply the fractions:

$$X \times 1'' = 2.54 \text{ cm} \times 58''$$

- Solve for X by dividing both sides of the equation by 1″ and cancelling units that appear in both the numerator and denominator:

$$\frac{X \times 1''}{1''} = \frac{2.54 \text{ cm} \times 58''}{1''}$$

$$X = 147.32 \text{ cm}$$

The patient measures 147.32 cm.

Real-world problems

Here are real-world examples using alternative measurement systems.

Calcium question

The following I.V. fluid has been prescribed for your patient: 2000 mg calcium gluconate in 500 ml of 10% glucose in water. The

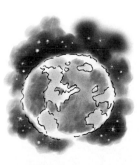

calcium gluconate is available in a vial containing 100 mg calcium gluconate per 1 ml. How many millilitres of calcium gluconate should you add to the glucose solution?
- Set up a proportion using X as the unknown quantity.

$$\frac{X}{2000 \text{ mg}} = \frac{1 \text{ ml}}{100 \text{ mg}}$$

- Cross-multiply the fractions:

$$X \times 100 \text{ mg} = 1 \text{ ml} \times 2000 \text{ mg}$$

- Find X by dividing both sides of the equation by 100 mg and cancelling units that appear in both the numerator and denominator:

$$\frac{X \times \cancel{100 \text{ mg}}}{\cancel{100 \text{ mg}}} = \frac{1 \text{ ml} \times 2000 \cancel{\text{ mg}}}{100 \cancel{\text{ mg}}}$$

$$X = 20 \text{ ml}$$

You should add 20 ml of calcium gluconate to the 500 ml of 10% glucose.

A tall order

Your patient's height is 68″. How many centimetres is this?
- Remember that 1″ = 2.54 cm so you can set up a proportion using X for the unknown quantity:

$$\frac{X}{68″} = \frac{2.54 \text{ cm}}{1″}$$

- Cross-multiply the fractions:

$$X \times 1″ = 2.54 \text{ cm} \times 68″$$

- Solve for X by dividing both sides of the equation by 1″ and cancelling units that appear in both the numerator and denominator:

$$\frac{X \times \cancel{1″}}{\cancel{1″}} = \frac{2.54 \text{ cm} \times 68\cancel{″}}{1\cancel{″}}$$

$$X = 172.72 \text{ cm}$$

The patient measures 172.72 cm.

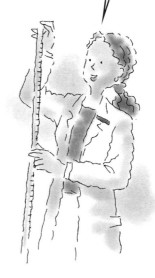

Looks like my patient has grown 7.62 cm since his last physical examination. What are they feeding teenagers these days?

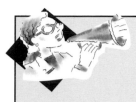

That's a wrap!

Alternative measurement systems review

Keep these important facts in mind when performing calculations with alternative measurement systems.

Unit conversions

- Insulin is the most common drug measured in units.
- Divide the units required by the amount of drug available in units.

Millimole conversions

- The millimole system is used to measure some electrolytes.

- Divide the amount of millimoles required by the amount of drug available in millimoles.

Commonly used conversions

- Pounds to kilograms: divide the number of pounds by 2.2.
- Kilograms to pounds: multiply the number of kilograms by 2.2.
- Inches to centimetres: multiply the number of inches by 2.54.
- Centimetres to inches: divide the number of centimetres by 2.54.

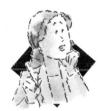

Quick quiz

1. Drugs that are measured in units include:
    A. phenoxymethylpenicillin, insulin and heparin
    B. co-trimoxazole
    C. cough medicine
    D. erythromycin and calcium

Answer: A. Phenoxymethylpenicillin, insulin and heparin are measured in units.

2. Electrolytes are measured in:
    A. grams
    B. milligrams
    C. millimoles
    D. millilitres

Answer: C. Most electrolytes, such as potassium chloride, are measured in millimoles.

3. When converting pounds to kilograms, you should:
    A   multiply by 2.54
    B. divide by 2.2
    C. divide by 2.54
    D. multiply by 2.2

Answer: B. One kilogram equals 2.2 lb. By dividing pounds by 2.2, you obtain kilograms.

4. The equivalent in millilitres of 55 units of insulin (U-100) is:
   A. 55 ml
   B. 5.5 ml
   C. 5 ml
   D. 0.55 ml

Answer: D. To do the conversion, set up the proportion:

$$\frac{X}{55 \text{ units}} = \frac{1 \text{ ml}}{100 \text{ units}}$$

Cross-multiply the fractions; then divide both sides of the equation by 100 units and cancel units that appear in both the numerator and denominator to get 0.55 ml:

$$\frac{X \times 100 \text{ units}}{100 \text{ units}} = \frac{1 \text{ ml} \times 55 \text{ units}}{100 \text{ units}}$$

$$X = 0.55 \text{ ml}$$

5. The equivalent of 43 inches in centimetres is:
   A. 109.22 cm
   B. 10.922 cm
   C. 1.0922 cm
   D. 2.54 cm

Answer: A. 109.22 cm. To do the conversion, set up a proportion using X for the unknown quantity. Remember 1″ is equivalent to 2.54 cm.

$$\frac{X}{43''} = \frac{2.54 \text{ cm}}{1''}$$

Cross-multiply the fractions:

$$X \times 1'' = 2.54 \text{ cm} \times 43''$$

Solve for X by dividing both sides of the equation by 1″ and cancelling units that appear in both the numerator and denominator:

$$\frac{X \times 1''}{1''} = \frac{2.54 \text{ cm} \times 43''}{1''}$$

$$X = 109.22 \text{ cm}$$

Scoring

☆☆☆ If you answered all five items correctly, fantastic! Reward yourself with a milligram of ice cream. (Okay, you can have a kilogram!)

☆☆ If you answered three to five items correctly, good job! Have a centilitre of champagne. (Enjoy every millilitre!)

☆ If you answered fewer than three items correctly, keep at it. In the meantime, have a gram of chocolate. (Savour every milligram!)

Part III

Recording drug administration

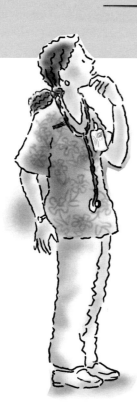

7 Prescriptions

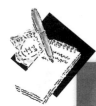

Just the facts

In this chapter, you'll learn:

♦ what a prescription consists of
♦ how to interpret prescriptions using standard abbreviations
♦ how to use the 24-hour clock
♦ what to do about unclear prescriptions.

A look at drug prescriptions

Administering drugs is one of your most critical nursing responsibilities. It's also the area with the smallest margin for error. How can you prevent drug errors? The best way is by knowing how to read and correctly interpret drug prescriptions. To do this, you need to understand what a drug prescription is and how it's used.

Direct handoff

In an outpatient setting, a doctor or other healthcare professional who's qualified to prescribe drugs writes a list of drugs on a prescription form and gives it directly to the patient.

Keyboard or form

The routine for prescribing drugs may be different in various inpatient facilities. There, a prescriber generates a drug prescription in one of two ways:
• by entering the drugs into a computer system that transmits it to the pharmacy and to the nurses' station
• by writing the drugs on a record sheet in the patient's chart.

What's in a drug prescription?

The drug record sheet in a patient's chart must include all patient information, so it's usually stamped with the patient's admission

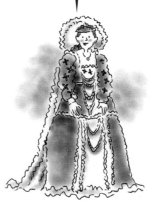

Drug prescriptions have become much more efficient since my day!

label. When writing the prescription, the information should include:
• date and time of the prescription
• the generic name of the drug (or occasionally the specific brand name)
• dosage form in appropriate measurement units (millimoles, metric units or International Units)
• route of administration (in some facilities, if the route isn't specified, the staff may assume that the oral route is preferred)
• administration schedule written as times per day or as number of hours between doses
• restrictions or specifications related to the prescription
• prescriber's signature, or name and code number in a computerised system (one signature, or name and code number, is sufficient after a group of prescribed drugs)
• doctor's registration number for controlled drugs, if applicable.

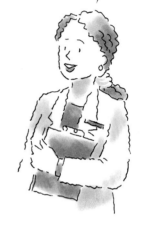

Being aware of standard guidelines will help you interpret prescriptions.

Following orders

Standard guidelines exist for writing prescriptions. Being aware of these guidelines will help you interpret these safely.
• The generic name of a drug is written entirely in lower-case letters.
• A specific brand name for a drug begins with a capital letter.
• Drug-related abbreviations are written entirely in capital letters; drug names should not be abbreviated, to avoid errors.
• Information is written in a standard sequence, including drug name first, then dose, administration route and lastly time and frequency of administration.

A brief look at abbreviating

Standard abbreviations are used to describe drug measurements, dosages, routes and times of administration, and related terms. When used correctly they can save time and reduce documentation.

However, it is important to recognise that abbreviations can also be misinterpreted easily, especially if they're written carelessly or quickly. If an abbreviation seems unusual or doesn't make sense to you, contact the prescriber for clarification. Then clearly write the correct term in your revision and transcription.

What a difference a day makes!

Some doctors and healthcare facilities require prescriptions and medication administration records to be written and transcribed using the 24-hour clock. For example, a prescription might read *furosemide 40 mg I.V. b.i.d. at 0900 and 2100 hours* (See *The 24-hour clock*.)

The 24-hour clock

Study the two clocks below to better understand the 24-hour clock. The clock on the left represents the hours from 1 a.m. (0100 hours) to noon (1200 hours). The clock on the right represents the hours from 1 p.m. (1300 hours) to midnight (2400 hours).

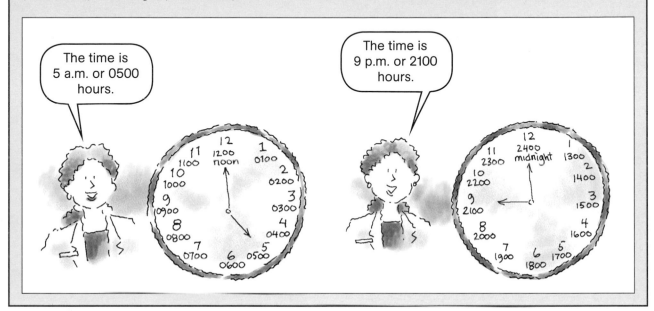

Simply confusing or confusingly simple?

The 24-hour clock might seem confusing at first, but it's actually simple to use. This method of time is based on a 24-hour system. Here's how it works:

• To write single-digit times from 1:00 a.m. to 12:59 p.m., put a zero before the times and remove the colon. For example, 1:00 a.m. is written 0100 hours.

• To write double-digit times from 1:00 a.m. to 12:59 p.m., just remove the colon. For example, 11:00 a.m. becomes 1100 hours.

• The minutes after the hour remain the same. For example, 4:45 a.m. becomes 0445 hours.

• To write times from 1:00 p.m. to 12 midnight, simply add 1200 to the hour and remove the colon. For example, 1:00 p.m. becomes 1300 hours (1:00 + 1200); 3:30 p.m. becomes 1530 hours (3:30 + 1200); and 12:00 a.m. (midnight) becomes 2400 hours (12:00 + 1200).

• To write the minutes between 12:01 a.m. and 12:59 a.m., start over with zero. For example, 12:33 a.m. becomes 0033 hours.

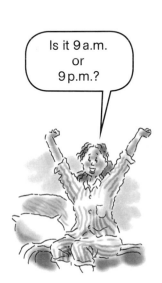

Dealing with prescriptions

After you determine that a prescription contains all the necessary information, you can begin to interpret it. Read on to find guidelines for dealing with illegible handwriting, timing of drug administration, renewing prescriptions and discontinued prescriptions. (See *Say it in English*.)

Hospital hieroglyphics

If any required information is missing or if the handwriting is illegible, check with the prescriber and clarify the prescription before signing the transcription. Also, ask the prescriber for clarification if non-standard abbreviations have been used.

When the prescription is clear, sign it and send a copy to the pharmacy where the drug will be dispensed according to the policy in your healthcare setting.

Calibrating the clinical clock

Although the prescription sheet tells you when to give a drug, the actual administration time depends on three things:

⓵ your facility's policy (for drugs that are given a specific number of times per day)

⓶ the nature of the drug

⓷ the drug's onset and duration of action.

Be sure to administer drugs within half an hour of the times specified on the prescription sheet. After giving a drug, record the actual time of administration on the medication administration record.

Re-evaluate, renew, reorder

Healthcare facilities also have policies for how often prescriptions must be renewed. For example, a prescription for opioids may need to be renewed every 24, 48 or 72 hours. This requirement allows healthcare professionals to re-evaluate the patient's need for the drug and to adjust the dosage or frequency of administration, if necessary.

Remember that I.V. fluids – such as normal saline solution, glucose and water, and total parenteral nutrition solutions – are considered drugs. Check all prescribed I.V. fluids carefully. Most healthcare facilities provide guidelines for the renewal of I.V. fluids as well as for other drugs.

> Drug administration time depends on your facility's policy and the nature of the drug, as well as its onset and duration.

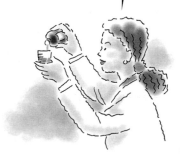

Say it in English

The following examples illustrate how to read and interpret a wide range of prescriptions.

Prescription	Interpretation
Flucloxacillin 250 mg P.O. q.i.d. a.c.	Give 250 mg of flucloxacillin by mouth four times per day before meals.
Promethazine hydrochloride 25 mg I.M. every 3 hours, p.r.n. anxiety	Give 25 mg of promethazine hydrochloride intramuscularly every 3 hours as needed for anxiety.
Increase morphine sulphate to 6 mg I.V. every 8 hours	Increase morphine sulphate to 6 mg intravenously every 8 hours.
Folic acid 5 mg P.O. daily	Give 5 mg of folic acid by mouth daily.
Prazosin 500 mcg P.O. every 8 hours, hold for sys BP < 120	Give 500 mcg of prazosin by mouth every 8 hours; withhold the drug if the systolic blood pressure falls below 120 mmHg.
Nifedipine 20 mg, sub-lingual t.i.d.	Give 20 mg of nifedipine sublingually three times per day.
Begin aspirin 300 mg P.O. daily	Begin giving 300 mg of aspirin by mouth daily.
Dipyridamole 100 mg P.O. t.i.d.	Give 100 mg of dipyridamole by mouth three times per day.
Doxazosin 1 mg P.O. daily	Give 1 mg of doxazosin by mouth daily.
1000 ml glucose 5% in water with KCl 20 mmol I.V. at 100 ml/hr	Give 1000 ml of glucose 5% in water with 20 millimoles of potassium chloride intravenously at a rate of 100 millilitres per hour.
D/C penicillin I.V., start benzylpenicillin 800,000 units P.O. every 6 hours	Discontinue intravenous penicillin; start 800 000 units of benzylpenicillin by mouth every 6 hours.
Lorazepam 1–2 mg P.O. at bedtime p.r.n. insomnia	Give 1 to 2 mg of lorazepam by mouth at bedtime as needed for insomnia.

Short-winded

Dipyrimadole 100 mg P.O. t.i.d.

Give 100 mg of dipyrimadole by mouth three times per day.

Long-winded

Stop! That's an order

If the prescriber decides to discontinue a drug before the prescription runs out, they must write a replacement. These instructions on the new prescription must also be precise. For example, if the instructions read 'discontinue K' and the patient is receiving vitamin K and potassium chloride, you'll need to contact the prescriber to clarify which medication they wish to discontinue.

Handling ambiguous prescriptions

All too often, prescriptions for drugs are unclear because of non-standard abbreviations, illegible handwriting, incorrect dosages or missing information. It helps if handwritten prescriptions are neat, with drugs showing the correct spelling (See *Don't struggle with difficult prescriptions*.)

Rule 1: Bad input equals bad output

Even if the prescriber enters a prescription into the computer system, your interpretation skills are still extremely important. Although computers solve the problem of illegible handwriting, they can't correct human error. A computer will accept the wrong drug, the wrong dose, the wrong route and the wrong frequency. It's up to you to verify the input.

Rule 2: Advocate appropriate administration

Your responsibility in interpreting prescriptions includes making sure that the prescribed drug is an appropriate treatment. Your role as patient advocate comes into play in this situation. To make sure the drug you're asked to administer is appropriate:
•   Think critically; don't be afraid about asking for clarification and justification.
•   Know the action of each drug you give, the purpose for which it's given and its possible adverse effects.

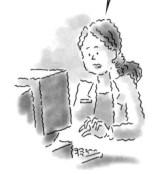

Computers aren't perfect. They won't correct an incorrect prescription. It's up to you!

Memory jogger

Repetition is key!

Use repetition to remember your responsibilities when it comes to drug administration. As you prepare to administer each drug, think of the actions you must take. To remember the steps in sequence, think of the phrase 'Until Clear, Ask Many Times':

Understand the drug and how it works.

Clarify the prescription as needed.

Administer the drug.

Monitor the patient for therapeutic response to the drug and for adverse effects.

Teach the patient about the drug as needed.

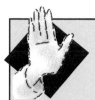

Before you give that drug!

Don't struggle with difficult prescriptions

The combination of poor handwriting and inappropriate abbreviations on a prescription can lead to confusion and medication errors. Ask the doctor to clarify a prescription that's difficult to understand or one that seems wrong.

FREEDOM HOSPITAL

PRESCRIPTION SHEET

UNIT NO. 290768 [4427]

NAME JOHN SMITH

ADDRESS 22 ACACIA AVENUE

CITY LONDON DOB 29/07/68

INSTRUCTIONS
1. For each prescription, detach top copy and send to pharmacy
2. Rule off unused lines after last copy (Pink) has been sent to pharmacy

DO NOT USE THIS SHEET UNLESS A NUMBER SHOWS 1

DATE	TIME	ORDERS	DOCTOR'S SIGNATURE	NURSE'S SIGNATURE

Discharge diagnoses in order of decreasing priority must be supplied at time of patient's discharge.

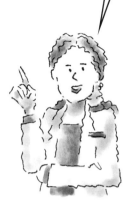

If you can't read something on the prescription, ask the doctor for clarification.

All this goes for I.V. fluids too!

- Know your patient. Drugs should be used with caution in very young or very old patients as well as those who are pregnant or who have known kidney or liver disease or diabetes.
- If a prescription seems questionable, use all available resources to check it. For example, ask the prescriber, the pharmacist and your colleagues, and refer to the *British National Formulary* or another drug handbook.
- Always check the five 'rights' before giving a drug. (See *Right on target*.)
- Check and recheck all your drug calculations.
- Never administer a drug that's improperly labelled or missing a label or that you personally didn't draw from a vial.
- Never use open or unmarked I.V. solution bags.

Advice from the experts

Right on target

No matter how careful you are when administering drugs, occasional errors can still occur. The pharmacy may even send the wrong drug. To avoid errors and keep your patient safe, never administer a drug without first checking off the five 'rights' at your patient's bedside.

  Right drug

 Right dose

 Right route

 Right time

Right patient

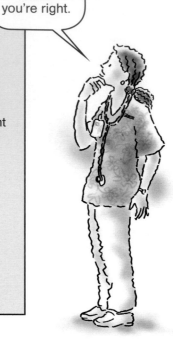

I think you're right.

Real-world problems

The following are examples of poorly written prescriptions that need to be clarified by the prescriber who wrote them. See if you can find the errors.

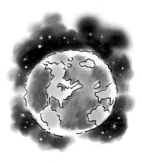

What?

K 40 mmol I.V. daily – It's unclear what drug is being prescribed. Is it vitamin K or potassium chloride (KCl)? If it's KCl, remember that this electrolyte must be diluted in a large volume of I.V. fluid before administration.

How?

Digoxin 0.25 mg, daily – The administration route is missing. Digoxin may be given orally as a pill or elixir or may be given intravenously.

When?

Nifedipine 10 mg, orally – The frequency of administration is missing. Nifedipine can be given in a single dose for hypertension, or it can be given on another schedule as a maintenance drug. In the latter case, it's usually given orally.

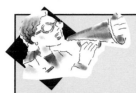

That's a wrap!

Prescriptions review

Here's a quick review of important points about prescriptions.

Reading and transcribing prescriptions

Make sure the drug prescription includes all of the following information:

- drug name
- dose
- administration route
- time and frequency of administration.

Using the 24-hour clock

- To write single-digit times from 1:00 a.m. to 12:59 p.m., put a zero before the time and remove the colon. (Example: 4:00 a.m. is 0400 hours.)
- To write double-digit times from 1:00 a.m. to 12:59 p.m., just remove the colon. (Example: 12:00 p.m., or noon, is 1200 hours.)
- To write times from 1:00 p.m. to 12 a.m. (midnight), add 1200 to the hour and remove the colon. (Example: 9:00 p.m. is 2100 hours.)
- Minutes after the hour remain the same. (Example: 10:36 p.m. is 2236 hours.)

Administering drugs

- Give within 30 minutes of the specified time.
- Record the actual administration time.
- If the drug is discontinued, make sure the doctor writes a new prescription or that the prescriber uses two lines to score out the drug, and initials the amendment.
- With each prescription, ensure that the appropriate drug is being administered.

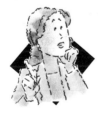

Quick quiz

1. Abbreviations for drugs should be written:
   A. in lower-case letters.
   B. in capital letters.
   C. should not be used.
   D. in print.

Answer: B. Drug abbreviations should be avoided in all situations.

2. The correct abbreviation for 'after meals' is:
   A. P.O.
   B. P.R.
   C. p.c.
   D. a.c.

Answer: C. P.O. stands for 'by mouth', P.R. stands for 'by rectum', and a.c. stands for 'before meals'. Again it is preferable to write out instructions in long-hand.

3.   Which abbreviation should never be used?
   A.   p.r.n.
   B.   p.o.
   C.   mcg.
   D.   S.C.

Answer: D. The abbreviation S.C. should not be used. Instead, write out subcutaneously.

4.   A prescription reads: *morphine 5 mg I.M. every 4 hours, p.r.n. pain, hold for respiratory rate < 12 BPM*. This means:
   A.   Give morphine 5 mg intramuscularly four times per day for pain; hold for respiratory rate less than 12 breaths per minute.
   B.   Give morphine 5 mg intramuscularly every 4 hours for pain; hold for respiratory rate greater than 12 breaths per minute.
   C.   Give morphine 5 mg intramuscularly every 4 hours as needed for pain; hold for respiratory rate less than 12 breaths per minute.
   D.   Give morphine 5 mg intramuscularly every 6 hours for pain; hold for respiratory rate greater than 12 breaths per minute.

Answer: C. The abbreviation p.r.n. means 'as needed', and the symbol '<' means 'less than'.

5.   'Give phenytoin 150 mg by mouth twice per day at 0900 hours and 2100 hours; draw phenytoin levels every other day' can be written on a prescription as:
   A.   Phenytoin 150 mg P.O. b.i.d. at 9:00 a.m. and 9:00 p.m., draw phenytoin levels every other day.
   B.   Phenytoin 150 mg P.O. t.i.d. at 9:00 a.m. and 9:00 p.m., draw phenytoin levels q.d.
   C.   Phenytoin 150 mp I.V. b.i.d. at 9:00 a.m. and 9:00 p.m., draw phenytoin levels q.o.d.
   D.   Phenytoin 150 mg P.R. b.i.d. at 0900 and 2100, draw phenytoin levels q.o.d.

Answer: A. In option B, t.i.d. means 'three times per day', and q.d., meaning daily, shouldn't be used. In option C, mp isn't a standard abbreviation, I.V. means 'intravenously', and 'q.o.d' shouldn't be used. In option D, 'P.R.' means 'per rectum' and 'q.o.d.' shouldn't be used.

Scoring

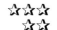   If you answered all five items correctly, wow! You're error-free!

   If you answered four items correctly, you're almost there! You can spot an incorrect prescription and read hospital hieroglyphics.

   If you answered fewer than four items correctly, keep going! You're acquiring the art of drug prescribing.

8 Administration records

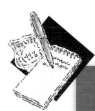

Just the facts

In this chapter, you'll learn:

♦ what types of medication administration record systems are used

♦ how to document patient information on the administration record

♦ how to record drug information on the administration record

♦ how to document administration of controlled substances.

A look at administration records

Maintaining accurate medication administration records is a vital nursing responsibility, for both legal reasons and patient safety. The liability risk of the healthcare provider may increase if medication administration isn't properly documented. Missing or inaccurate documentation can lead to drug errors that may compromise your patient's health.

Record-keeping systems

Two main types of medication administration record systems are used today: the medication administration record (MAR) and computer charting.

The MAR

A widely used system, the MAR is a standard form that goes into the patient's chart. It also may be kept in the medication room on the medication trolley or may be attached to the patient's chart or

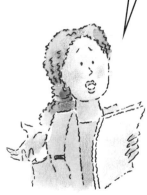

Missing or inaccurate documentation may compromise your patient's health.

clipboard while the patient is hospitalised. On discharge, the MAR is placed in the patient's chart with the other MARs already used for that patient. Some units use the MAR in combination with another system that uses index cards.

Computer charting

Another system – computer charting – is being used increasingly by more healthcare facilities. Information is entered into a computer that automatically generates a list of administration times for all scheduled medications. Computer systems cut the risk of drug errors caused by illegible handwriting. (See *Record keeping in the computer age*.)

Record keeping in the computer age

As healthcare facilities purchase or develop computer systems, manufacturers offer increased choices among medication-monitoring programs.

From simple...

Computerised record systems range from simple to sophisticated. In the simplest systems, the computer is used as a word processor or typewriter.

...to sophisticated

In more sophisticated systems, doctors can request drugs from the pharmacy by typing the drug's name, or they can select specific drugs by searching through various listings, such as pharmacological categories, pharmacokinetic categories and disease-related uses.

   The computer indicates whether the pharmacy has the drug. The prescription then goes into the pharmacy's computer for filing. The request also generates a copy of the patient's record, on which the nurse can document medication administration. In some cases, the nurse can document medication administration right onto the computer.

Benefits bit by bit

Computer systems offer the following advantages:

- When drug prescriptions are changed, the pharmacy receives immediate notification, so drugs arrive on the unit faster.
- The pharmacy's computer can immediately confirm or deny a drug's availability.
- Nurses can document on medication administration records quickly and easily.
- Nurses can see at a glance which drugs have been administered and which still must be given.
- Errors from misinterpreted handwriting are eliminated.
- Records can be stored electronically in addition to, or instead of, paper copies.

Now we're cooking with gas! Changing orders by computer means instant notification – and less delay.

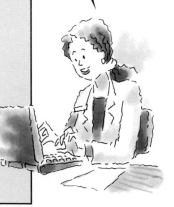

Different forms, same info

The medication administration record below illustrates the kind of information required on all types of medication administration forms. Although different facilities may use different forms, virtually all require the patient information, date, drug information, time of administration and the nurse's initials after administering the drug.

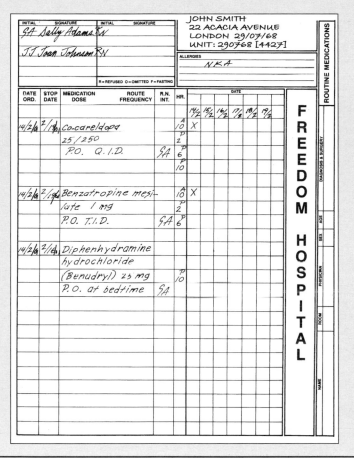

INITIAL	SIGNATURE	INITIAL	SIGNATURE
SA	Sally Adams RN		
JJ	Joan Johnson RN		

R = REFUSED　O = OMITTED　F = FASTING

JOHN SMITH
22 ACACIA AVENUE
LONDON 29/07/68
UNIT: 290768 [4427]

ALLERGIES
NKA

ROUTINE MEDICATIONS

DATE ORD.	STOP DATE	MEDICATION DOSE ROUTE FREQUENCY	R.N. INT.	HR.	DATE 14/2	15/2	16/2	17/2	18/2	19/2			
14/2/81	2/18/81	Co-careldopa 25/250 P.O. Q.I.D.	SA	A10 P2 P6 P10	X								
14/2/81	2/18/81	Benzatropine mesilate 1 mg P.O. T.I.D.	SA	A10 P2 P6	X								
14/2/81	2/18/81	Diphenhydramine hydrochloride (Benudryl) 25 mg P.O. at bedtime	SA	P10									

FREEDOM HOSPITAL

DIAGNOSIS & SURGERY

AGE　SEX　PHYSICIAN　ROOM

NAME

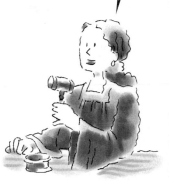

My ruling: keep good records!

See you in court

No matter what type of medication charting system your healthcare setting uses, you must still record certain standard information. Standardisation allows medication administration records to be used as legal documents if it ever becomes necessary to prove that a drug dose was given. (See *Different forms, same info*.)

Documentation

In general, documentation reflects the tasks, assessments and procedures that nurses perform. Documenting on the administration record indicates that the prescription has been fulfilled.

Does that say subcutaneous or subcuticular?

Before transcribing prescriptions, make sure that they're complete, clear and correct. If you detect a problem, contact the prescriber before sending the prescription to the pharmacy. If you detect a problem after it has gone to the pharmacy, contact both the prescriber and the pharmacy.

Is that 1 mg I.V. over 10 minutes or 10 mg over 1 minute?

Information recorded on an MAR must be written legibly in ink. Most facilities require the use of blue or black ink to allow for clear reproduction of the record. All handwritten or computerised administration records must contain patient information, drug information and signatures. *Remember:* transcribing prescriptions requires close attention because even a small discrepancy can cause a major drug error.

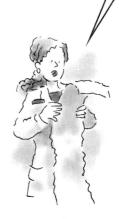

Before transcribing the prescription, make sure that it's complete, clear and correct!

Recording patient information

If your facility uses a computerised system, you don't need to transcribe patient information onto the administration record. It's already there because the admissions office enters the patient information into the system, and the pharmacy adds information, such as the patient's height, weight and allergies. In some systems, however, nurses may also enter this information.

   If you use an MAR, label the form with the patient's admission data. If these aren't available, copy the information from the patient's identification bracelet.

Identification, please

Record the patient's full name, hospital identification number, unit number, bed assignment and allergies, even those that aren't drug-related. If the patient doesn't have any known allergies, record this too. Transcribe the information exactly as it appears on the bracelet.

Recording drug information

Next, transcribe from the prescription sheet complete information about every drug the patient is taking. Include dates and drug names, dosages, strengths, dosage forms, administration routes and administration times.

It's a date!

You must always record these dates on the administration record: the date the prescription was written; the date the drug should begin, if this is different from the original prescription date; and the date the drug should be discontinued.

At some facilities, the time and date the drug should begin are recorded together. This serves as a reference for the time to discontinue a drug when a limited period is indicated. Many facilities also have a standard length of time that a drug may be given before it is automatically discontinued.

Full name, please

Record the drug's full generic name. If the drug has been prescribed using a proprietary (trade or brand) name, record this name as well. Don't use abbreviations, chemical symbols, research names or special facility names. Doing so can cause medication errors or delay therapy.

Working on your strength

When recording drug strength, be sure to write the actual amount of the drug to be administered. If the dose you administer varies in any way from the strength or amount prescribed, note this in a special area on the administration record, or, if there isn't an administration record, in the patient's progress notes.

For example, document whether the patient refused to take a drug, consumed only part of a drug or vomited shortly after taking a drug.

As a matter of form...

Also record the drug dosage form that was prescribed. Then decide whether the form is appropriate, considering the patient's special needs.

For example, if sustained-action theophylline tablets are prescribed for a patient with a nasogastric tube, he won't be able to take the tablets orally. You may have to crush them before administering them through the tube.

However, crushing sustained-action tablets destroys the drug's integrity and alters its therapeutic action. So, you'll need to contact the prescriber and discuss an alternative drug dosage form. Generally, the crushing of tablets should be avoided.

A lot of important information needs to be transcribed... prescriber, drug name, dosage and administration route and time.

Be sure to record the dosage form and strength, too.

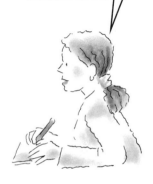

Tracking the route

Recording the route of administration is especially critical for drugs that may be given by two different routes. For example, paracetamol can be given orally or rectally. Other drugs can be given by only one correct route; for example, isophane insulin may be given subcutaneously but not intravenously.

If you administer a drug by a different route from that which it has been prescribed, indicate that change, along with the reason and authorisation for the change. Also document whether a special administration technique, such as a Z-track I.M. injection, was used.

Citing the site

When administering a drug by a parenteral route, record the injection site to facilitate site rotation. Most administration forms include a numbered list of recognised sites, allowing you to record the site by its number. However, if necessary, describe anatomical landmarks used to locate the specific site.

Schedule scheme

The prescription should also include an administration schedule, such as t.i.d. (three times daily) or q.q.h. (every four hours). Transcribe the schedule onto the administration record; then convert it into actual times based on your facility's policy and the drug's availability, characteristics, onset and duration of action.

For example, t.i.d. may mean 9 a.m., 1 p.m. and 5 p.m. in one setting and 10 a.m., 2 p.m. and 6 p.m. in another. Similarly, b.i.d. may be 10 a.m. and 6 p.m. or 10 a.m. and 10 p.m.

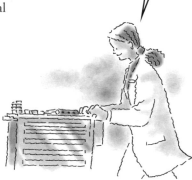

Recording the administration route is especially critical for drugs that may be given by two or more different routes.

Working around the clock

Remember that time notations are based on a 24-hour clock, unless otherwise specified. This means that the hour appearing first on a 24-hour clock should appear first in the time notation.

In other words, if an administration schedule is 2-10-2-10, the first 2 represents 2 a.m., or 0200 hours; the first 10 represents 10 a.m., or 1000 hours; the second 2 is 2 p.m., or 1400 hours; and the second 10 is 10 p.m., or 2200 hours.

Under special circumstances

Some facilities have separate administration records or specially designated areas of the regular administration record for recording single items or special drugs. Special drugs include those given p.r.n., large-volume parenteral drugs, and dermatological and ophthalmic medications dispensed in bottles or tubes.

Regulation of controlled substances

Current legislation regulates the dispensing, administration and documentation of controlled substances. When these substances are issued to a unit, they are accompanied by a perpetual inventory record, commonly called a controlled inventory record.

A paper trail

If the doctor prescribes a controlled substance for your patient, document its administration on the administration record and the perpetual inventory record. When you remove a dose from the locked storage site, note this information on the perpetual inventory record:

- date and time the dose is removed
- amount of the drug remaining in the locked storage site
- patient's full name
- doctor or prescriber's name
- drug dose
- your signature.

If you have to discard any of the dose, have another nurse verify the amount discarded and ask him or her to sign the form, too.

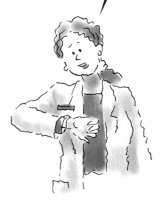

A nurse really has to keep track of time!

Other facilities put single items or special drugs on the regular administration record. If this is the case where you work, be careful to distinguish these drugs from those that are regularly scheduled. All facilities have special forms for recording controlled substances. (See *Regulation of controlled substances*.)

Time is of the essence

Immediately after giving a drug, document the time of administration to prevent you from mistakenly giving the drug again. For scheduled drugs, you'll usually initial the appropriate time slot for the date that the drug is administered.

Scheduled drugs are considered on time if they're given within half an hour of the prescribed time. For unscheduled drugs, such as single doses and p.r.n. drugs, record the exact time of administration in the appropriate slot.

If you don't give a drug on time or if you miss a dose, document the reason on either the administration record or the patient's progress notes. Facility policy may require you to initial and circle the particular time missed on the administration record to draw attention to it.

Your signature here

Every time you document on the administration record, you must sign it. First, initial the record after transcribing from the prescription. Many facilities also require the nurse to perform a chart check and initial the prescription on a line after the last prescribed drug. This indicates that all drugs have been transcribed correctly onto the administration record.

If someone other than a nurse transcribes the prescription, a nurse must co-sign the prescription and the administration record.

Initiate initialling

You also need to sign the administration record after giving a drug. Put your initials in the appropriate space on the form. Make sure that they're legible and always sign them the same way. If another nurse on your unit has the same initials or name, use your middle initial to avoid confusion.

In addition, write your full name, title and initials in the signature section of the administration record. This information must appear on every record you initial when administering drugs.

Real-world problems

Here are some examples of administration record problems you may encounter in the real world.

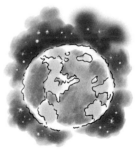

Nil by mouth

Your patient receives oral potassium chloride supplements. You're due to give a dose but the patient was made 'nil by mouth' (NBM) for a test, so you withheld the dose. How do you record this?

In most facilities still using written charts, you record a withheld dose by placing your initials in the appropriate time slot on the MAR, and then circle them. You can dictate the reason you withheld the dose (in this case, the patient was made NBM) in the progress notes.

In control

Your patient needs a dose of morphine sulphate, a controlled substance. You only need 2 mg of the 4-mg prefilled syringe available. On the record, how do you indicate that the extra morphine was discarded appropriately?

First, ask another nurse to watch as you appropriately discard the extra medication. Then, have her sign the controlled inventory record (or follow your facility's policy) to verify this process.

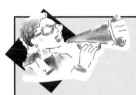

That's a wrap!

Administration records review

Keep these important points about administration records in mind.

Drug administration record systems

- MAR
  - Uses a form to record medication administration
  - Widely used
  - Sometimes used in combination with an index card system
- Computer charting
  - Medication administration information entered into a computer
  - Automatic, computer-generated list of scheduled medications and their administration times
  - Used increasingly over other systems

Documenting drug administration

- Write legibly in blue or black ink.
- Record allergy information if it isn't already documented, using 'NKA' if no allergies are known.
- Transcribe from the prescription complete information about each drug (dates and drug names, dosages, strengths, dosage forms, administration routes and administration times).
- If parenteral, record the injection site.
- Immediately document the times of all administrations.
- If unscheduled, record the exact time the drug was given.
- If given late or not at all, document the reason.
- Always sign any documentation on the administration record.

Recording controlled-substance administration

- Include the date and time that the dose is removed from the locked storage area.
- Include the amount of drug remaining in the locked storage area.
- Record the patient's full name.
- Document the doctor's full name.
- Enter the drug dose given.
- Include your full signature.
- If any part of the drug was discarded, obtain the signature of another nurse who verified the amount discarded.

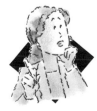

Quick quiz

1. You may be required to circle and initial the time slot of a medication if:
    A. you missed the dose or gave it late.
    B. the administration time has changed.
    C. another nurse forgot to administer a drug.
    D. the medication has been discontinued.

Answer: A. Circling and initialling the time slot signals to the next nurse that the dose was missed or late. The nurse then refers to the single-item or p.r.n. section of the MAR to find the actual administration time. That way, the next dose should not be mistakenly administered too soon.

2. The abbreviation NKA stands for:
   A. no known adverse reactions.
   B. no known administraton.
   C. no known alteration.
   D. no known allergies.

Answer: D. Allergy information should always be recorded. If there are no known allergies, document NKA or, preferably, write it out in long-hand.

3. To avoid confusion, nurses with the same initials should sign the administration record with:
   A. their identification numbers.
   B. pens with different colors of ink.
   C. their middle initials.
   D. their birth dates.

Answer: C. Middle initials should be used. In addition, be sure to write legibly and always sign the same way.

4. Immediately after you administer a drug, you should:
   A. document its effectiveness.
   B. document the time of administration.
   C. order the next dose of the drug from the pharmacy.
   D. take the patient's vital signs.

Answer: B. Documenting the time of administration immediately after you give the drug prevents you from mistakenly giving the drug again.

Scoring

☆☆☆ If you answered all four items correctly, amazing! You've been voted best nurse at the Administration Academy Awards!

☆☆ If you answered three items correctly, fantastic! Here's your Oscar for best supporting nurse!

☆ If you answered fewer than three items correctly, keep your chin up! You're still a record setter!

9 Preventing drug errors

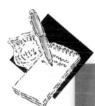

Just the facts

In this chapter, you'll learn:

♦ the types and causes of common drug errors
♦ how to prevent drug errors
♦ how to report drug errors.

A look at drug errors

Drug errors cause thousands of injuries and are responsible for many deaths in healthcare settings every year. In 2006, over 40 000 drug-related errors were reported in UK hospitals, of which approximately 2000 were responsible for serious injury. Of these serious incidents between 40 and 50 contributed to the death of patients. Because only about 1 out of every 10 drug errors is reported, no one knows exactly how many errors actually occur. Despite such discouraging statistics, finding better ways to safeguard patients against these kinds of errors has become a National Health Service priority.

Are you legal?

Depending on where you practise nursing, several different healthcare professionals, including doctors, nurse prescribers and dentists, may be legally permitted to prescribe, dispense and administer medications. Usually, however, doctors prescribe medications, pharmacists prepare and dispense the drugs, and nurses administer them to patients.

An integral team player

As a nurse, you're almost always on the front line when it comes to medication administration. That means you also bear a major share of the responsibility in protecting patients from all types of drug errors.

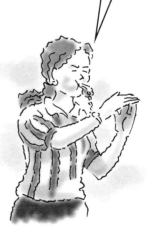

Time-out called to review that drug play!

Doing your part

Many kinds of drug errors can occur in everyday nursing practice. Consequently, each institution has its own set of guidelines for how and when to properly administer drugs to patients, and each nurse is responsible for knowing what those guidelines are. Besides following your facility's administration policies faithfully, you can help prevent drug errors by studying and avoiding the common slip-ups that allow them to happen. (See *Common drug errors*.)

As you can see, many things can go wrong. It pays to be extra careful and to follow your facility's guidelines when administering drugs.

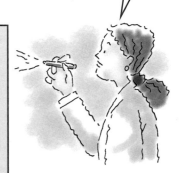

Common drug errors

Certain situations or activities can place nurses at high risk for making a drug error. Some of the most common types and causes of errors are highlighted here.

Types of error

- Giving the wrong drug
- Giving the wrong dose
- Using the wrong diluent
- Preparing the wrong concentration
- Missing a dose or failing to give a prescribed drug
- Giving the drug at the wrong time
- Administering a drug to which the patient has an allergy
- Infusing the drug too quickly
- Giving the drug to the wrong patient
- Administering the drug by the wrong route

Causes

- Insufficient knowledge
- Chaotic work environment
- Use of floor stock medications
- Failure to follow facility policies and procedures
- Incorrect preparation or administration techniques
- Use of I.V. solutions that aren't premixed
- Failure to verify drug and dosage instructions
- Following oral, not written, orders
- Inadequate staffing
- Typographical errors
- Use of acronyms or erroneous abbreviations
- Calculation errors
- Poor handwriting
- Failure to check dosages for high-risk drugs or paediatric medications

Medication errors in practice

In addition to dosage calculation errors (which account for roughly 7% of all reported drug errors), common errors include mistakes with drug or patient names, missed allergy alerts, errors compounded by two or more practitioners, errors involving routes of administration, misinterpreted abbreviations, misinterpreted prescriptions, preparation errors and errors caused by stress.

Drug name errors

Drugs with similar-sounding names are easy to confuse. Even different-sounding names can look similar when written out rapidly by hand. Remember, if the patient's prescription doesn't seem right for their diagnosis, call the prescriber for clarification. (See *Look-alike and sound-alike drug names*.)

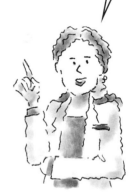

If a prescribed drug doesn't seem right for the patient's diagnosis, don't hesitate to call the prescriber to clarify the order.

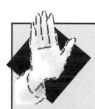

Before you give that drug!
Look-alike and sound-alike drug names

The drug names listed here resemble each other in terms of spelling or sound. Always double-check the prescription sheet carefully before administering one of them to your patient. If you have any doubt about the appropriateness of the drug, consult the prescriber, the pharmacist or a drug reference:

- amiodarone *and* amiloride
- benzatropine *and* bromocriptine
- calciferol *and* calcitriol
- cimetidine *and* simeticone
- codeine *and* chloroquine
- desmopressin *and* vasopressin
- dexamethasone *and* dexamfetamine
- digoxin *and* doxepin
- adrenaline (epinephrine) *and* noradrenaline (norepinephrine)
- flunisolide *and* fluocinonide

- hydromorphone *and* morphine
- imipramine *and* distamine
- levothyroxine *and* liothyronine
- naloxone *and* naltrexone
- nifedipine *and* nicardipine
- pentostatin *and* Pentostam
- Ritalin *and* Rifadin
- sulfasalizine *and* sulfadiazine
- vinblastine *and* vincristine
- Xanax *and* Zantac
- Zyvesca *and* Zyprexa.

Morphing the name

For example, a prescription for diamorphine hydrochloride can be easily confused with one for hydromorphone hydrochloride. Both drugs are available, and both cause respiratory depression. However, diamorphine hydrochloride has a greater effect on a patient's respiratory status. If you administer the wrong drug, the patient could develop respiratory depression or even respiratory arrest.

Posting prevention

To prevent errors, consider posting a notice prominently on your unit where opioids are kept, to warn the staff about this potential mix-up.

Patient name errors

Drug names aren't the only names subject to confusion. Sometimes, patient names can cause trouble as well, especially when nurses don't verify each patient's identity before administering medications. Caring for two patients with the same or similar first or last name can further complicate matters. Consider the following scenario.

A tale of two Bobs

Five-year-old Robert Brown is hospitalised with chronic gastro-oesophageal reflux. Robert Black, also age 5, is admitted to the same paediatric unit after a severe asthma attack. The boys are assigned to adjacent rooms. Each has a non-productive cough.

The nurse caring for Robert Brown enters his room to give him an expectorant. As the nurse is about to administer the drug, the child's mother informs her that someone else came into the room a few minutes ago to give Robert a medication that he inhaled by mask. The nurse quickly determines that another nurse mistakenly gave Robert Black's medication (acetylcysteine, a mucolytic) to Robert Brown.

Fortunately, no harmful adverse effects developed. However, if the other nurse had checked the patient's identity more carefully, this error would never have occurred.

Check and double-check

Always check each patient's full name by comparing it against the patient's chart and the identification bracelet issued by your facility at the time of admission. Teach the patient (or parents if the patient is a

Preventing drug errors through teaching

Drug errors aren't limited to hospital settings. Patients sometimes make drug errors when taking their medications at home. To prevent such errors, take the time to educate your patient thoroughly about each medication they will be taking. Be sure to cover these points:

- drug's name (generic and trade name)
- drug's purpose
- correct dosage and how to calculate it (such as breaking scored tablets or adding or mixing liquids when necessary)
- how to take the drug
- when to take the drug
- what to do if a dose is missed
- how to monitor the drug's effectiveness (for example, checking blood glucose levels when taking a hypoglycaemic drug)
- potential drug interactions (including the need to avoid certain over-the-counter and herbal medicines)
- required dietary changes (including the use of alcohol)
- possible adverse effects and what to do if they occur
- proper storage, handling and disposal of the drug or supplies (such as syringes)
- required follow-up.

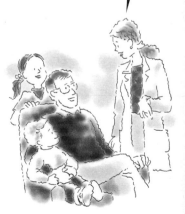

We need to take a few minutes to go over Bobby's medication regimen.

child) to offer his or her identification bracelet for inspection and to state his or her first and last name when anyone arrives to administer medication. Also, urge patients to tell you or another nurse whenever an identification bracelet falls off, is removed or becomes misplaced. Then, replace it or substitute a new one immediately.

Patients can also be taught what their medications look like, how they're given and at what times they should take them. That way, they know what they should be receiving while in hospital and are prepared to use the drug safely after discharge. (See *Preventing drug errors through teaching*.)

Missed allergy alerts

After you've verified your patient's full name, check to see if they are wearing allergy identification, such as MedicAlert jewellery. All allergy identification tags or jewellery should have the name of the specific allergen conspicuously written or embossed on them. This same allergy information should be recorded on the front of the patient's chart and on their medication record. Always double-check the information against the chart. Regardless of whether the patient is wearing allergy identification, take the time to ask the patient directly about drug allergies – even if the patient is in distress.

> Can you please state and spell your first and last name? … Are you allergic to any medications, Mr. Stanley?

A distressing situation

Consider this example. The doctor prescribes chlorpromazine, stat, for a distressed patient. By the time the nurse arrives with the drug, the patient has grown more visibly distressed. Unnerved by the patient's demeanor, the nurse quickly administers the drug – without checking the patient's allergy bracelet or medication administration record first, and without documenting the order. The patient has an immediate allergic reaction.

Because the patient's allergy bracelet clearly stated a known allergy, and this same information was clearly indicated on the chart and medication administration record, this error was fully preventable.

Resisting temptation

Any time you're in a tense situation with a patient who needs or wants medication fast, resist the temptation to act first and document later. Skipping this crucial step can easily lead to a medication error.

Not just talking peanuts

Certain medications should never be given to patients allergic to peanuts, soy or sulfa compounds. Keep these tips in mind to help prevent allergic reactions in these patients:
- A patient who's severely allergic to peanuts or soy may have an anaphylactic reaction (a severe, life-threatening reaction) to ipratropium bromide aerosol given by metered-dose inhaler. Ask the patient (or parents) whether they are allergic to peanuts or soy before giving this drug. If you find that they have such an allergy, you'll need to use the nasal spray or inhalation solution (nebuliser) form of the drug. Because neither form contains soy lecithin (an emulsifier used in the metered-dose formula), it's safe for patients allergic to peanuts or soy.
- Patients allergic to sulfa drugs shouldn't receive sulfonylurea hypoglycaemic agents, such as chlorpropamide, glybenclamide and glipizide.

> Be especially alert for the possibility of an anaphylactic reaction when a patient is allergic to peanuts, soy or sulfa compounds.

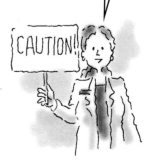

Compound errors

For a drug to be given correctly, each member of the healthcare team must fulfil an appropriate role: the prescriber must choose the right medication for the patient, then write the prescription correctly and legibly. The pharmacist must interpret the prescription, determine whether it's complete and prepare the drug using precise measurements. Finally, the nurse must evaluate whether the medication is appropriate for the patient, then administer it correctly according to facility guidelines.

Never break the chain

A breakdown along this chain of events can easily lead to a medication error – an error that's further compounded because of the number of people who could have prevented it. That's why it's vital for all healthcare providers to work together as a team, supporting and helping each other to promote the best patient care. In some cases, working as a team may be as simple as asking for further clarification or as complicated as double-checking another practitioner's action and calling them to task.

Calling all pharmacists

For instance, the pharmacist can help clarify the number of times a drug must be given each day. He can also help you label drugs in the most appropriate way. Furthermore, the pharmacist can remind you to always return unused or discontinued medications to the pharmacy.

I can see clearly now

As a nurse, you're responsible for clarifying a prescription that doesn't seem clear or correct. You must also correctly handle and store multidose vials obtained from the pharmacist, and administer only those drugs that you've prepared personally. Never give a drug with an ambiguous label or no label at all. Here's an example of what could happen if you do.

Medication mix-up

The nurse places an unlabelled syringe of phenol (used as a rectal sclerosant) next to a measure of guanethidine monosulphate (a post-ganglionic-blocking drug) on the bedside table of a patient

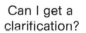

Go team!

Can I get a clarification?

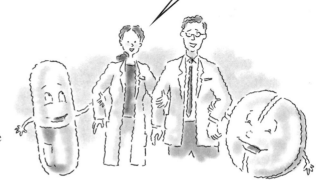

scheduled for a guanethidine injection. The doctor enters the room, examines the patient, and accidentally injects phenol into the patient's arm, causing severe tissue damage. The patient requires emergency surgery and later develops neurological complications from receiving the wrong, unlabelled injection.

Obviously, this was a compound medication error. The nurse should have labelled each syringe clearly, and the doctor should never have given an unlabelled drug to the patient.

Litres versus grams

In another example of a compound error, a nurse working in the neonatal intensive care unit prepares a dose of aminophylline to administer to an infant. No one bothers to check the nurse's calculations. Shortly after receiving the drug, the infant develops tachycardia and other signs of theophylline toxicity and later dies. The nurse thought that the prescription read 7.4 ml of aminophylline. Instead, it read 7.4 mg.

This tragedy might have been avoided if the doctor had written a clearer prescription, if the nurse had clarified the prescription before administering it, if the pharmacist had prepared and dispensed the drug or if another nurse had double-checked the dosage calculation. To avoid this type of problem, many facilities require pharmacists to prepare and dispense all non-emergency parenteral doses whenever commercial unit doses aren't available.

Would you mind going over my maths one more time? This calculation was a little tricky.

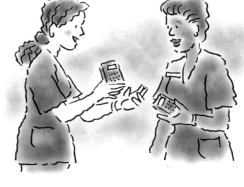

Take necessary precautions to breathe easier

Here's another example: a nurse mistakenly leaves a container of 5% acetic acid (used to clean tracheostomy tubing) near nebulisation equipment in the room of a 10-month-old infant. A respiratory therapist mistakes the liquid for normal saline solution and uses it to dilute salbutamol for the child's nebuliser treatment. During the treatment, the child experiences bronchospasm, hypercapneic dyspnoea, tachypnoea and tachycardia.

Leaving dangerous chemicals near patient-care areas is extremely risky, especially when container labels don't warn of toxicity. To prevent such problems, always read the label on every drug you prepare, and never administer a drug or solution that isn't labelled or that's labelled poorly. Ideally, you should not administer a drug that you have not been involved in preparing or have checked immediately before its administration.

Never administer a drug or solution that isn't labelled or is labelled poorly.

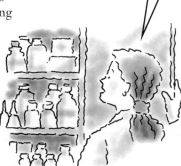

Route errors

Many drug errors stem, at least in part, from problems involving the route of administration. The risk of error increases when a patient has several lines running for different purposes, as illustrated in the following scenario.

Crossing the line

A nurse prepares a dose of digoxin elixir for a patient with a central I.V. line and a ileostomy tube in place. The nurse mistakenly administers the oral drug into the central I.V. line. Fortunately, the patient suffers no adverse effects.

To help prevent similar mix-ups in the route of administration, prepare all oral medications in a syringe that has a tip small enough to fit an abdominal tube but too large to fit a central line. Some facilities even use designated tubing for enteral feedings, so that it cannot be inadvertently connected to an I.V. line.

Clearing the air

Here's another error that could have been avoided: to clear air bubbles from a 9-year-old patient's insulin infusion, the nurse disconnects the tubing and raises the pump rate to 200 ml/hour, flushing the bubbles through quickly. She then reconnects the tubing and restarts the infusion, but she forgets to reset the drip rate back to 2 units/hour. The child receives 50 units of insulin before the nurse detects the error.

To prevent this kind of mistake, *never* increase the drip rate to clear bubbles from a line. Instead, remove the tubing from the pump, disconnect it from the patient and use the flow-control clamp to establish gravity flow of the I.V. fluid to purge the air from the line.

Misinterpreted abbreviations

Some commonly used abbreviations are known to contribute significantly to drug errors. For example, in a prescription reading levothyroxine 50 µg by mouth, daily, the µg (meaning micrograms) may be easily misinterpreted to mean milligrams. The patient could mistakenly receive 50 mg of levothyroxine, or 1000 times the prescribed dose. The internationally accepted abbreviation for microgram is currently mcg. Local policies should be consulted with respect to the use of abbreviations; the *British National Formulary* (or *BNF*) documents currently acceptable abbreviations. However,

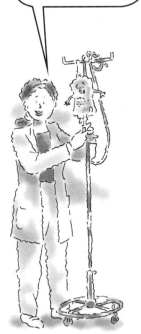

To clear bubbles from an I.V. line, always remove the tubing from the pump, disconnect it from the patient and use the flow-control clamp to establish gravity flow.

Dangerous abbreviations

Although difficult to enforce, the use of abbreviations in clinical documentation should be actively discouraged because of the potential for confusion and misinterpretation. Examples of errors commonly associated with abbreviations are detailed below.

Abbreviation	Potential problem	Preferred term
U (for unit)	Mistaken as 0 (zero), 4 (four) or cc	Write *unit*.
IU (for international unit)	Mistaken as I.V. (intravenous) or 10 (ten)	Write *international unit*.
Trailing zero (as in X.0 mg), absence of leading zero (as in .X mg)	Inaccuracies with numbers or values due to missed decimal point	Never write a zero by itself after a decimal point (X mg), and always use a zero before a decimal point (0.X mg).
MS, MSO_4, $MgSO_4$	Confused for one another (can mean morphine sulphate or magnesium sulphate)	Write *morphine sulphate* or *magnesium sulphate*.
μg (for microgram)	Mistaken for mg (milligrams), resulting in a thousand-fold overdose	Write *mcg* or *microgram*.
S.C. (for subcutaneous)	Mistaken as SL (for sublingual) or as 5 every...	Write *subcutaneously*.
D/C (for discharge)	Misinterpreted as discontinue (followed by drug name, typically discharge medication)	Write discharge.
cc (for cubic centimetre)	Mistaken for U (units) when written poorly	Write *ml* for *millilitres*.
a.s., a.d., a.u. (Latin abbreviation for left, right or both ears); o.s., o.d., o.u. (Latin abbreviation for left, right or both eyes)	Mistaken for each other (such as a.s. for o.s., a.d. for o.d. or a.u. for o.u.)	Write *left ear*, *right ear* or *both ears*; *left eye*, *right eye* or *both eyes*.

it should be noted that there are proposals introduce legistation to stop the use of all medically related abbreviations within the UK. (See *Dangerous abbreviations*.)

Shorthand for shortsighted

Abbreviating or using a shorthand version of a drug name is equally risky, as shown in this example: Epoetin alfa (commonly abbreviated as EPO) is a synthetic form of erythropoietin that's sometimes used by anaemic cancer patients to stimulate red blood cell production. In one case, a doctor wrote, 'May take own supply of EPO' on the discharge documentation of a patient whose cancer was in remission. However, the patient wasn't anaemic.

Sensing that something was wrong with prescribing epoetin alfa for a patient who wasn't anaemic, the pharmacist interviewed the patient, who confirmed that 'EPO', or evening primrose oil, was being taken to lower their cholesterol level. Fortunately, the pharmacist became aware of his misinterpretation of the abbreviation before an error could occur in this situation.

To avoid this type of error, ask prescribers to spell out all drug names.

Misinterpreted prescriptions

As a rule of thumb, if you're unfamiliar with a drug that has been prescribed, always consult a drug reference, such as the *BNF*, before administering the medication to the patient. Also, ask the prescriber to clarify vague or ambiguous terms. Don't assume that you'll get it right on your own.

Guessing is always wrong

Here's an example. A patient was supposed to receive one dose of the anti-neoplastic drug lomustine to treat brain cancer. (Lomustine is typically given as a single oral dose once every 4–6 weeks.) The doctor's prescription read, 'Administer at night'. Because the evening shift nurse misinterpreted the prescription to mean 'every night' when the doctor meant 'at bedtime', the patient received three daily doses of a drug he should have only received once, developed severe thrombocytopenia and neutropenia, and then died.

Remember to clarify confusing prescriptions with the prescriber, and to read each prescription carefully. Also remember to look up in a drug reference any drugs you're unfamiliar with – doing so may prevent an error and save a life.

Did I hear you right?

In rare cases, you may need to follow a doctor's verbal instructions to administer a drug. These situations typically involve emergencies, such as resuscitation of a patient, when there's no time to write out a prescription. If you find yourself in this type of situation, be sure to listen closely to the instruction, repeating it back to the doctor as necessary to ensure you've heard correctly, before administering the drug. Then promptly document the prescription and the details of the incident in the patient's chart. Make sure that the doctor reviews and signs all prescriptions as necessary as soon as the patient has stabilised.

It's extremely important to know your facility's policy on accepting and documenting this type of prescription. Be aware that many facilities have started phasing out both verbal and telephone prescriptions because of the prevalence of computers at nurse's stations and other key units allowing prescriptions to be entered and retrieved quickly from virtually any location.

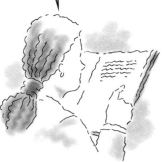

Let me see… this reference says, 'For adults and paediatric patients, give 130 mg/m^2 by mouth, as a single dose…'

Even in an emergency, make sure the prescription is complete, clear and correct!

EMERGENCY

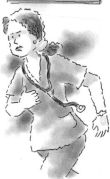

Preparation errors

Sometimes the incorrect selection of a drug compound or solution strength when preparing a medication can be harmful, even fatal, to the patient. With practice, nurses can develop a sharp eye for this type of error, as illustrated in the following situations. In both cases, the alert nurses noticed that anti-neoplastics prepared in the pharmacy appeared suspiciously different and took the appropriate action.

The sleuthing Holmes...

The first case involves a 6-year-old child who was to receive 12 mg of methotrexate intrathecally. The pharmacist handling the prescription mistakenly selected a 1-g vial of methotrexate instead of a 25-mg vial and reconstituted the drug with 10 ml of normal saline solution. The preparation containing 100 mg/ml was incorrectly labelled as containing 2 mg/ml, and 6 ml of the solution was drawn into a syringe. Although the syringe label indicated 12 mg of methotrexate, the syringe actually contained 600 mg of the drug.

The nurse who received the syringe observed that the drug's colour didn't appear correct, and returned it to the pharmacy for verification. The pharmacist retrieved the vial used to prepare the dose and withdrew the remaining solution into another syringe. The solutions in both syringes were compared and, noting that they matched, the pharmacist concluded that the colour change was due to a change in the manufacturer's formula. No one noticed the vial's 1-g label.

The child received the 600-mg dose and experienced seizures 45 minutes later. A pharmacist responding to the emergency detected the error. The child received an appropriate antidote and soon recovered.

...and Dr. Watson

In a similar case, a 20-year-old patient with leukaemia was supposed to receive mitomycin instead of mitoxantrone. These drugs are both anti-neoplastic antibiotics; however, mitoxantrone is a dark blue liquid.

Upon receiving the medication from the pharmacy, the nurse noticed the unusual bluish tint of what was labelled mitomycin and immediately questioned the pharmacist. The pharmacist assured her that the colour difference was due to a change in manufacturer, so she administered the drug. Upon further investigation, however, it was discovered that the pharmacist had mislabelled a solution of

> Astute observation is key for any good detective or nurse!

mitoxantrone as mitomycin. Fortunately, the patient suffered no harmful effects.

It's elementary!

If a familiar drug seems to have an unfamiliar appearance, investigate the cause. If the pharmacist cites a manufacturing change, ask them to double-check whether they've received verification from the manufacturer. Always document the appearance discrepancy, your actions and the pharmacist's response in the patient record.

Stress-related errors

No one will argue that nursing is sometimes a difficult, stressful occupation, even under the best circumstances. Clearly, nurses carry a great deal of responsibility in drug administration, ensuring that the right patient gets the right drug, in the right concentration, at the right time and by the right route.

Recognising stressors

Too much stress – whether personal, job-related or environmental – can cause or contribute to drug errors. Avoiding stress, or at least learning to recognise and minimise it, will help lower your risk of making errors and maximise the therapeutic effects of your patients' drug regimen.

Added stress from error

Committing a serious medication error can cause enormous stress that might cloud your judgement. If you're administering a medication and realise that you've made a mistake, seek help immediately instead of trying to remedy the situation yourself, as in the following situation.

A nurse just gave the sedative midazolam to the wrong patient. Discovering the error, the nurse reaches for what is thought to be a vial of the antidote, flumazenil, then withdraws 2.5 ml of the drug and administers it to the patient. When the patient fails to respond, the nurse realises that a vial of ondansetron (an antiemetic) was picked up by mistake. The nurse quickly calls for another practitioner, who assists with proper I.V. administration of flumazenil. The patient recovers unharmed.

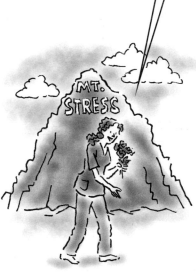

When there's too much stress, sometimes you just have to step away from the situation and take time to smell the roses.

Ensuring quality and preventing errors

Each healthcare setting has its own method of tracking errors in drug administration. Unfortunately, many errors aren't documented because the administering nurses are afraid to report them or may not recognise the event as an error. What they fail to realise, however, is that tracking and documenting errors allows the performance-improvement (quality-assurance) team to recommend ways to prevent future episodes, thereby benefiting both nurses and patients.

Stepping up to the challenge

On a more personal level, you can take several steps to help decrease your risk of making drug errors. Perhaps the easiest way is to strictly adhere to your facility's policies, suggested safety precautions and performance-improvement recommendations.

Other measures you can take include being especially careful when transcribing prescribed drugs from the prescription sheet to the administration record, being aware of your right to refuse administering potentially dangerous drugs, and maintaining a calm, professional demeanor.

Follow policies
Transcribe with care
Know legal rights
Keep a cool head
Report promptly

Overcoming your fear

Keep in mind that, despite the best intentions and circumstances, mistakes are bound to happen. You may very well find yourself in a situation where you caused or contributed to a medication error. If this occurs, you'll need to swallow your fear, take the proper measures and report the incident promptly.

Transcribe carefully

Taking the time to carefully document prescriptions is one of the easiest ways to prevent errors. To avoid transcription errors, follow these guidelines:
• Transcribe all prescribed drugs from the prescription to the administration record in a quiet area, where you can concentrate without interruption.
• Before signing the prescription and initialling the administration record, carefully check both forms to make sure that you've copied the prescription accurately.

- Follow your facility's policy for reviewing prescriptions. Some require nurses to check all patient charts for newly prescribed drugs several times each shift. Others require checking all prescriptions written within the past 24 hours. (In many cases, this responsibility falls on the night shift.)

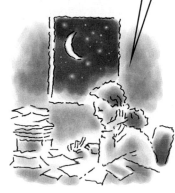

Is it me, or does this job always seem to fall on the night shift?

Know your rights

On rare occasions, you may be asked to administer a drug that you know you would feel uncomfortable giving. Be aware that you can legally refuse to administer a drug under these circumstances:
- if you think the dosage prescribed is too high
- if you think the drug might interact dangerously with other drugs the patient is taking, including alcohol
- if you think the patient's physical condition contraindicates use of the drug.

The right way to just say 'No'

When you refuse to administer prescribed drugs, follow these steps:

Notify your immediate supervisor so they can make alternative arrangements (such as assign a new nurse or clarify the prescription).

Notify the prescriber, if your supervisor hasn't already done so.

Document that the drug wasn't given and explain why (if your facility requires you to do so).

Keep a cool head

Many drug errors occur because nurses are in a hurry, are under a great deal of stress or are unfamiliar with a drug. Try to take your time, and do what you can to avoid distractions and stress. Remember that many drugs are derivatives of other drugs, so they have similar names. If a drug is new to you, use available resources, such as drug references and online medical services, to find out all you can about it. (See *Conquering confusion*.)

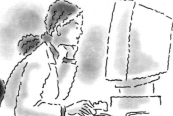

Let's see what the *BNF* says about this drug!

Report drug errors promptly

Whenever you're involved in a drug error – regardless of whether you or someone else caused the mistake – you need to report it immediately and document meticulously what occurred.

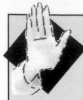

Before you give that drug!

Conquering confusion

Before giving a drug, remind yourself of these essential tactics.

Remember the five rights

Check that you're giving the right drug, at the right dose, by the right route, at the right time, to the right patient.

Double-check the calculations

You can never be too safe. Go over your calculations at least twice to make sure they are correct.

Look at the label

Examine drug labels closely – many of them look alike.

Notice the name

Pay attention! Many drugs have similar-sounding or similar-looking names.

The right response

If you make an error, follow these steps:

Notify the prescriber immediately.

Consult the pharmacist, who can provide information about drug interactions, solutions to dose-related problems (such as what to do about an overdose or an omitted dose) and an antidote (if needed).

Follow your facility's policy for documenting drug errors. You may have to complete an incident report for legal purposes. If so, clearly document what happened, without defending your actions or placing blame. Record the names and functions of everyone involved and what actions they took to protect the patient after the error was discovered.

Consider reporting the error to a professional body which can then use this information to help improve patient safety through the development of educational programmes to prevent future errors of the same nature.

Real-world problem

Here's a complex scenario involving some of the medication errors discussed in this chapter. See if you can unravel what went wrong.

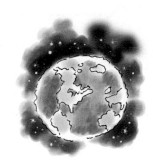

All the wrong moves

The nurse pages the doctor to ask for a prescription of an antiemetic for a patient who's complaining of nausea. The doctor calls the nurse back from the hospital cafeteria, giving a verbal prescription for the antiemetic prochlorperazine. The nurse documents the prescription on a patient chart; however, it's the wrong patient's chart. The nurse then receives a call to report to the emergency department and asks another nurse to administer the drug before leaving the unit.

The second nurse reads the chart with the prescription for prochloperazine and administers the drug to the wrong patient. Fortunately, the patient was not harmed after taking the prochlorperazine; however, the patient who should have received it continued to suffer from nausea until the nurse administered their dose of the medication.

No hits, no runs... and how many errors?

This situation shows how carelessness and failure to follow proper procedures can lead to various errors, in this case involving two patients: one who received a drug that they shouldn't have, and another who failed to receive a drug that was needed.

Starting from the beginning of the scenario, the verbal prescription should never have been accepted from the doctor, because this clearly wasn't an emergency. Having the doctor write the prescription on the patient's chart or enter it into the computer system could have prevented the medication error.

This case also involved a transcription error; no matter how busy the nurse was, time should have been taken to make sure that the correct patient's chart was being documented. It also demonstrates a compound error because of the number of practitioners involved, each of whom could have taken an extra step to reduce the likelihood of error.

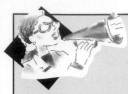

That's a wrap!

Preventing drug errors review

These bullets outline important points about preventing drug errors.

Common drug errors

- Dosage calculation errors
- Drug name errors
- Patient name errors
- Missed allergy alerts
- Compound errors
- Route errors
- Misinterpreted abbreviations
- Misinterpreted prescriptions
- Preparation errors
- Stress-related errors

Avoiding transcription errors

- Transcribe prescriptions in a quiet area.
- Carefully check your work before signing.
- Follow your facility's policy for reviewing prescriptions.

Refusing to dispense a prescription

- Notify your supervisor.
- Notify the prescribing doctor.
- Document according to your facility's policy.

The five 'rights' of drug administration

- Right drug
- Right dose
- Right route
- Right time
- Right patient

In case of error

- Notify the prescriber.
- Consult the pharmacist.
- Assess the patient throughout.
- Follow your facility's drug error-documentation policy.
- If you desire, report the error to a relevant professional body.

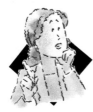

Quick quiz

1. Remembering the five 'rights' of drug administration will help:
   - A. save time.
   - B. increase drug awareness.
   - C. ensure compliance with the drug regimen.
   - D. prevent drug errors.

   Answer: D. The five 'rights' (right drug, dose, patient, time and route) help prevent drug errors, thereby promoting patient safety.

2. A nurse is preparing to administer a dose of chlorpropamide to a patient with type 2 diabetes. Checks for allergies are made and the nurse notices that the patient is wearing an allergy alert

bracelet indicating allergies to sulfa drugs. Which action should the nurse take?
- A.   Administer the drug as prescribed.
- B.   Notify the nursing supervisor immediately.
- C.   Withhold administering the drug and notify the prescriber.
- D.   Confirm that the dosage is correct, then administer the drug.

Answer: C. Patients who are allergic to sulfa drugs shouldn't receive sulphonylurea hypoglycaemic drugs, such as chlorpropamide, because of the possibility of an allergic reaction. The nurse should withhold the drug and notify the prescriber, who can authorise an alternative treatment.

3.   The nurse must administer a bolus dose of glucose 10% in water to a patient. Another nurse drew the solution into a syringe and left it at the patient's bedside, but forgot to label the syringe. What action should the nurse take?
- A.   Administer the medication in the unlabelled syringe.
- B.   Verbally confirm the contents of the syringe with the other nurse before administering it.
- C.   Discard the unlabelled syringe.
- D.   Call the pharmacist.

Answer: C. By discarding this unlabelled syringe, the nurse eliminates the risk of giving the wrong drug or solution to the patient. Never administer unlabelled syringes or solutions. If you do, there's no way to be certain that you're giving the right drug. Even if the other nurse confirms the syringe's contents, it's possible that the syringe became mixed up with another one at the bedside. It's best to be safe – draw up and label a new syringe with glucose 10% in water, to administer to the patient.

4.   Professional bodies are interested in nurses reporting drug errors to:
- A.   prevent future errors.
- B.   place blame on the nurse.
- C.   use the information in future legal cases.
- D.   discredit non-compliant healthcare facilities.

Answer: A. Currently, it's difficult to assess fully the incidence of drug errors and how and why they occur. Many nurses fear that reporting their errors will allow them to be blamed, disciplined or worse. However, by reporting actual or potential errors directly to these agencies, which often ensure confidentiality and anonymity, nurses can help to identify the types and causes of errors, track their incidence and initiate educational programmes to prevent future occurrences.

Scoring

☆☆☆   If you answered all four items correctly, fantastic! You haven't misinterpreted a thing.

☆☆   If you answered three items correctly, wonderful! You're avoiding mistakes and calculating your responses well.

☆   If you answered fewer than three items correctly, keep on trying! Dwelling on your errors will only compound the problem.

Part IV

Oral, topical and rectal drugs

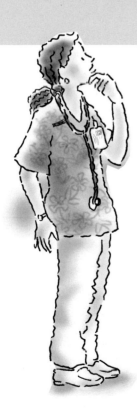

⑩ Calculating oral drug dosages

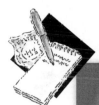

Just the facts

In this chapter, you'll learn:

♦ how to read drug labels to obtain accurate information for calculations

♦ how to administer drugs safely

♦ the correct way to calculate oral dosages of tablets, capsules and liquids

♦ how to calculate dosages using different measurement systems.

A look at oral drugs

Drugs that are administered orally are usually in tablet, capsule or liquid form. Most oral drugs are available in a limited number of strengths or concentrations. Therefore, your ability to calculate prescribed dosages for various drug forms and strengths is an important skill.

Reading oral drug labels

Before you can administer an oral drug safely, you must make sure that it's the correct drug and the correct dosage. Your first step is to read the label carefully, noting the drug's name, dose strength and expiration date.

Drug name

When reading a drug label, check the generic name first. If the drug has two names, the generic name typically

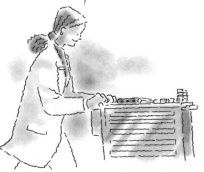

With all the drugs that are out there, make sure you read the labels!

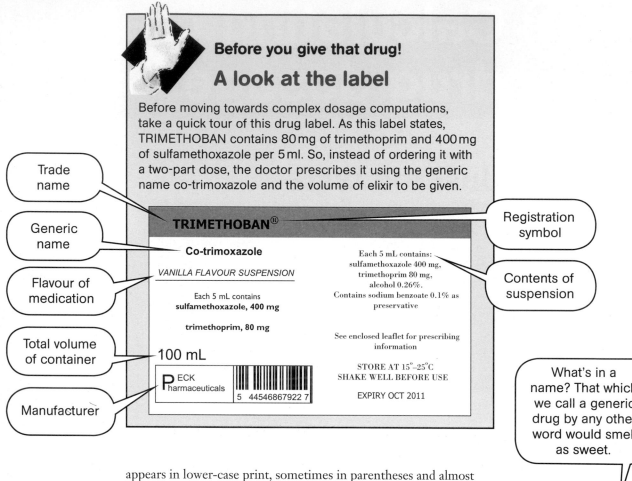

Before you give that drug!

A look at the label

Before moving towards complex dosage computations, take a quick tour of this drug label. As this label states, TRIMETHOBAN contains 80 mg of trimethoprim and 400 mg of sulfamethoxazole per 5 ml. So, instead of ordering it with a two-part dose, the doctor prescribes it using the generic name co-trimoxazole and the volume of elixir to be given.

Trade name

Generic name

Flavour of medication

Total volume of container

Manufacturer

TRIMETHOBAN®

Co-trimoxazole

VANILLA FLAVOUR SUSPENSION

Each 5 mL contains
sulfamethoxazole, 400 mg

trimethoprim, 80 mg

100 mL

Pᴇᴄᴋ
harmaceuticals

5 44546867922 7

Registration symbol

Contents of suspension

Each 5 mL contains:
sulfamethoxazole 400 mg,
trimethoprim 80 mg,
alcohol 0.26%.
Contains sodium benzoate 0.1% as
preservative

See enclosed leaflet for prescribing
information

STORE AT 15°–25°C
SHAKE WELL BEFORE USE

EXPIRY OCT 2011

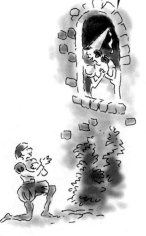

What's in a name? That which we call a generic drug by any other word would smell as sweet.

appears in lower-case print, sometimes in parentheses and almost always under the manufacturer's trade name. The generic name is the accepted non-proprietary name, which is a simplified form of the drug's chemical name.

Next, note the drug's trade name, also called the *brand* or *proprietary* name. This name, given by the manufacturer, typically appears prominently on the label – usually above or before the generic name with at least the first letter capitalised, followed by the registration symbol. (See *A look at the label*.)

Two in one

Some oral medications contain two drugs. The labels for these combination drugs list both generic names and their doses. These drugs are also prescribed by the generic name and the number of capsules or tablets or the volume of suspension/elixir to be given – for example, *co-amoxiclav 5 ml, t.d.s.*

The name game

A drug may have several trade names, but it has only one generic name. For example, the generic drug procyclidine hydrochloride goes, in various forms, by the trade names Arpicolin and Kemadrin. The generic drug glyceryl trinitrate in transdermal patch form goes by the trade names Deponit, Minitran and Trintek, among others.

Unless there are specific reasons, such as bioavailability issues, generic names should always be used in prescribing. This enables any suitable product to be dispensed, thereby saving delay to the patient. The exception to this rule follows where, for example, bioavailability issues may be important, and the patient must receive the same brand. In such cases, the trade name should also be stated.

Worth a second glance

Whether a generic or trade name is used, be extra careful when reading the label to avoid errors.

Meeting the standard

The initials *B.P.* may appear after the drug name. They stand for a legally recognised standard for drugs: *British Pharmacopeia*. These initials mean that a drug has met standards of purity, potency and storage, which are enforced by government agencies.

Dose strength

After checking the drug name, look for the dose strength on the label. Pay close attention: the labels and containers for different concentrations of the same drug may look exactly alike except for the listing of the drug's concentration. (See *Look-alike labels: oral solutions.*)

Expiration date

Lastly, check the expiration date. This vital information is commonly overlooked. Expired drugs may be chemically unstable or may no longer provide the correct dose. If a drug has expired, return it to the pharmacy so that it can be disposed of properly and a new batch of the drug released.

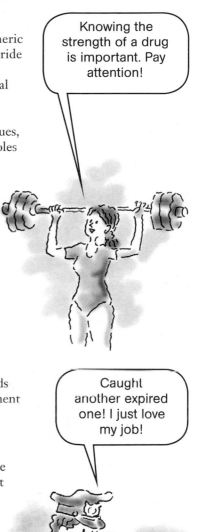

Knowing the strength of a drug is important. Pay attention!

Caught another expired one! I just love my job!

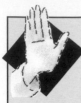

Before you give that drug!

Look-alike labels: oral solutions

The oral solution labels below are examples of look-alikes that you're likely to encounter. Reading labels carefully can help you avoid medication errors.

CO-AMOXICLAV 125 mg/5 mL

AMOXICILLIN/CLAVULANIC ACID

FOR ORAL SUSPENSION

When reconstituted, each 5 mL contains
AMOXICILLIN, 125 mg
As trihydrate
CLAVULANIC ACID, 31.25 mg
as clavulanate potassium

100 mL (when reconstituted)

PECK
Pharmaceuticals

5 44546832152 7

Directions for mixing: Invert bottle until powder flows freely. Add approximately 2/3 total water for reconstitution

Total = 95 mL

Shake well to wet powder. Add remaining water and shake well. See enclosed leaflet for prescribing information

KEEP REFRIDGERATED
DISCARD AFTER 10 DAYS

EXPIRY OCT 2011

> This one is Co-amoxiclav 125 mg/5 ml.

CO-AMOXICLAV 250 mg/5 mL

AMOXICILLIN/CLAVULANIC ACID

FOR ORAL SUSPENSION

When reconstituted, each 5 mL contains
AMOXICILLIN, 250 mg
As trihydrate
CLAVULANIC ACID, 62.5 mg
as clavulanate potassium

100 mL (when reconstituted)

PECK
Pharmaceuticals

5 44546832162 8

Directions for mixing: Invert bottle until powder flows freely. Add approximately 2/3 total water for reconstitution

Total = 95 mL

Shake well to wet powder. Add remaining water and shake well. See enclosed leaflet for prescribing information

KEEP REFRIDGERATED
DISCARD AFTER 10 DAYS

EXPIRY OCT 2011

> This label reads 250 mg/5 ml of Co-amoxiclav – double the concentration of the other one.

Administering oral drugs safely

The first rule in ensuring the safest possible administration of drugs is to check the five 'rights' of medication administration – right drug, right route, right dose, right time, right patient. Another important rule is to triple-check drug labels and prescriptions. Safe drug administration requires you to compare the prescription as transcribed on the medication administration record against the drug label three times. (See *Say it three times: check prescriptions and labels*.)

Proceed with caution

Your patient has been prescribed *150 mg ranitidine b.i.d., by mouth.* Before giving the drug, follow this procedure to the letter:

Open the patient's medication drawer, find the drug labelled *ranitidine 150 mg*, and note that it's in oral tablet form.

Place the labelled drug next to the transcribed drug on the administration record and carefully compare each part of the label to the prescription.

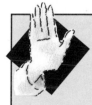

Before you give that drug!

Say it three times: check prescriptions and labels

The secret of drug safety is to check, check and check again. Before giving a drug, carefully compare the drug's label with each part of the medication administration record, holding the label next to the administration record to ensure accuracy. The example below walks you through the steps for administering generic *furosemide 40 mg, by mouth*.

Check drug names

- Read the drug's generic name on the administration record and compare it with the generic name on the label. They both should say *furosemide*.

Check the dosage, route and record

- Read the dosage on the administration record and compare it with the dose on the label. They both should say *40 mg*.
- Read the route specified on the administration record and note the dose form on the label. The record should say *by mouth*, and the label should say *oral tablet*.
- Note any special considerations on the administration record, such as

'aspiration precautions (head of bed elevated to 45 degrees for all oral intake)', 'patient is hard of hearing' or 'patient is visually impaired'.

Check prescriptions and labels three times

Follow this routine three times before giving the drug. Do it the first time when you obtain the drug from floor stock or from the patient's supply. Do it the second time before placing the drug in the medication cup or other administration device. Lastly, do it the third time before replacing the stock drug bottle or removing the drug from the unit-dose package at the patient's bedside.

Check the expiry date on the container and check that the prescription has been signed and dated.

If the drug is supplied in bulk or in a stock bottle, transfer one tablet from the supply to a medication container, pouring from the supply to the lid and then into the container without handling the tablet.

Before returning the supply to the drawer or shelf, once again compare the label to the prescription on the administration record, and note whether this is the right administration time. *When you've removed a drug from its container, you can't ever be certain that it's the correct drug unless you've carefully compared the label with the administration record while pouring.*

Now, go to the patient's bedside, check their identification bracelet, and do your third drug check, comparing the label with the prescription and checking the administration time again. Ask the patient if they have any allergies and check whether this has been recorded on the prescription and administration record. Then give the drug.

If the drug comes in a unit-dose packet, do not remove it from the packet until you are at the patient's bedside and ready to administer it. Then do your third drug check. Remove the drug from the packet and give it to the patient, using the packet label for comparison when recording your administration information. (See *Unit-dose packaging.*)

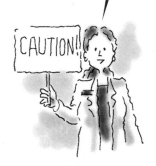

Here are seven essential steps for safe oral drug administration.

Unit-dose packaging

Tablets or capsules in unit doses may be dispensed on a card with the drugs sealed in bubbles or in strips with each drug separated by a tear line. Unit doses of liquids may be packaged in small sealed cups with identifying information on the cover.

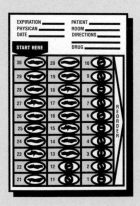

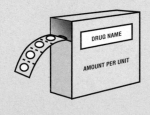

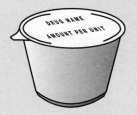

Discovering discrepancies

If you notice discrepancies between the medication administration record and the drug label, check them out. For example, suppose the medication administration record specifies *Disaclor* and the drug packet is labelled *cefaclor*. Check your drug handbook and you'll find that Distaclor is a trade name for cefaclor.

Or, suppose the drug packet is labelled *Ceclor 250 mg* and the dose on the medication administration record is *500 mg*. In this case, you need to calculate the required dose. Scrupulous attention to details like these will help ensure safe, error-free drug administration.

Unit-dose systems

Many facilities use the unit-dose system, which provides prepackaged drugs in single-dose containers and decreases the need for dosage calculations. (See *Save time with the unit-dose system*.)

Save time with the unit-dose system

Using the unit-dose drug distribution system gives you more time for evaluating patient responses to drugs and for teaching patients about their drug regimens.

More exact (that's a fact)

This time-saving system provides the exact dose of medication needed for each patient. The pharmacist computes the number of tablets or the volume of liquid and prepares the proper dose for administration. Errors are decreased because the drug remains in its labelled container until you give it to the patient.

Don't throw away your calculator yet

Does this mean your dosage calculation days are over? Not by a long shot. Some facilities don't use the unit-dose system, and others have systems that don't operate 24 hours per day. So your dosage calculation skills are still vitally important.

Calculating dosages

Despite the prevalence of unit-dose systems, calculations are still necessary in many patient situations. For example, you may have to determine individualised dosages for special patients. You also must know how to convert between measurement systems to determine how many tablets, capsules or other dosage forms to administer. (See *Special delivery drug dosages*.)

You'll often use ratios and fractions in proportions to calculate drug dosages and to convert between measurement systems. The following section reviews these mathematical concepts and shows step-by-step calculations.

Advice from the experts

Special delivery drug dosages

Even if your facility uses the unit-dose system, you'll still need to calculate dosages for some patients. For example, patients on critical care units, paediatric patients and geriatric patients require individualised medication dosages that may be unusually large or small.

The nearest milligram

Some patients need dosages that are calculated to the nearest milligram instead of the nearest 10 mg. For them, the correct calculation of the exact dosage can mean the difference between an underdose or overdose and the correct dose. A few examples of drugs that are measured to the nearest milligram or microgram are digoxin, levothyroxine sodium and many paediatric drugs.

Changing the delivery route

Some people can't handle drugs that are delivered by the usual route because their ability to absorb, distribute, metabolise or excrete drugs is impaired. Some patients can't absorb drugs from

the gastrointestinal (GI) tract because of upper-GI disorders or surgery; deficiencies of gastric, pancreatic or intestinal secretions; or passive congestion of GI blood vessels from severe heart failure. These patients need drugs in parenteral form in larger-than-average oral doses. Smaller doses of a drug can be used when the drug is given by the I.V. route because it may be delivered to the bloodstream more efficiently and is more readily absorbed.

Don't forget these special patients

Other patients who need individualised dosages include those with conditions that cause abnormal drug distribution from the GI tract or from parenteral sites to the sites of action. Premature infants and patients with low serum protein levels or severe liver or kidney disease who can't metabolise or excrete drugs as readily as normal patients also require special drug dosages. You can help individualise drug regimens for these patients by assessing their kidney or liver function, monitoring blood levels of drugs and calculating exact dosages.

Using ratios, fractions and proportions

Ratios and fractions are two ways to express the numerical relationship between things. A proportion expresses equality between two ratios or fractions. Proportions may be written using ratios, as in:

$$1 : 3 :: 2 : 6$$

or using fractions, as in:

$$\frac{1}{3} = \frac{2}{6}$$

When proportions are expressed using ratios, the product of the means (the inside numbers) equals the product of the extremes (the outside numbers):

$$2 : 4 :: 1 : 2$$

means

extremes

so,

$$4 \times 1 = 2 \times 2$$

When proportions are expressed as fractions, their cross products are equal.

$$\frac{3}{6} \times \frac{6}{12}$$

so,

$$3 \times 12 = 6 \times 6$$

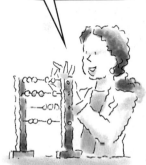

Learning ratios and fractions can be tough, but at least we don't have to use this thing anymore!

Equally mean and extreme

When a proportion is expressed using ratios, the units of the mean on one side of the proportion must match the units of the extreme on the other side, and vice versa:

$$mg : tablet :: mg : tablet$$

When a proportion is expressed using fractions, the units of measure in the numerators must be the same, and the units of measure in the denominators must be the same:

Denominators are the same.

$$\frac{mg}{tablet} = \frac{mg}{tablet}$$

Numerators are the same.

Four rules for calculating drug dosages

To help you prevent calculation and medication errors and simplify your calculations, remember these four rules. (See *Helpful hints to minimise calculation errors*.)

Rule 1: use correct units of measure

Using the incorrect unit of measure is one of the most common dosage calculation errors. When calculating doses, matching units of measure in the numerator and denominator cancel each other, leaving the correct unit of measure in the answer. Here's an example:

How many milligrams of a drug are in two tablets if one tablet contains 5 mg of the drug?

State the problem as a proportion:

$$5 \text{ mg} : 1 \text{ tablet} :: X : 2 \text{ tablets}$$

Remember that the product of the means equals the product of the extremes:

> **Multiply the means.**

$$1 \text{ tablet} \times X = 5 \text{ mg} \times 2 \text{ tablets}$$

> **Multiply the extremes.**

Solve for X. Divide each side of the equation by the known value, 1 tablet, and cancel units that appear in both the numerator and denominator:

$$\frac{1 \text{ tablet} \times X}{1 \text{ tablet}} = \frac{5 \text{ mg} \times 2 \text{ tablets}}{1 \text{ tablet}}$$

$$X = 10 \text{ mg}$$

Rule 2: double-check decimals and zeros

An error in the number of decimal places or zeros in a dosage calculation can cause a ten-fold or greater dosage error. Here's an example using decimals and zeros: your patient has been prescribed *0.05 mg levothyroxine by mouth*, but the only levothyroxine on hand is in tablets that contain 0.025 mg each. How many tablets should you give?

- State the problem as a proportion:

$$0.025\,\text{mg} : 1\,\text{tablet} :: 0.05\,\text{mg} : X$$

- The product of the means equals the product of the extremes:

$$1\,\text{tablet} \times 0.05\,\text{mg} = 0.25\,\text{mg} \times X$$

- Solve for X by dividing each side of the equation by 0.025 mg and cancelling units that appear in both the numerator and denominator, checking decimal placement carefully:

$$\frac{1\,\text{tablet} \times 0.05\,\cancel{\text{mg}}}{0.025\,\cancel{\text{mg}}} = \frac{0.025\,\cancel{\text{mg}} \times X}{0.025\,\cancel{\text{mg}}}$$

$$X = 2\,\text{tablets}$$

Rule 3: question strange answers

Be especially careful to recheck suspicious-looking calculations. For example, if a dosage calculation suggests giving 25 tablets or 200 ml of suspension, assume that you've made an error and check your figures. If you're still unsure about your results, have another nurse check your calculation.

Rule 4: get out the calculator

An electronic calculator can *improve* the accuracy and speed of your calculations, but it can't *guarantee* accuracy. You still must set up proportions carefully and double-check units of measure and decimal places.

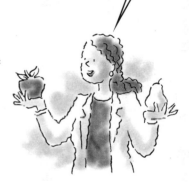

This is mighty suspicious… how did I end up with apples when I started with pears? Better double-check my calculations.

Special considerations

Occasionally when administering oral drugs, you may come across unusual situations that require you to take a few extra steps.

Divided doses

Most tablets, capsules and similar dose forms are available in only a few strengths. Usually, you'll administer one tablet or one-half of a scored tablet.

Breaking a scored tablet in portions smaller than one-half usually creates inaccurate doses. If a dose smaller than one-half of a scored tablet or any portion of an unscored tablet is needed, you should

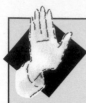

Before you give that drug!

Be cautious with tablets and capsules

Before you break or crush a tablet or capsule, call the pharmacist to see if the drug is available in smaller dosage strengths or in liquid form for patients who have difficulty swallowing. Also check your drug handbook – or check with the pharmacist – to see whether altering the drug will affect its action. Drugs that shouldn't be broken or crushed include:

- sustained-release drugs, also called extended-release, timed-release or controlled-release (suffixes such as 'SR', 'CR', 'DUR' and 'LA' in a drug name usually indicate that the drug is sustained-release)
- capsules that contain tiny beads of medication, although you may empty the contents of some of these capsules into a food or beverage
- enteric-coated tablets, which have a hard coating (usually shiny or glossy) that's designed to protect the upper GI tract from irritation
- buccal and sublingual tablets.

Tips for crushing and breaking

Crushing or cutting tablets is not recommended. If you are required to administer a smaller dose that available, smaller-dose tablets should be requested from the pharmacy.

However, if you need to crush a tablet, use a chewable form, which is softer. The easiest method is to crush the tablet while it's still in its package, using a haemostat or pill crusher. Or you can remove it from the package and crush it with a mortar and pestle.

If you need to break a tablet, use one that's scored. Carefully cut the tablet on the score line with a scalpel or pill cutter. Enlist the pharmacist's help when you need to break a tablet into smaller pieces than the score allows or when you must administer a portion of a capsule. If you need to break an unscored tablet, have the pharmacist crush, weigh and dispense it in two equal doses.

---

substitute a commercially available solution or suspension or have one prepared by the pharmacist.

You can also ask the pharmacist to crush the tablet and measure an exact dose. However, some oral preparations shouldn't be opened, broken, scored or crushed because those actions change the drug's effect. (See *Be cautious with tablets and capsules*.)

All things being equianalgesic

At times, you may need to convert a dose of an analgesic from the parenteral route to the oral route. If so, equianalgesic charts provide the information you need to recalculate the dose necessary to produce the desired pain control. These charts use morphine sulphate as the gold standard for comparing pain control. (See *Equianalgesic charts: a painless path for converting dosages*.)

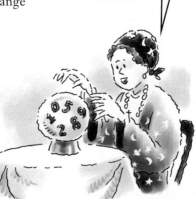

Don't leave half-doses to chance. Be exact!

Equianalgesic charts: a painless path for converting dosages

When substituting one analgesic for another, equianalgesic charts provide the information you need to calculate the dose necessary to produce the desired pain control (equianalgesic effect).

These charts use morphine sulphate as the *gold standard* for comparison. On most charts, doses for many drugs are listed; each dose provides pain relief equivalent to 10 mg of I.M. morphine. Here's an example of an equianalgesic chart.

Medication	P.O. dose	I.M. dose
Morphine	10 mg	30 mg
Codeine	1.5 mg	7.5 mg
Hydromorphone	2 mg	4 mg

Remember: every dose on the equianalgesic chart provides an equivalent amount of pain control, and any change in medication requires a new prescription.

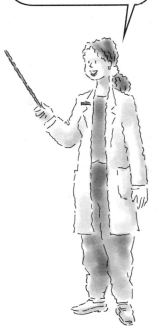

An equianalgesic chart can help you calculate the correct dose when changing the route of administration or when substituting one analgesic for another. But don't forget the prescription!

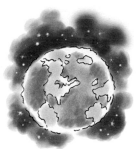

Real-world problems

When calculating the number of tablets to administer, use proportions. Set up the first ratio or fraction with the known tablet strength. Set up the second ratio or fraction with the prescribed dose and the unknown quantity of tablets or capsules. Then solve for *X* to determine the correct dose. To illustrate, here are some typical patient situations.

The paracetamol poser

A patient has been prescribed *1 g of paracetamol by mouth*, *stat*, but the drug is available only in 500-mg tablets. How many tablets should you give?

Here's the calculation using ratios:

• Set up the first ratio with the known tablet strength:

500 mg : 1 tablet

- Set up the second ratio with the desired dose and the unknown number of tablets, bearing in mind that 1 g is equivalent to 1000 mg:

$$1000\,mg : X$$

- Put these ratios into a proportion:

$$500\,mg : 1\,tablet :: 1000\,mg : X$$

- Set up the equation by multiplying the means and extremes:

$$1\,tablet \times 1000\,mg = 500\,mg \times X$$

- Solve for X by dividing both sides of the equation by 500 mg and cancelling units that appear in both the numerator and denominator:

$$\frac{1\,tablet \times 1000\,\cancel{mg}}{500\,\cancel{mg}} = \frac{\cancel{500\,mg} \times X}{\cancel{500\,mg}}$$

$$X = 2\,tablets$$

The clozapine clue

Your patient is prescribed *250 mg of clozapine, by mouth, daily*. How many tablets should he take if each tablet contains 100 mg?

Here's the calculation using ratios:

- Set up the first ratio with the known tablet strength:

$$100\,mg : 1\,tablet$$

- Set up the second ratio with the desired dose and the unknown number of tablets:

$$250\,mg : X$$

- Put these ratios into a proportion:

$$100\,mg : 1\,tablet :: 250\,mg : X$$

- Multiply the means and the extremes:

$$1\,tablet \times 250\,mg = 100\,mg \times X$$

- Divide each side of the equation by 100 mg and cancel units that appear in both the numerator and denominator:

$$\frac{1\,tablet \times 250\,\cancel{mg}}{100\,\cancel{mg}} = \frac{\cancel{100\,mg} \times X}{\cancel{100\,mg}}$$

$$X = 2\tfrac{1}{2}\,tablets$$

Gliding through glimepiride

The patients prescription reads *glimepiride 1.5 mg 3 tablets, by mouth, daily*. What's the total dose in milligrams?

Here's the solution using fractions:

- Set up the first fraction with the known tablet strength:

$$\frac{1.5 \text{ mg}}{1 \text{ tablet}}$$

- Set up the second fraction with the desired dose and the unknown number of milligrams:

$$\frac{X}{3 \text{ tablets}}$$

- Put these fractions into a proportion:

$$\frac{X}{3 \text{ tablets}} = \frac{1.5 \text{ mg}}{1 \text{ tablet}}$$

- Cross-multiply the fractions:

$$X \times 1 \text{ tablet} = 3 \text{ tablets} \times 1.5 \text{ mg}$$

- Divide both sides of the equation by 1 tablet and cancel units that appear in both the numerator and denominator:

$$\frac{X \times \cancel{1 \text{ tablet}}}{\cancel{1 \text{ tablet}}} = \frac{3 \cancel{\text{ tablets}} \times 1.5 \text{ mg}}{\cancel{1 \text{ tablet}}}$$

$$X = 4.5 \text{ mg}$$

Calculating liquid dosages

In addition to administering tablets to your patients, you'll also give them liquid medications in suspension or elixir form. Before calculating a dosage, read the label carefully to identify the dose strength in a specified amount of solution. Then check the label for the expiration date.

> Doing *liquid* dosage calculations is probably more fun than any other kind of calculation I can think of.

More real-world problems

In each of the following problems, use the proportion method to calculate the amount of solution. Set up the first ratio or fraction with the known solution strength, and set up the second ratio or fraction with the desired dose and the unknown quantity. Then solve for X to find the correct dose.

Here are some typical patient situations.

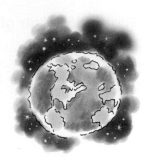

Pay attention to the suspension

Your patient is receiving 500 mg of ceflaclor oral suspension for a severe infection. The label reads *ceflaclor 250 mg/5 ml*, and the bottle contains 100 ml. How many millilitres of ceflaclor should you give?

Here's the solution using fractions:

• Set up the first fraction with the known solution strength:

$$\frac{5\ \text{ml}}{250\ \text{mg}}$$

• Set up the second fraction with the desired dose and the unknown number of millilitres:

$$\frac{X}{500\ \text{mg}}$$

• Put these fractions into a proportion:

$$\frac{X}{500\ \text{mg}} = \frac{5\ \text{ml}}{250\ \text{mg}}$$

• Cross-multiply the fractions:

$$X \times 250\ \text{mg} = 5\ \text{ml} \times 500\ \text{mg}$$

• Solve for X by dividing both sides of the equation by 250 mg and cancelling units that appear in both the numerator and denominator:

$$\frac{X \times 250\ \cancel{\text{mg}}}{250\ \cancel{\text{mg}}} = \frac{5\ \text{ml} \times 500\ \cancel{\text{mg}}}{250\ \cancel{\text{mg}}}$$

$$X = \frac{2500\ \text{ml}}{250}$$

$$X = 10\ \text{ml}$$

Erythromycin enigma

Your patient needs 400 mg of erythromycin oral suspension. The label reads *erythromycin 200 mg/5 ml*. How many millilitres should you give?

Here's the calculation using ratios:

• Set up the first ratio with the known solution strength:

$$5 \, ml : 200 \, mg$$

• Set up the second ratio with the unknown number of millilitres and the desired dose:

$$X : 400 \, mg$$

• Put these ratios into a proportion:

$$5 \, ml : 200 \, mg :: X : 400 \, mg$$

• Set up an equation by multiplying the means and extremes:

$$X \times 200 \, mg = 5 \, ml \times 400 \, mg$$

• Solve for X by dividing both sides of the equation by 200 mg and cancelling units that appear in both the numerator and denominator:

$$\frac{X \times \cancel{200 \, mg}}{\cancel{200 \, mg}} = \frac{5 \, ml \times 400 \, \cancel{mg}}{200 \, \cancel{mg}}$$

$$X = \frac{2000 \, ml}{200}$$

$$X = 10 \, ml$$

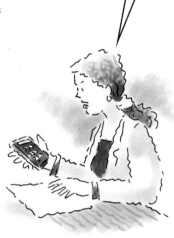

Once I set up my proportion, it's all about multiplication and division — that's where you come in, my friend!

Don't fall over flucloxacillin

Your patient has been prescribed *100 mg flucloxacillin, oral solution, t.i.d.* by the doctor. The label reads *flucloxacillin 125 mg/5 ml*. How many millilitres should you give?

Here's the calculation using ratios:

• Set up the first fraction with the known solution strength:

$$5 \, ml : 125 \, mg$$

• Set up the second fraction with the unknown number of millilitres and the desired dose:

$$X : 100 \, mg$$

• Put these ratios into a proportion:

$$X : 100 \, mg :: 5 \, ml : 125 \, mg$$

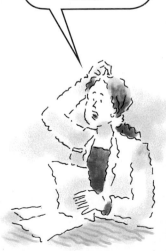

To set up a proportion, I need to know what I want, what I have and what I don't know.

- Set up an equation by multiplying the means and extremes:

$$100\,mg \times 5\,ml = 125\,mg \times X$$

- Solve for X by dividing each side of the equation by 125 mg and cancelling units that appear in both the numerator and denominator:

$$\frac{100\,\cancel{mg} \times 5\,ml}{125\,\cancel{mg}} = \frac{125\,\cancel{mg} \times X}{125\,\cancel{mg}}$$

$$\frac{500\,ml}{125} = X$$

$$X = 4\,ml$$

Diluting powders

Some oral drugs become unstable when they're stored as liquids, so they're supplied in powder form. Before giving these drugs, dilute them with the appropriate diluent, usually tap water. Read the drug labels carefully to see how much diluent to add.

After adding the diluent and mixing thoroughly, read the labels again to determine the dose strengths contained in the volumes of fluid. To calculate the dosages, use the ratio or fraction and proportion method.

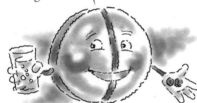

Don't forget to read the labels *after* you mix as well as before!

Weighing in

The dose concentration in oral solutions is expressed as the weight – or dose strength – of the drug contained in a volume of solution. For example, furosemide oral solution is provided as 4 mg/ml. So the solution contains 4 mg of furosemide (drug weight) in 1 ml (solution volume).

Measuring oral solutions

To administer an oral solution accurately, measure it with a medicine cup, dropper or syringe.

Good to the last drop

Medicine cups are usually calibrated to measure solutions in millilitres. For accuracy, hold the cup at eye level while pouring the solution. Also, hold the solution container with the medication label turned toward the palm of your hand so that solution doesn't drip over the label when poured.

For good measure

Drugs that are prescribed in drops are usually packaged with a dropper. If they aren't, use a standard dropper. They can be used to measure solutions in millilitres. After measuring and administering a drug from a multiple-dose container, store it as directed on the drug label.

Syringe cringe

Syringes are handy for drawing up and measuring solutions accurately. However, never use a syringe to administer an oral drug. If you leave the plastic tip on by mistake, the patient can swallow or aspirate it.

Two-step dosage calculations

Most dosage calculations require more than one equation. For example, the doctor may prescribe a drug in millimoles, but it may be available only in tablet, capsule or liquid form in milligrams. When this happens, you need to convert from one measurement system to another before determining how much medication to administer. (See *When you need a new measure*.)

Keeping in step

When converting between measurement systems, first consult a conversion table to find the standard equivalent value – the equivalent between the two measurement systems. Then use the ratio and proportion or fraction method to calculate the correct dose. Put the standard equivalent values in the first ratio or fraction, and put the quantity prescribed and the unknown quantity in the second ratio or fraction.

Still more real-world problems

The following example shows how to convert from one measurement system to another and then how to calculate the correct dose.

Digoxin dilemma

Your patient receives a prescription for *62.5 mcg of digoxin elixir, by mouth, daily*. The elixir label reads *0.05 mg/ml*. How many millilitres of digoxin should you give?

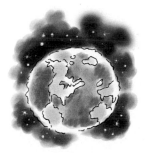

Here's how to solve this problem using ratios:
- Convert micrograms to milligrams. Recall that 1000 mcg equals 1 mg.
- Set up the first ratio with the standard equivalent value:

$$1\,mg : 1000\,mcg$$

- Set up the second ratio with the unknown quantity in the appropriate position:

$$X : 62.5\,mcg$$

- Put these ratios into a proportion:

$$1\,mg : 1000\,mcg :: X : 62.5\,mcg$$

- Multiply the means and the extremes:

$$X \times 1000\,mcg = 1\,mg \times 62.5\,mcg$$

- Solve for X by dividing both sides of the equation by 1000 mcg and cancelling units that appear in both the numerator and denominator:

$$\frac{X \times \cancel{1000\,mcg}}{\cancel{1000\,mcg}} = \frac{1\,mg \times 62.5\,\cancel{mcg}}{1000\,\cancel{mcg}}$$

$$X = \frac{62.5\,mcg}{1000}$$

$$X = 0.0625\,mg$$

- The prescribed dose is 62.5 mcg, or 0.0625 mg. Calculate the number of millilitres to be given by setting up a proportion:

$$0.0625\,mg : X :: 0.05\,mg : 1\,ml$$

- Set up an equation by multiplying the means and extremes:

$$X \times 0.05\,mg = 1\,ml \times 0.0625\,mg$$

- Solve for X by dividing each side of the equation by 0.05 mg and cancelling units that appear in both the numerator and denominator:

$$\frac{X \times \cancel{0.05\,mg}}{\cancel{0.05\,mg}} = \frac{1\,ml \times 0.0625\,\cancel{mg}}{0.05\,\cancel{mg}}$$

$$X = 1.25\,ml$$

The dose to be given is 1.25 ml.

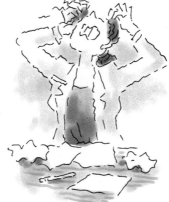

Remembering to multiply means and extremes can be extremely frustrating!

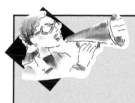

That's a wrap!

Calculating oral drug dosages review

Keep these important facts in mind when calculating doses of oral drugs.

Reading oral drug labels

- First, check the drug's generic name (and trade name if required). Remember that combination drugs are more usually prescribed using a trade name.
- Then check the dose strength.
- Lastly, check the expiration date.

Safe oral drug administration

- Check the five 'rights' of medication administration.
- Check drug names.
- Check the dosage, route and medication administration record.
- Check prescriptions and labels three times.

Dosage calculation key

- Use correct units of measure.
- Double-check units of measure and decimal places.

- Check answers that seem wrong.
- Use a calculator to check your calculation.

Liquid dosages

- Read drug labels carefully: the drug concentration is expressed as the dose strength contained in a volume of solution.
- Dilute powders with the appropriate fluid (usually tap water for oral preparations).
- Measure oral solutions with a medicine cup, dropper or syringe.

Calculating with different systems

- First, find the standard equivalent value with a conversion table.
- Then calculate the dosage using the ratio and proportion method.
- The standard equivalent values equal the unknown quantity over the quantity ordered.

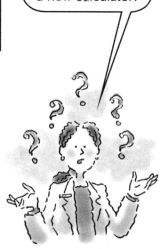

This chapter is a great reason to go out and buy a new calculator!

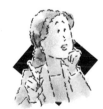

Quick quiz

1.   If a patient needs 100 mcg of levothyroxine, by mouth, and the available dose is 25 mcg/tablet, the number of tablets to give is:

    A.   2
    B.   3
    C.   4
    D.   6

Answer: C. If 1 tablet provides 25 mcg, divide 100 by 25 to get the answer: 4 tablets.

2. If *300 mg of griseofulvin* is prescribed for a patient, but only 100-mg tablets are available, you should give:
- A. 1 tablet
- B. 2 tablets
- C. 3 tablets
- D. 6 tablets

Answer: C. By dividing 300 by 100, you get 3 tablets.

3. Some oral drugs become unstable when they're supplied in powder form. Therefore, you usually must dilute them in which diluent before administration?
- A. tap water
- B. sterile water
- C. normal saline solution
- D. Ringer-lactate solution

Answer: A. Drugs that become unstable when they're stored as liquids are usually diluted with tap water before administration.

4. A patient needs 4 mg of chlorphenamine solution, by mouth, stat, and the bottle label reads *chlorphenamine 2 mg/5 ml*. You should give:
- A. 5 ml
- B. 10 ml
- C. 15 ml
- D. 20 ml

Answer: B. Use fractions to solve for X. The known factor is 2 mg equals 5 ml.

Scoring

☆☆☆ If you answered all four items correctly, excellent! Expressed as a ratio, it's 10 : 10 :: 100 : 100 (in other words, perfect).

☆☆ If you answered three items correctly, good job! Your calculation skills are almost perfect! (But, remember, a good calculator never hurt anybody.)

☆ If you answered fewer than three items correctly, don't worry! Keep on calculating (a little practice goes a long way).

11 Calculating topical and rectal drug dosages

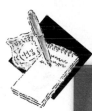

Just the facts

In this chapter, you'll learn:

♦ how to interpret topical and rectal drug labels

♦ what types of drugs are given topically and rectally and how they work

♦ how to perform dosage calculations for topical and rectal drugs.

A look at topical and rectal drugs

Some types of drugs must be administered by the topical, or dermal, route. These drugs include creams, lotions, ointments and powders, which are commonly used for dermatological treatment or wound care, or patches, which have various uses, including treating angina. Topical drugs are applied to the skin and absorbed through the epidermis into the dermis.

Drugs may also be given rectally. This route may be best for patients who can't take drugs orally, such as those with nasogastric tubes, nausea or vomiting. It may also be used for unconscious patients who can't swallow and to achieve specific local and systemic effects. Rectal drugs include enemas and suppositories.

Are you label able?

When you read the labels on topical and rectal drugs, look for the same information you would look for on oral and parenteral drug labels. (See *Labelling a successful administration*.)

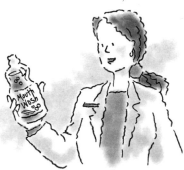

Always remember to check the expiration date. Make sure you look closely!

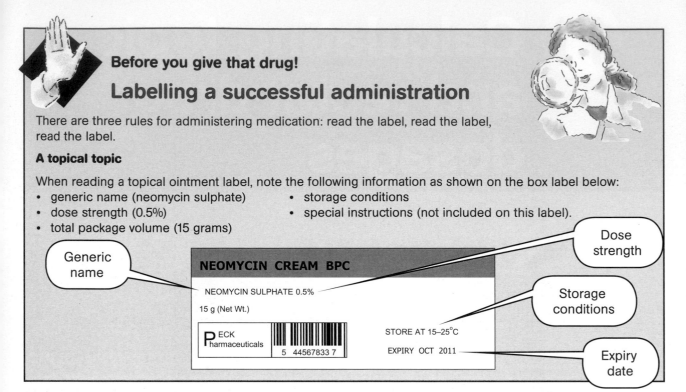

Before you give that drug!

Labelling a successful administration

There are three rules for administering medication: read the label, read the label, read the label.

A topical topic

When reading a topical ointment label, note the following information as shown on the box label below:
- generic name (neomycin sulphate)
- dose strength (0.5%)
- total package volume (15 grams)
- storage conditions
- special instructions (not included on this label).

Generic name

Dose strength

Storage conditions

Expiry date

NEOMYCIN CREAM BPC

NEOMYCIN SULPHATE 0.5%

15 g (Net Wt.)

P ECK
harmaceuticals

5 44567833 7

STORE AT 15–25°C

EXPIRY OCT 2011

The trade name appears first, followed by the generic name, the dose strength and the total volume of the package. Labels may also contain special administration instructions. Sometimes, the print on the labels is quite small, so look carefully. (See *Combination product alert*.)

Transdermal patches

In the past, topical drugs were used almost solely for their local effects. Today, however, several topical drugs, such as transdermal patches, are used for their systemic effects as well.

I've got you under my skin

Transdermal patch drugs penetrate the outer layers of the skin by way of passive diffusion at a constant rate; then the drugs are absorbed into the circulation. Patches are a good way to administer drugs that aren't absorbed well in the GI tract as well as those that are metabolised and eliminated too quickly to be effective.

Patches are convenient and easy to use, and they maintain consistent blood levels of the drug. However, they also have disadvantages. Their onset of action is slow, so a therapeutic blood level takes hours or even days to achieve. Patches must also be checked frequently, especially if the patient is active, because they may

Before you give that drug!

Combination product alert

Topical preparations may contain more than one drug. For example, Cicatrin cream contains bacitracin zinc, neomycin sulphate, cysteine, glycine and threonine. Carefully note all ingredients when checking labels and make sure that your patient isn't allergic to any of them.

Prescribed patches

These transdermal drugs allow you to topically administer systemic drugs.

Glycerol trinitrate

Transdermal glyceryl trinitrate provides prophylactic treatment of chronic angina. Available brands include Deponit, Nitro-Dur, Transderm-Nitro and Trintek. A new patch is applied daily (usually in the morning) and removed after 12 to 14 hours to prevent the patient from developing a tolerance to the drug.

Nicotine

Transdermal nicotine is used to treat smoking addiction. Brands include Nicorette and NiQuitin CQ. These drugs should be used only as adjuncts to behavioural therapy programmes. A new patch is applied daily. Nicorette should be removed after 16 hours, but NiQuitin CQ should stay on for 24 hours.

Fentanyl

Transdermal fentanyl is administered to treat severe chronic pain. Its brand name is Duragesic. Each patch may be worn up to 72 hours.

Estradiol

Transdermal estradiol provides hormone replacement to oestrogen-deficient women. The brand names include Climara, Evorel and Femapak. It is administered on an intermittent cyclic schedule (3 weeks of therapy followed by discontinuation for 1 week).

Testosterone

Transdermal testosterone provides hormone replacement for men with testosterone deficiency. Brand names include Andropatch. The testosterone-replacement patch is applied once daily to clean, hairless scrotal skin, which is the only skin that's thin enough to allow adequate blood levels to be achieved.

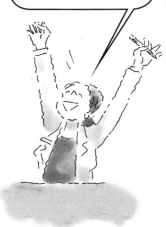

What a break! No calculations needed for this transdermal patch prescription. Just apply the patch and remove it in 24 hours!

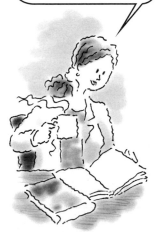

Nicotine and contraceptive patches have been getting a lot of publicity lately, but patches are available for a variety of conditions.

become displaced. In addition, reversing the toxic effects of patches can be difficult because the drug takes so long to be metabolised.

Release me

Drug concentrations in transdermal patches vary depending on the design of the patch, but the concentration isn't as important as the drug's rate of release. Two patches containing the same drug in different concentrations may actually release the same amount of drug per hour. (See *Prescribed patches*.)

Batches of patches

Patches are available for many conditions, including glyceryl trinitrate patches to prevent angina, estradiol patches used in hormone-replacement therapy and a fentanyl patch to manage chronic pain.

The fentanyl transdermal system, or Duragesic patch, is an example of a transdermal drug used systemically. It's held in a reservoir behind a membrane that allows controlled drug absorption through the skin. These patches are available in doses of 12, 25, 50, 75 and 100mcg/hour, with the higher doses for use with opioid-resistant patients. To ensure that the patient receives the correct dose, change the patch every 72 hours and check the label to verify the fentanyl dosage.

Topical drug dosages

Determining topical drug dosages requires very little calculating. As discussed previously, transdermal patches are changed at regular intervals to ensure that the patient receives the correct dose. To apply a patch, simply remove the old patch and replace it with a new one at the appropriate time, following the manufacturer's guidelines.

Applying your judgement (along with the ointment)

When ointment is prescribed as part of wound care or dermatological treatment, the amount to be applied is usually left up to the patient. However, the prescriber may give general guidance, such as 'use a thin layer' or 'apply thickly'. When an ointment contains a drug intended for a systemic effect, more specific administration guidelines are necessary.

Measuring a topical dose

To measure a specified amount of ointment from a tube, squeeze the prescribed length of ointment in centimetres or inches onto a paper ruler like the one shown here. Then use the ruler to apply the ointment to the patient's skin at the appropriate time, following the manufacturer's guidelines for administration.

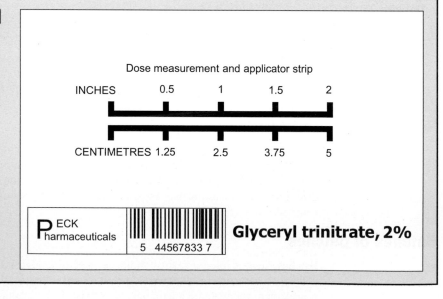

Many ointments, including glyceryl trinitrate, are available in tubes. To apply ointment from a tube, use a paper ruler applicator to measure the correct dose. (See *Measuring a topical dose*.)

Rectal drug dosages

Rectal drugs include enemas and suppositories. Suppositories are the most common form of rectal drugs.

To calculate the number of suppositories to give, use the proportion method with ratios or fractions. These drugs are usually prescribed in the dose provided by one suppository, but occasionally you may need to insert two suppositories. (See *Check and check again*.)

Real-world problems

These problems illustrate how to calculate suppository dosages.

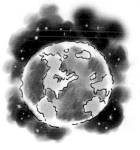

A paracetamol poser

Your paediatric patient needs 250 mg of paracetamol by suppository. The package label reads *paracetamol suppositories 125 mg*. How many suppositories should you give?

This is how to solve this problem using fractions:

- Set up the first fraction with the known suppository dose:

$$\frac{1 \text{ supp}}{250 \text{ mg}}$$

- Set up the second fraction with the desired dose and the unknown number of suppositories:

$$\frac{X}{250 \text{ mg}}$$

- Put these fractions into a proportion:

$$\frac{1 \text{ supp}}{125 \text{ mg}} = \frac{X}{250 \text{ mg}}$$

- Cross-multiply the fractions:

$$125 \text{ mg} \times X = 1 \text{ supp} \times 250 \text{ mg}$$

- Solve for X by dividing each side of the equation by 125 mg and cancelling units that appear in both the numerator and denominator:

$$\frac{125 \cancel{\text{ mg}} \times X}{125 \cancel{\text{ mg}}} = \frac{1 \text{ supp} \times 250 \cancel{\text{ mg}}}{125 \cancel{\text{ mg}}}$$

$$X = 2 \text{ suppositories}$$

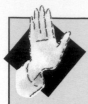

Before you give that drug!

Check and check again

Occasionally you may need to insert more than one or a portion of one suppository. Here's what to do.

More than one

Do your dosage calculations indicate a need for more than one suppository? If so, check your figures and ask another nurse to check them, too. Then ask the pharmacist whether the suppository is available in other dosage strengths.

More than two

If more than two suppositories are needed, confirm the dose with the doctor. Then check with the pharmacist, who may be able to give you one suppository with an adequate amount of the drug.

A portion of one

If less than one suppository is needed, check your calculations and have another nurse do the same. Then ask the pharmacist if the dose is available in one suppository. This ensures the most accurate dose.

Battling with bisacodyl bedlam

The patient's prescription states *bisacodyl 10 mg per rectum at 6 a.m.* You only have 5-mg suppositories on hand. How many suppositories should you give this patient?

This is how to solve this problem using fractions:

- Set up the first fraction with the known suppository dose:

$$\frac{1 \text{ supp}}{5 \text{ mg}}$$

- Set up the second fraction with the desired dose and the unknown number of suppositories:

$$\frac{X}{10 \text{ mg}}$$

- Put these fractions into a proportion:

$$\frac{1 \text{ supp}}{5 \text{ mg}} = \frac{X}{10 \text{ mg}}$$

- Cross-multiply the fractions:

$$1 \text{ supp} \times 10 \text{ mg} = X \times 5 \text{ mg}$$

- Solve for X by dividing each side of the equation by 5 mg and cancelling units that appear in both the numerator and denominator:

$$\frac{1 \text{ supp} \times 10 \text{ \cancel{mg}}}{5 \text{ \cancel{mg}}} = \frac{X \times 5 \text{ \cancel{mg}}}{5 \text{ \cancel{mg}}}$$

$$X = 2 \text{ suppositories}$$

Pacing through another paracetamol problem

Your patient is prescribed a 125-mg paracetamol suppository. The pharmacy is closed, and the only paracetamol on hand contains *250 mg per suppository*. How many suppositories should you give?

This is how to solve this problem using ratios:

- Set up the first ratio with the known suppository dose:

$$1\,supp : 250\,mg$$

- Set up the second ratio with the desired dose and the unknown number of suppositories:

$$X : 125\,mg$$

- Put these ratios into a proportion:

$$1\,supp : 250\,mg :: X : 125\,mg$$

- Multiply the means and the extremes:

$$250\,mg \times X = 125\,mg \times 1\,supp$$

- Solve for X by dividing each side of the equation by 250 mg and cancelling units that appear in both the numerator and denominator:

$$\frac{\cancel{250\,mg} \times X}{\cancel{250\,mg}} = \frac{125\,\cancel{mg} \times 1\,supp}{250\,\cancel{mg}}$$

$$X = \tfrac{1}{2}\ suppository$$

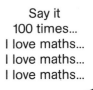

Say it
100 times...
I love maths...
I love maths...
I love maths...

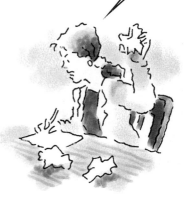

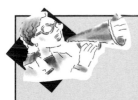

That's a wrap!

Topical and rectal drug dosages review

Review these key facts before giving topical and rectal drugs.

Transdermal patches

- Transdermal patch drugs penetrate the outer layers of the skin by passive diffusion and then are absorbed into the circulation.
- These drugs have a slow onset of action, so it may take hours or even days to achieve a therapeutic drug level.

Topical drug calculations

- Use your own judgement in accordance with the doctor's general instructions.
- Follow specific guidelines for drugs prescribed for a systemic effect.

Rectal drug calculations

- Use the proportion method with ratios or fractions.
- A dose is typically prescribed to be provided in one suppository (occasionally two).

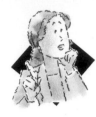

Quick quiz

1. Transdermal patches used to relieve chronic pain are effective for many hours due to:

    A. controlled absorption through the skin.
    B. an enhanced effect on local tissue.
    C. rapid then slow release of analgesics.
    D. sustained-release dosing.

Answer: A. These drugs are slowly released and absorbed through the skin over time.

2. A commonly used transdermal drug is:

    A. intraconazole.
    B. glyceryl trinitrate.
    C. levothyroxine.
    D. morphine sulphate.

Answer: B. Glyceryl trinitrate patches are used to prevent angina.

3. If a drug label reads *Stemetil (prochlorperazine) suppositories 5 mg, Castlemead, for rectal use only,* the drug's proprietary name is:

    A. Stemetil.
    B. prochlorperazine.
    C. Castlemead.
    D. suppositories.

Answer: A. The proprietary name, or trade name, usually appears first on a drug label, just before or above the generic name.

4. A patient is prescibed *Percutol Ointment 2.5 cm, t.i.d.* You should measure this dose:

    A. on a paper ruler applicator.
    B. by using your own judgement to approximate 2.5 cm of ointment.
    C. by holding a ruler to the patient's skin to measure the ointment.
    D. by dispensing it into a syringe.

Answer: A. Percutol Ointment comes with its own paper ruler. Squeeze the prescribed length of ointment onto the ruler and then use the ruler to apply the ointment to the patient's skin.

5. If a patient needs 500 mg of paracetamol by suppository, but all you have are 250-mg suppositories, you should insert:

    A. 1 suppository.
    B. 2 suppositories.
    C. 3 suppositories.
    D. 4 suppositories.

Answer: B. A simple calculation tells you that the patient needs 2 suppositories. However, because more than 1 suppository is needed, you should check your calculations, have another nurse do the same and then call the pharmacy to see if a 500-mg dose is available.

6. When an antibiotic ointment for a finger laceration has been prescribed, you should:

    A. ask the prescriber to state the amount to be applied.
    B. use a paper applicator to apply the ointment.
    C. use your own judgement about the amount of ointment to apply.
    D. call the pharmacist for the recommended amount of ointment to apply.

Answer: C. Unless the ointment has a systemic effect, the prescriber will usually leave the amount to apply up to you.

7. If a child needs 2.5 mg of prochlorperazine, and the package label reads *prochlorperazine suppositories 5 mg*, you should give:

    A. 2 suppositories.
    B. 1½ suppositories.
    C. 1 suppository.
    D. ½ suppository.

Answer: D. By setting up a proportion and solving for X, you'll find that the child needs ½ of a 5-mg suppository.

8. Your patient is receiving transdermal glyceryl trinitrate to treat angina. Which action is necessary when administering this drug?

    A. Remove the patch after 7 days.
    B. Remove the patch after 72 hours.
    C. Remove the patch after 12 to 14 hours.
    D. Remove the patch after 1 to 2 hours.

Answer: C. Transdermal glyceryl trinitrate should be removed after 12 to 14 hours to prevent the patient from developing a tolerance to the drug.

Scoring

☆☆☆ If you answered all eight items correctly, wow! You know your routes better than the RAC!

☆☆ If you answered six or seven items correctly, all right! You'll soon be top dog in topical drug administration.

☆ If you answered fewer than six items correctly, keep at it! You're absorbing information at an incredible rate.

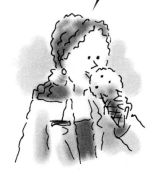

Another chapter bites the dust.... Let's see how well I can do with this ice cream cone!

Part V

Parenteral administration

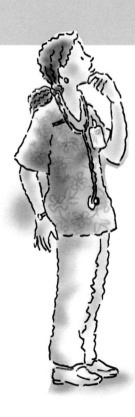

12 Calculating parenteral injections

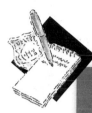

Just the facts

In this chapter, you'll learn:

♦ about calculating intradermal, subcutaneous and intramuscular injections
♦ about different types of syringe and needle
♦ how to interpret parenteral drug labels
♦ how to administer insulin and other unit-based drugs
♦ how to reconstitute powders.

A look at parenteral injections

Parenteral is a term that refers to 'outside the intestines'. Drugs may be administered parenterally through direct injection into the skin, subcutaneous tissue, muscle or vein. They may be supplied as liquids or as powders that require reconstitution. When using either form, you need to perform calculations to determine the amount of liquid medication to inject.

This chapter shows how to use the ratio or fraction and proportion method to calculate liquid parenteral dosages as well as how to reconstitute powdered drugs. Another parenteral drug administration route – I.V. infusion – is discussed in the next chapter. I.V. injections are discussed in Chapter 16, Calculating critical care dosages.

My point is…you gotta stay sharp and focused when giving parenteral drugs. (Just trying to *inject* a little humour into the situation!)

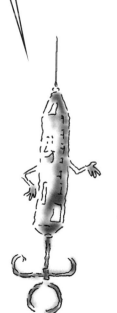

Types of injection

Parenteral drugs are administered by four types of injection:
* intradermal
* subcutaneous

- intramuscular (I.M.)
- intravenous (I.V.). (See Chapter 13, Calculating I.V. infusions.)
  Giving parenteral drugs safely depends on choosing the right type of injection for the patient's condition and the right syringe and needle for the type of injection.

Intradermal injections

In an intradermal injection, medication is injected into the dermis – the layer of skin beneath the epidermis, or the outermost layer of skin. This type of injection is used to anaesthetise the skin for invasive procedures and to test for allergies, tuberculosis, histoplasmosis and other diseases.

I've got you intra my skin

The volume of a drug that's given by intradermal injection is less than 0.5 ml. A 1-ml syringe, calibrated in 0.01-ml increments, is usually used, along with a 25- to 27-gauge (G) needle that's approximately 1 to 1.75 cm long.

To perform an intradermal injection, use this basic procedure:

Clean the skin thoroughly.

Stretch the skin taut with one hand.

With your other hand, insert the needle quickly at a 10- to 15-degree angle to a depth of about 0.5 cm.

Inject the drug. A small wheal forms where the drug is injected into the skin.

> Make sure that the patient's skin is good and clean!

Subcutaneous injections

In a subcutaneous injection, the drug is injected into the subcutaneous tissue, which is beneath the dermis and above the muscle. Drugs are absorbed faster in this layer than in the dermis because the subcutaneous layer has more capillaries. Insulin, heparin, tetanus toxoid and some opioid analgesics are injected through this route.

More than skin deep

Only 0.5 to 1 ml of a drug can be injected subcutaneously. The needles used for subcutaneous injections are 23 to 28G and approximately 1.25 to 1.75 cm long. Subcutaneous injection sites include the:
- lateral areas of the upper arms and thighs
- abdomen (above, below and lateral to the umbilicus)
- upper back.

To perform a subcutaneous injection, use this basic procedure:
• Choose the injection site.
• Clean the skin.
• If the patient is thin, pinch the skin between your index finger and thumb, and insert the needle at a 45-degree angle.
• If the patient is obese, insert the needle into the fatty tissue at a 90-degree angle.
• Aspirate for blood to make sure that the needle isn't in a vein (unless injecting insulin or heparin).
• Administer the injection.
• Massage the site after removing the needle; this may enhance absorption. Don't massage the site if you're giving heparin or insulin.

Intramuscular injections

An I.M. injection, which goes into a muscle, is used for drugs that need to be absorbed quickly, that are given in a large volume, or that irritate the tissues if given by a shallow route. The volume for these injections ranges from 0.5 to 3 ml. I.M. injection sites include the:
• dorsogluteal, ventral gluteal or vastus lateralis muscle (for 3-ml injections)
• rectus femoris or deltoid muscle (for injections of less than 3 ml).
  The choice of injection site depends on the patient's muscle mass and overlying tissue and the volume of the injection. The needles are approximately 2.5 to 7.5 cm long and are 18 to 23G in diameter.

The choice of I.M. injection site depends on the patient's muscle mass, among other things.

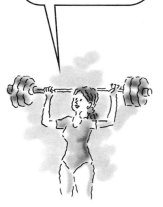

Use a little muscle

To administer an I.M. injection, use this basic procedure:
• Choose the injection site.
• Clean the skin.
• Using a quick, dart-like action, insert the needle at a 75- to 90-degree angle.
• Before injecting the drug, aspirate for blood to make sure that the needle isn't in a vein.
• Push the plunger and keep the syringe steady.
• After the drug is injected, pull the needle straight out and apply pressure to the site.

Syringes and needles

The many types of syringe and needle used to administer parenteral drugs are designed for specific purposes.

Types of syringe

To measure and administer parenteral drugs, three basic types of hypodermic syringe are used, including:

- standard syringes
- tuberculin syringes
- prefilled syringes.

Although these syringes are sometimes calibrated in cubic centimetres, the drugs they're used to measure are commonly prescribed in millilitres. (Recall that 1 cc equals 1 ml and that millilitres and cubic centimetres are used interchangeably.)

Standard syringes

Standard syringes are available in 1, 2, 3, 5, 10, 20, 30, 50 and 60 ml. Each syringe consists of a plunger, a barrel, a hub, a needle and dead space. The dead space holds fluid that remains in the syringe and needle after the plunger is completely depressed. Some syringes, such as insulin syringes, don't have dead space. (See *Anatomy of a syringe.*)

Marked for good measure

The calibration marks on syringes allow you to measure drug doses accurately. The 3-ml syringe, the most commonly used, is calibrated in tenths of a millilitre. It has large marks for every 0.5 ml on the right. The larger-volume syringes are calibrated in 2- to 10-ml increments.

Anatomy of a syringe

Standard syringes come in many different sizes, but each syringe has the same components. This illustration shows the parts of a standard syringe.

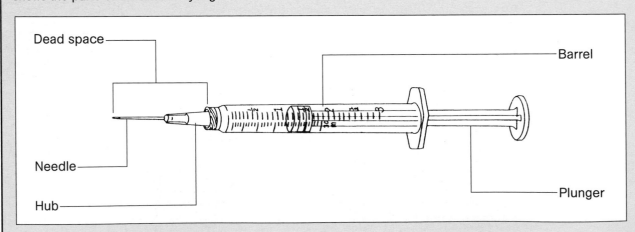

Dead space

Barrel

Needle

Hub

Plunger

To administer a drug, remember the five 'rights' of medication administration – right drug, right route, right dose, right time, right patient – and then follow these basic steps:
- Use aseptic technique.
- Calculate the dose.
- Draw the drug into the syringe.
- Pull the plunger back until the top ring of the plunger's black portion aligns with the correct calibration mark.
- Double-check the dose measurement.
- Administer the drug.

Double the fun (well, not exactly fun)

Parenteral drugs come in various dose strengths or concentrations so that the usual adult dose can be contained in 1 to 3 ml of solution. If a patient needs a dose larger than 3 ml, give it in two injections at two different sites to ensure proper drug absorption.

Tuberculin syringes

Tuberculin syringes are commonly used for intradermal injections and to administer small amounts of drugs, such as those given to paediatric patients or those on intensive care units. Each syringe is calibrated in hundredths of a millilitre, allowing you to administer doses as small as 0.25 ml accurately. Tuberculin syringes are also marked for alternate tenths of a millilitre: 0.2, 0.4, 0.6 and 0.8 ml. (See *Touring a tuberculin syringe*.)

Read the fine print

Measure drugs in a tuberculin syringe as you would those in a standard syringe. Take extra care when reading the dose, however, because the measurements on the tuberculin syringe are very small.

Prefilled syringes

A sterile syringe filled with a premeasured dose of drug is called a prefilled syringe. These syringes usually come with a cartridge-needle unit and require a special holder that enables the release of the drug from the cartridge. Each cartridge is calibrated in tenths of a millilitre and has larger marks for half and full millilitres. (See *Perusing a prefilled syringe*.)

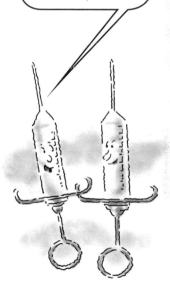

If a patient needs a dose larger than 3 ml, give it in two injections at different sites to ensure proper absorption

Touring a tuberculin syringe

A tuberculin syringe has the same components as a standard syringe. However, the size and calibration of the syringe are distinct. Because the measurements on the tuberculin syringe are so small, take extra care when reading the dose.

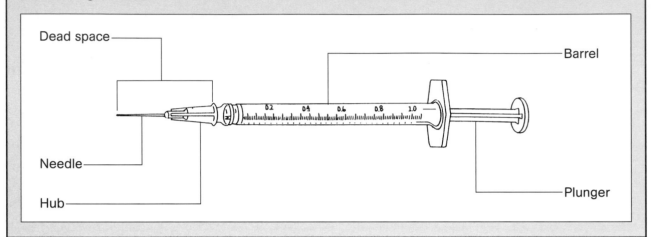

Dead space

Needle

Hub

Barrel

Plunger

First, the good news...

Prefilled syringes have many advantages over multiple-dose vials. They're labelled with the drug name and dose, so preparation time is reduced and so is the risk of drug errors. This labelling also makes it easier to record the amount of drug used and eliminates the need to figure out how much drug is left in a vial after you've given an injection.

The most obvious advantage of prefilled syringes is that you don't have to measure each drug dose. The manufacturer has already done this and placed the dose in the syringe. However, be aware that most manufacturers add a little extra drug to the syringe in case some is wasted when the syringe is purged of air.

...Now, the bad news

Unfortunately, prefilled syringes aren't available in all doses. When the prescribed dose doesn't match the amount in the prefilled syringe, you'll need to calculate the correct amount of drug needed.

Before giving the injection, discard the extra drug by expelling it from the syringe.

If you're using a prefilled syringe, be aware that most manufacturers add a little extra drug to the syringe in case some is wasted when purging the syringe of air.

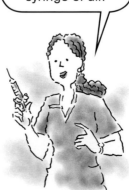

Perusing a prefilled syringe

This illustration shows the parts of a prefilled syringe. Note the holder on the right.

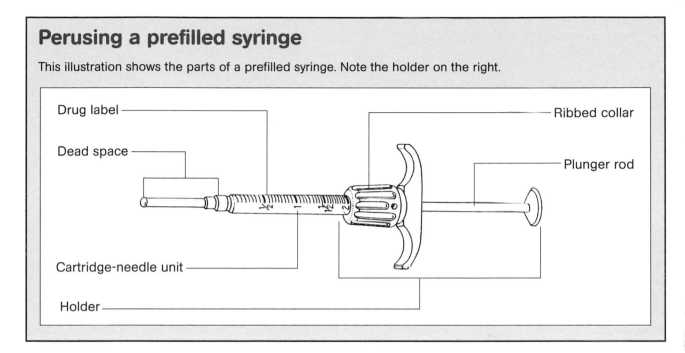

Drug label

Dead space

Cartridge-needle unit

Holder

Ribbed collar

Plunger rod

Closed-system devices

Another type of prefilled syringe – a closed-system device – comes with a needle and syringe in place and a separate prefilled drug chamber. Emergency drugs, such as atropine and lidocaine, may come in this type of prefilled syringe.

To prepare a closed-system device, hold the drug chamber in one hand and the syringe and needle in the other. Flip the protective caps off both ends. Insert the drug chamber into the syringe section. Then remove the needle cap and expel air and extra medication.

Types of needle

Five types of needle are used to inject drugs: intradermal, subcutaneous, I.M., I.V. and filter. Each type of needle is designed for a different purpose. (See *Choosing the right needle*.)

When choosing a needle, consider the gauge, bevel and length:
• Gauge refers to the inside diameter of the needle; the smaller the gauge, the larger the diameter. For example, a 14G needle has a larger diameter than a 25G needle.
• Bevel refers to the angle at which the needle tip is opened. The bevel may be short, medium or long.
• Length describes the distance from needle tip to needle hub. It ranges from approximately 1 to approximately 7.5 cm.

Choosing the right needle

When choosing a needle, consider its purpose as well as its gauge, bevel and length. Use this selection guide to choose the right needles for your patients.

Intradermal needles

Intradermal needles are approximately 1 to 1.75 cm long, usually have short bevels, and are 25 to 27G in diameter.

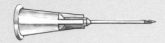

Subcutaneous needles

Subcutaneous needles are approximately 1.25 to 1.75 cm long, have medium bevels, and are 23 to 28G in diameter.

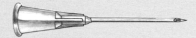

I.M. needles

I.M. needles are approximately 2.5 to 7.5 cm long, have medium bevels, and are 18 to 23G in diameter.

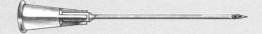

I.V. needle

I.V. needles are approximately 2.5 to 7.5 cm long, have long bevels, and are 14 to 25G in diameter.

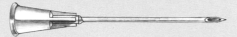

Filter needles

Filter needles are used for preparing a solution from a vial or ampoule and shouldn't be used for injections. They're approximately 3.75 cm long, have medium bevels, and are 20G in diameter.

Microscopic pieces of rubber or glass can enter the solution when you puncture the diaphragm of a vial with a needle or snap open an ampoule. You can use a filter needle with a screening device in the hub to remove minute particles of foreign material from a solution. Remember: after the medication is prepared, discard the filter needle!

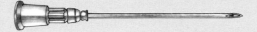

Real-world problems

The following examples show how to use the ratio or fraction and proportion method to calculate doses given by injection.

Prefilled painkiller problem

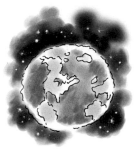

Your patient requires *40 mg of I.M. triamcinolone* for an inflammatory disorder. The drug is available in a 2-ml prefilled syringe containing 40 mg of triamcinolone. How many millilitres of triamcinolone should you discard?

This is how to solve this problem using fractions:

• Set up the first fraction using the known triamcinolone concentration, remembering the volume available is 2 ml:

$$\frac{80 \text{ mg}}{2 \text{ ml}}$$

- Set up the second fraction with the desired dose and the unknown amount of triamcinolone:

$$\frac{40 \text{ mg}}{X}$$

- Put these fractions into a proportion:

$$\frac{80 \text{ mg}}{2 \text{ ml}} = \frac{40 \text{ mg}}{X}$$

- Cross-multiply the fractions:

$$80 \text{ mg} \times X = 40 \text{ mg} \times 2 \text{ ml}$$

- Solve for X by dividing each side of the equation by 80 mg and cancelling units that appear in both the numerator and denominator:

$$\frac{80 \text{ mg} \times X}{80 \text{ mg}} = \frac{40 \text{ mg} \times 2 \text{ ml}}{80 \text{ mg}}$$

$$X = \frac{80 \text{ ml}}{80}$$

$$X = 1.0 \text{ ml}$$

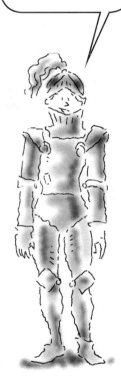

Divide and cancel. Sounds like a good plan!

- The amount of triamcinolone to give the patient is 1 ml. To calculate the amount to be wasted, subtract the prescribed dose from the entire contents of the syringe:

$$
\begin{array}{r}
2.0 \text{ ml} = 80 \text{ mg triamcinolone} \\
-1.0 \text{ ml} = 40 \text{ mg triamcinolone} \\
\hline
1.0 \text{ ml} = 40 \text{ mg triamcinolone}
\end{array}
$$

The amount of triamcinolone to be discarded is 1 ml.

Milligram mystery

A patient has been prescribed *100 mg methylprednisolone I.M. t.i.d.* for an asthmatic condition. The vial contains 125 mg/ml. How much drug should you give?

Here's how to solve this problem using ratios:
- Set up the first ratio with the known methylprednisolone concentration:

$$125 \text{ mg} : 1 \text{ ml}$$

- Set up the second ratio with the desired dose and the unknown amount of methylprednisolone:

$$100 \text{ mg} : X$$

- Put these ratios into a proportion:

$$125\,mg : 1\,ml :: 100\,mg : X$$

- Set up an equation by multiplying the means and extremes:

$$100\ mg \times 1\ ml = 125\ mg \times X$$

- Solve for X by dividing each side of the equation by 125 mg and cancelling units that appear in both the numerator and denominator:

$$\frac{100\ \cancel{mg} \times 1\ ml}{125\ \cancel{mg}} = \frac{\cancel{125\ mg} \times X}{\cancel{125\ mg}}$$

$$\frac{100\ ml}{125} = X$$

$$X = 0.8\ ml$$

You should give the patient 0.8 ml of methylprednisolone.

Vial trial

The doctor prescribes *100 mg of gentamicin I.M.* for your patient. The vial available contains 40 mg/ml. How much gentamicin should you give?

Here's how to solve this problem using ratios:

- Set up the first ratio with the known gentamicin concentration:

$$40\,mg : 1\,ml$$

- Set up the second ratio with the desired dose and the unknown amount of gentamicin:

$$100\,mg : X$$

Memory jogger

When you're working with ratios and proportions, the trick is to keep like units in the same position on both sides of the proportion:

$$120\,mg : 1\,ml :: 100\,mg : X\,ml$$

Remember to multiply the means and extremes:

means = **m**iddle numbers

extremes = **e**nd numbers.

Finally, isolate X to solve the problem:

Divide each side of the equation by the number you want to eliminate so that X is by itself, then cancel units that appear in both the numerator and denominator.

- Put these ratios into a proportion:

$$40\,mg : 1\,ml :: 100\,mg : X$$

- Set up an equation by multiplying the means and extremes:

$$1\,ml \times 100\,mg = 40\,mg \times X$$

- Solve for X by dividing each side of the equation by 40 mg and cancelling units that appear in both the numerator and denominator:

$$\frac{1\,ml \times 100\,\cancel{mg}}{40\,\cancel{mg}} = \frac{\cancel{40\,mg} \times X}{\cancel{40\,mg}}$$

$$\frac{100\,ml}{40} = X$$

$$X = 2.5\,ml$$

You should give the patient 2.5 ml of gentamicin.

Interpreting drug labels

Before you can safely administer a parenteral drug, you must know how to read its label. (See *A close look at a label*.) Parenteral drugs are packaged in glass ampoules, in single- or multiple-dose vials with rubber stoppers, and in prefilled syringes and cartridges. The packaging will state clearly that the drugs are used for injection.

Practising dosage calculations will make you look like you can do magic!

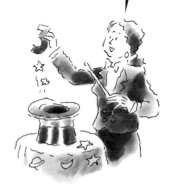

A close look at a label

The label below shows the information you need to know to safely administer a parenteral drug.

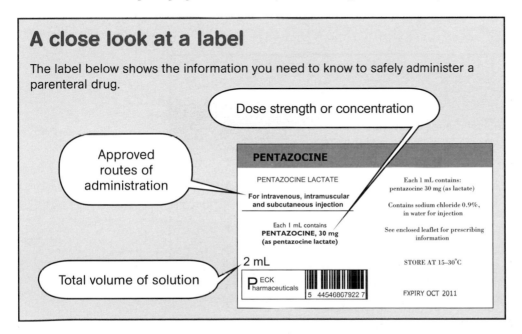

Dose strength or concentration

Approved routes of administration

Total volume of solution

PENTAZOCINE

PENTAZOCINE LACTATE

For intravenous, intramuscular and subcutaneous injection

Each 1 mL contains
PENTAZOCINE, 30 mg (as pentazocine lactate)

2 mL

Each 1 mL contains: pentazocine 30 mg (as lactate)

Contains sodium chloride 0.9%, in water for injection

See enclosed leaflet for prescribing information

STORE AT 15–30°C

EXPIRY OCT 2011

PECK Pharmaceuticals

5 44546807922 7

Looking at labels

Reading the label of a parenteral solution is a lot like reading an oral solution label. Here's the information you'll see:

- trade name
- generic name
- total volume of solution in the container
- dose strength or concentration (drug dose present in a volume of solution)
- approved routes of administration
- expiration date
- special instructions, as needed.

Solution components

A *solute* is a liquid or solid form of a drug. A *solution* is a liquid that contains a solute dissolved in a *diluent* or *solvent*, most commonly sterile water for parenteral injections. Normal saline solution is a solution of salt (the solute) in purified water (the solvent).

Solution strengths

Solutions come in different strengths, which are expressed on the drug label as percentage solutions or ratio solutions. (See *Interpreting percentage solutions*.)

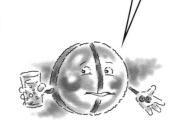

Here's the problem…how to fit a large pill like me into this tiny glass of sterile water…I hope the solution presents itself quickly!

Interpreting percentage solutions

You can determine the contents of a weight per volume (W/V) or volume per volume (V/V) percentage solution by reading the label, as shown here.

What the label says	What the solution contains
0.9% (W/V) NaCl	0.9 g of sodium chloride in 100 ml of finished solution
5% (W/V) boric acid solution	5 g of boric acid in 100 ml of finished solution
5% (W/V) glucose	5 g of glucose in 100 ml of finished solution
2% (V/V) hydrogen peroxide	2 ml of hydrogen peroxide in 100 ml of finished solution
70% (V/V) isopropyl alcohol	70 ml of isopropyl alcohol in 100 ml of finished solution
10% (V/V) glycerol	10 ml of glycerol in 100 ml of finished solution

Percentage solutions: always part of 100

A clear way to label or describe a solution is as a percentage. Providing information in percentages makes it easy to make dosage calculations, dilutions or alterations.

On the label, a solution may be expressed either as weight per volume (W/V) or volume per volume (V/V).

In a W/V solution, the percentage or strength refers to the number of grams (the weight) of solute per 100 ml (the volume) of finished, or reconstituted, solution. With a V/V solution, the percentage refers to the number of millilitres of solute per 100 ml of finished solution.

Here's how to express these two relationships mathematically:

$$\% = \frac{\text{weight}}{\text{volume}} \text{ grams solute/100 ml finished solution}$$

$$\% = \frac{\text{volume}}{\text{volume}} \text{ milliliters solute/100 ml finished solution}$$

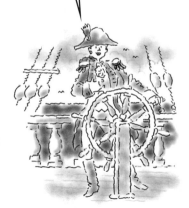

Remember, me hearties, in a ratio solution, the colon separates the amount of drug (the first number) from the finished solution (the second number, always expressed in millilitres).

Horatio ratio solutions: parts one and two

Another way to label or describe a solution is as a ratio. (See *Interpreting ratio solutions*.) The strength of a ratio solution is usually expressed as two numbers separated by a colon. In a weight per volume (W:V) solution, the first number signifies the amount of a drug in grams. In a volume per volume (V:V) solution, the first number signifies the amount of drug in millilitres; the second signifies the volume of finished solution in millilitres.

This relationship is expressed as:

$$\text{ratio} = \text{amount of drug : amount of finished solution}$$

Interpreting ratio solutions

You can determine the contents of a weight per volume (W:V) or volume per volume (V:V) ratio solution from the label, as shown here.

What the label says	What the solution contains
benzalkonium chloride 1 : 750 (W:V)	1 g of benzalkonium chloride in 750 ml of finished solution
silver nitrate 1 : 100 (W:V)	1 g of silver nitrate in 100 ml of finished solution
hydrogen peroxide 2 : 100 (V:V)	2 ml of hydrogen peroxide in 100 ml of finished solution
glycerol 10 : 100 (V:V)	10 ml of glycerol in 100 ml of finished solution

Insulin and unit-based drugs

Some drugs, such as heparin, insulin and benzylpenicillin, are measured in units. The unit system is based on an international standard of drug potency, not on weight. The number of units appears on the drug label. (See *Look for the unit label*.)

Insisting on insulin

The body needs insulin – a potent hormone produced by the pancreas – to regulate carbohydrate metabolism. The effect of insulin's activity is reflected in blood glucose levels. A lack of insulin or insulin resistance causes diabetes. (See *Differentiating diabetes*.)

There are approximately 2 million patients with diabetes in the UK. Chances are, at some point, you'll need to give an insulin injection or to teach a patient how to self-administer their medication.

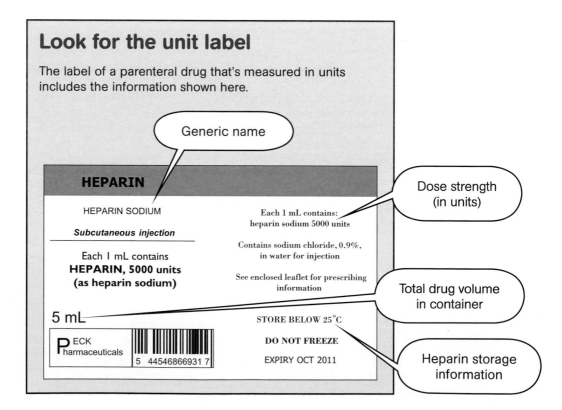

Look for the unit label

The label of a parenteral drug that's measured in units includes the information shown here.

Generic name

HEPARIN

HEPARIN SODIUM

Subcutaneous injection

Each 1 mL contains
**HEPARIN, 5000 units
(as heparin sodium)**

5 mL

Each 1 mL contains:
heparin sodium 5000 units

Contains sodium chloride, 0.9%,
in water for injection

See enclosed leaflet for prescribing
information

STORE BELOW 25°C

DO NOT FREEZE

EXPIRY OCT 2011

P ECK
Pharmaceuticals

5 44546866931 7

Dose strength
(in units)

Total drug volume
in container

Heparin storage
information

Differentiating diabetes

Diabetes is classified according to two major types: type 1 and type 2.

Type 1

In type 1 diabetes (also known as juvenile or insulin-dependent diabetes), the pancreas makes little or no insulin. Patients are typically diagnosed before age 20 and require long-term insulin therapy.

Type 2

In type 2 diabetes, the pancreas produces some insulin, but it's either too little or ineffective. This type of diabetes (also known as adult-onset or non-insulin-dependent diabetes) commonly affects patients older than age 40, although the incidence among children is rising. Type 2 diabetes can be controlled by diet and oral anti-diabetic agents; however, insulin may be needed to stabilise blood glucose levels.

Before you give that drug!

Heparin hazards

Heparin comes in many concentrations. Make sure that the heparin concentration is appropriate for the intended use.

Dosage calculation errors with heparin can cause excessive bleeding or under-treatment of a clotting disorder.

Insulin is injected subcutaneously in patients with chronic diabetes or I.V. in patients with acute diabetic ketoacidosis. You must calculate and administer insulin doses carefully because even a small error can cause a hypoglycaemic or hyperglycaemic reaction.

Hip to heparin

The anticoagulant heparin is used in moderate doses to prevent thrombosis and embolism, and in large doses to treat these disorders. Like insulin, it requires careful calculation and administration to prevent complications. (See *Heparin hazards*.)

Types of insulin

Several types of insulin are available. The prescriber chooses a particular type based on the patient's diet and activity level and disease severity.

Deducing the derivation

Insulin is classified according to its origin (human or animal) and action time. Some insulins are derived from porcine pancreas and differ from human insulin by only two amino acids. Others are identical to human insulin and are produced by enzymic conversion

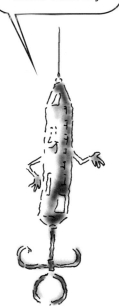

Remember to read insulin labels carefully

Insulin action times

Insulin preparations are modified through combination with larger insoluble protein molecules to slow absorption and prolong activity. An insulin preparation may be rapid-acting, intermediate-acting or long-acting, as shown in the table below.

Drug	Route	Onset	Peak	Duration
Rapid-acting				
regular insulin	I.V.	½ hour	2 to 4 hours	6 to 8 hours
lispro insulin	subcutaneous	<½ hour	½ to 1½ hours	<6 hours
Intermediate-acting				
insulin zinc suspension	subcutaneous	1 to 3 hours	6 to 15 hours	18 to 24 hours
isophane insulin suspension (NPH)	subcutaneous	1 to 2 hours	4 to 12 hours	18 to 24 hours
isophane 70%, regular insulin 30%	subcutaneous	½ hour	2 to 12 hours	24 hours
isophane 50%, regular insulin 50%	subcutaneous	½ hour	4 to 8 hours	24 hours
Long-acting				
extended insulin zinc suspension	subcutaneous	4 to 6 hours	10 to 30 hours	24 to 36 hours
insulin glargine	subcutaneous	1 hour	None	24 hours

of porcine insulin or by recombinant deoxyribonucleic acid (DNA) techniques. The origin appears on the drug label.

Each in its own time

Insulin preparations are modified by combination with larger, insoluble protein molecules to slow absorption and prolong activity. Thus, the different types of insulin vary in pharmacokinetic properties (See *Insulin action times*.)

What dose do U want?

Insulin doses, expressed in units, are available in two concentrations. U-100 insulin, which contains 100 units of insulin per millilitre, is called universal because it's the most common concentration. U-500 insulin, which contains 500 units/ml, is used on rare occasions when a patient needs an unusually large dose.

Selecting an insulin syringe

These syringes are examples of the different dose-specific insulin syringes that are available. The 1-ml U-100 syringe delivers up to 100 units of insulin. The low-dose 0.3- and 0.5-ml syringes deliver up to 30 or 50 units of U-100 insulin.

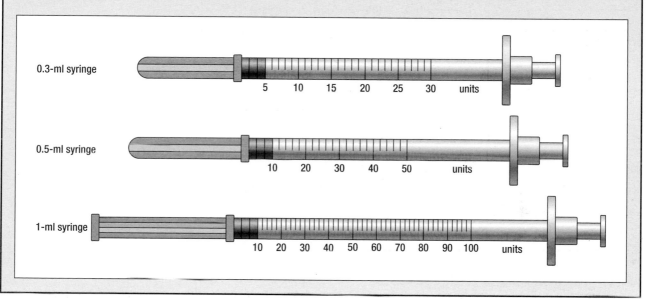

Insulin syringes

A U-100 syringe – the only type of insulin syringe available in the UK – is calibrated so that 1 ml holds 100 units of insulin. A low-dose U-100 syringe, holding 50 units of insulin or less, is also used for some patients. Another low-dose U-100 syringe holds 30 units of insulin or less.

Because no syringes are made for it, U-500 insulin must also be administered with a U-100 syringe. Therefore, exercise caution when administering this drug. (See *Selecting an insulin syringe*.)

Reading insulin prescriptions

Sometimes insulin doses are based on home monitoring of the patient's blood glucose values with glucometers. When a diagnosis of diabetes is first made, however, the patient undergoes tests to determine blood and urine glucose levels. Usually, the patient is enrolled in an outpatient centre where they can be educated about diet, exercise, monitoring blood glucose levels and insulin administration. Blood and urine glucose baselines are established.

Based on these determinations, small doses of rapid-acting insulin may be prescribed for administration at set times, such as every 4 hours or before meals and at bedtime, for several days. After a stable 24-hour dosage has been determined, dosage adjustments may be prescribed, such as one or two daily doses of intermediate-acting insulin, possibly accompanied by small doses of rapid-acting insulin. (See *Insulin action times*.)

Insulin on a sliding scale

For a newly diagnosed, ill or unstable diabetic patient, a prescription may be written on a sliding scale. This type of prescription individualises the insulin doses and administration times according to the patient's age, activity level, work habits, desired degree of blood glucose level control and response to insulin preparations.

This is an example of such a prescription:

Start regular insulin sliding scale:

Blood glucose value:	*Insulin dose:*
<10 mmol/l	*No insulin*
10.1 to 15 mmol/l	*10 units regular insulin subcutaneously*
15.1 to 20 mmol/l	*20 units regular insulin subcutaneously*
>20 mmol/l	*Call the prescriber for medical directions.*

Making connections with the dots

When reading insulin prescriptions, check closely for decimal points that indicate unusual doses.

If a prescription doesn't include the dose strength, then administer U-100 insulin, the universal strength. If U-500 insulin is needed, the prescriber will specify this on the prescription.

Combining insulins

Sometimes a prescription may be given for regular insulin mixed with isophane insulin to be injected together at the same site. When you receive an prescription for these drugs, draw them into the same syringe, following this procedure:

• Read the insulin prescription carefully.
• Read the vial labels carefully, noting the type, concentration, source and expiration date of the drugs.
• Roll the NPH vial between your palms to mix it thoroughly.
• Choose the appropriate syringe.
• Clean the tops of both vials of insulin with alcohol swabs.
• Inject air into the NPH vial equal to the amount of insulin you need to give. Withdraw the needle and syringe, but don't withdraw any NPH insulin.

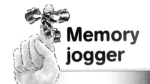

Memory jogger

If you have trouble remembering which insulin to draw first, think of the phrase 'clear before cloudy'. (Who doesn't prefer a clear day to a cloudy day?)

This phrase also reminds you how these drugs work: a clear day seems short, but a cloudy day seems to go on forever. Clear, regular insulin is short-acting and cloudy, insulin glargine is long-acting.

- Inject into the regular insulin vial an amount of air equal to the dose of the regular insulin. Then invert or tilt the vial and withdraw the prescribed amount of regular insulin into the syringe. Draw the clear, regular insulin first to avoid contamination by the cloudy, longer-acting insulin.
- Clean the top of the NPH vial again. Then insert the needle of the syringe containing the regular insulin into the vial, and withdraw the prescribed amount of NPH insulin.
- Mix the insulins in the syringe by pulling back slightly on the plunger and tilting the syringe back and forth.
- Recheck the drug prescription.
- Have a second nurse verify the withdrawn dose and co-sign the medication administration record.
- Administer the insulin immediately.

More real-world problems

Before drawing up and administering insulin, heparin or other drugs measured in units, check all your calculations for accuracy. The following examples show how to use the proportion method and a sliding scale to calculate insulin and heparin doses.

Help! How much heparin?

A patient has been prescribed *7000 units of heparin, subcutaneously, b.i.d.* The heparin you have available contains 10 000 units/ml. How many millilitres of heparin should you give?

This is the calculation using ratios:

- Set up the first ratio with the known heparin concentration:

$$10\,000\,\text{units} : 1\,\text{ml}$$

- Set up the second ratio with the desired dose and the unknown amount of heparin:

$$7000\,\text{units} : X$$

- Put these ratios into a proportion:

$$10\,000\,\text{units} : 1\,\text{ml} :: 7000\,\text{units} : X$$

- Set up an equation by multiplying the means and extremes:

$$1\,\text{ml} \times 7000\,\text{units} = 10\,000\,\text{units} \times X$$

- Solve for X by dividing each side of the equation by 10 000 units and cancelling units that appear in both the numerator and denominator:

$$\frac{1 \text{ ml} \times 7000 \text{ units}}{10\ 000 \text{ units}} = \frac{10\ 000 \text{ units} \times X}{10\ 000 \text{ units}}$$

$$X = 0.7 \text{ ml}$$

You should give the patient 0.7 ml of heparin.

U-nsure about insulin?

The nurse prescriber has determined that your patient requires *20 units of U-100 neutral insulin*. The only syringe on hand is a 1-ml tuberculin syringe. How many millilitres should you administer?

This is the calculation using fractions:

- Set up the first fraction with the known insulin concentrations:

$$\frac{100 \text{ units}}{1 \text{ ml}}$$

- Set up the second fraction with the unknown amount of insulin in millilitres and the desired dose:

$$\frac{20 \text{ units}}{X}$$

- Put these fractions into a proportion:

$$\frac{100 \text{ units}}{1 \text{ ml}} = \frac{20 \text{ units}}{X}$$

- Cross-multiply the fractions:

$$100 \text{ units} \times X = 20 \text{ units} \times 1 \text{ ml}$$

- Solve for X by dividing each side of the equation by 100 units and cancelling units that appear in both the numerator and denominator:

$$\frac{100 \text{ units} \times X}{100 \text{ units}} = \frac{20 \text{ units} \times 1 \text{ ml}}{100 \text{ units}}$$

$$X = 0.2 \text{ ml}$$

You should give the patient 0.2 ml of regular insulin.

Insulin sliding scale

Insulin doses may be based on blood glucose levels, as shown in this table.

Blood glucose level	Insulin dose
< 10 mmol/l	No insulin
10.1 to 12.5 mmol/l	2 units regular insulin
12.6 to 15 mmol/l	4 units regular insulin
15.1 to 17.5 mmol/l	6 units regular insulin
17.6 to 20 mmol/l	8 units regular insulin
20.1 to 22.5 mmol/l	10 units regular insulin
> 22.5 mol/l	Call prescriber for instructions.

Insulin on a sliding scale

Your patient's blood glucose is 18.3 mmol/l. Based on the sliding scale above, how much insulin should you give him? (See *Insulin sliding scale*.)

You should administer 8 units of regular insulin.

Reconstituting powders

Some drugs – such as levothyroxine sodium and penicillins – are manufactured and packaged as powders because they become unstable quickly when they're in solution. When such a drug is prescribed, either you or the pharmacist must reconstitute it before it can be administered.

The strength of one or many

Powders come in single-strength or multiple-strength formulations. A single-strength powder – such as levothyroxine sodium – may be reconstituted to only one dose strength per administration route, as specified by the manufacturer. A multiple-strength powder – such as penicillin – can be reconstituted to various dose strengths by adjusting the amounts of diluent.

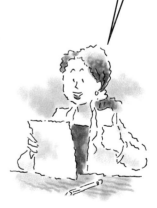

Another dosage calculation under my belt!

When reconstituting a multiple-strength powder, check the drug label or package insert for the dose-strength options and choose the one that's closest to the prescribed dose.

How to reconstitute

Follow the general guidelines described here when reconstituting a powder for injection.

Learn from the label

Begin by checking the label of the powder container. The label tells you the quantity of drug in a vial or ampoule, the amount and type of diluent to add to the powder, and the strength and expiration date of the resulting solution.

Fluid out exceeds fluid in

When a diluent is added to a powder, the fluid volume increases. That's why the label calls for less diluent than the total volume of the prepared solution. For example, the instructions may say to add 1.7 ml of diluent to a vial of powdered drug to obtain 2 ml of prepared solution.

Check out the chambers

Some drugs that need reconstitution are packaged in vials with two chambers separated by a rubber stopper. The upper chamber contains the diluent, and the lower chamber contains the powdered drug. (See *Two chambers (one's a powder room!)*.)

When you depress the top of the vial, the stopper dislodges, allowing the diluent to flow into the lower chamber, where it can mix with the powdered drug. Then you can remove the correct amount of solution with a syringe.

Say it with an equation

To determine how much solution to give, refer to the drug label for information about the dose strength of the prepared solution. For example, to give 500 mg of a drug when the dose strength of the solution is 1 g (or 1000 mg)/10 ml, set up a proportion with fractions as follows:

$$\frac{X}{500 \text{ mg}} = \frac{10 \text{ ml}}{1000 \text{ mg}}$$

Two chambers (one's a powder room!)

Some drugs that require reconstitution are packaged in vials with two chambers separated by a rubber stopper. In the illustration below, note that the upper chamber contains the diluent and the lower chamber contains the powder. The plunger is depressed to inject the diluent into the powder.

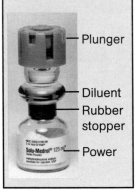

- Plunger
- Diluent
- Rubber stopper
- Power

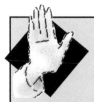

Before you give that drug!

Inspect the insert

The package inserts that are included with drugs commonly provide a great deal of information that may not be on the outer label. For example, the drug label for ceftazidime provides no information about reconstitution, but the package insert does. These are the possible diluent combinations as they appear in the package insert that comes with this drug.

Vial size	Diluent to be added	Approximate available	Approximate average concentration
I.M. or I.V. direct (bolus) injection			
1 g	3 ml	3.6 ml	280 mg/ml
I.V. infusion			
1 g	10 ml	10.6 ml	95 mg/ml
2 g	10 ml	11.2 ml	180 mg/ml

If information about a drug's dose strength isn't on the label, check the package insert. The label or insert will also list the type and amount of diluent needed, the dose strength after reconstitution and special instructions about administration and storage after reconstitution. (See *Inspect the insert*.)

Special considerations

When you reconstitute a powder that comes in multiple strengths, be especially careful in choosing the most appropriate strength for the prescribed dose.

Label logic

After you have reconstituted a drug, make sure you label it with the following information:
• your initials
• reconstitution date
• expiration date
• dose strength.

Yet more real-world problems

The following problems show how to calculate the amount of reconstituted drug to give a patient.

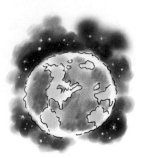

Penicillin puzzler (the solution is in the solution)

The doctor prescribes *100 000 units of penicillin* for your patient, but the only available vial holds 1 million units. The drug label says to add 4.5 ml of normal saline solution to yield 1 million units/5 ml. How much solution should you administer after reconstitution?

Here's how to solve this problem using fractions:

• First, dilute the powder according to the instructions on the label. Then set up the first fraction with the known penicillin concentration:

$$\frac{1\ 000\ 000\ units}{5ml}$$

• Set up the second fraction with the desired dose and the unknown amount of solution:

$$\frac{100\ 000\ units}{X}$$

• Put these fractions into a proportion:

$$\frac{1\ 000\ 000\ units}{5ml} = \frac{100\ 000\ units}{X}$$

• Cross-multiply the fractions:

$$5\ ml \times 100\ 000\ units = X \times 1\ 000\ 000\ units$$

• Solve for X by dividing each side of the equation by 1 million units and cancelling units that appear in both the numerator and denominator:

$$\frac{5\ ml \times 100\ 000\ \cancel{units}}{1\ 000\ 000\ \cancel{units}} = \frac{X \times \cancel{1\ 000\ 000\ units}}{\cancel{1\ 000\ 000\ units}}$$

$$X = \frac{500\ 000\ ml}{1\ 000\ 000}$$

$$X = 0.5\ ml$$

The amount of solution that yields 100 000 units of penicillin after reconstitution is 0.5 ml.

Deciphering diluents

Your patient needs *25 mg of gentamicin I.M.* The label says to add 1.3 ml of sterile diluent to yield 50 mg/1.5 ml. How many millilitres of reconstituted solution should you give the patient?

Here's how to solve this problem using ratios:
- First, dilute the powder according to the label instructions. Then set up the first ratio with the known gentamicin concentration:

$$50\,mg : 1.5\,ml$$

- Set up the second ratio with the desired dose and the unknown amount of solution:

$$25\,mg : X$$

- Put these ratios into a proportion:

$$50\,mg : 1.5\,ml :: 25\,mg : X$$

- Set up an equation by multiplying the means and extremes:

$$1.5\,ml \times 25\,mg = X \times 50\,mg$$

- Solve for X. Divide each side of the equation by 50 mg and cancel units that appear in both the numerator and denominator:

$$\frac{1.5\,ml \times 25\,\cancel{mg}}{50\,\cancel{mg}} = \frac{X \times 50\,\cancel{mg}}{50\,\cancel{mg}}$$

$$X = \frac{37.5\,ml}{50}$$

$$X = 0.75\,ml$$

The patient should receive 0.75 ml of the solution.

Attaining the ampicillin answer

Your patient has been prescribed *500 mg ampicillin.* A 1-g vial of powdered ampicillin is available. The label says to add 4.5 ml sterile water to yield 1 g/5 ml. How many millilitres of reconstituted ampicillin should you give?

Here's how to solve this problem using fractions:
- First, dilute the powder according to the instructions on the label. Then set up the first fraction with the known ampicillin concentration (recall that 1 g equals 1000 mg):

$$\frac{1000\,mg}{5\,ml}$$

- Set up the second fraction with the desired dose and the unknown amount of solution:

$$\frac{500\,mg}{X}$$

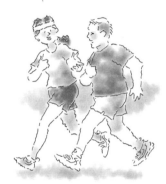

But Dr. Walker, I thought you said it was time for a constitutional, not time to reconstitute it all in a solution!

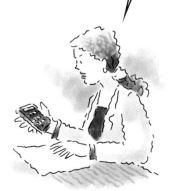

Dilute and then compute. Here we go!

- Put these fractions into a proportion, making sure the same units of measure appear in both numerators. In this case, the units must be grams or milligrams. If you use milligrams, the proportion would be:

$$\frac{1000 \text{ mg}}{5 \text{ml}} = \frac{500 \text{ units}}{X}$$

- Cross-multiply the fractions:

$$1000 \text{ mg} \times X = 500 \text{ mg} \times 5 \text{ ml}$$

- Solve for X by dividing each side of the equation by 1000 mg and cancelling units that appear in both the numerator and denominator:

$$\frac{\cancel{1000 \text{ mg}} \times X}{\cancel{1000 \text{ mg}}} = \frac{500 \cancel{\text{mg}} \times 5 \text{ ml}}{1000 \cancel{\text{mg}}}$$

$$X = \frac{2500 \text{ ml}}{1000}$$

$$X = 2.5 \text{ ml}$$

You should give the patient 2.5 ml of the solution, which will deliver 500 mg of ampicillin.

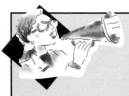

That's a wrap!

Calculating parenteral injections review

Keep these important points in mind when giving parenteral injections.

Intradermal injections

- This route is used to anaesthetise the skin for invasive procedures and to test for allergies, tuberculosis, histoplasmosis and other diseases.
- Amount of drug injected is <0.5 ml.
- Syringe and needle are a 1-ml syringe with a 25 to 27G needle that's approximately 1.25 to 3.75 cm long.

Subcutaneous injections

- Drugs commonly given subcutaneously include insulin, heparin, tetanus toxoid and some opioids.
- Amount of drug injected is 0.5 to 1 ml.
- Needle is 23 to 28G and approximately 1.25 to 1.75 cm long.
- When injecting insulin or heparin, don't aspirate for blood and don't massage the site.

Calculating parenteral injections review *(continued)*

I.M. injections

- This route is used for drugs that require quick absorption or those that are irritating to tissue.
- Amount of drug injected is 0.5 to 3 ml.
- Needles are 18 to 23G and approximately 2.5 to 7.5 cm long.
- Before injection, aspirate for blood to make sure that the needle isn't in a vein.

Syringe types

- Standard syringes come in a variety of sizes (1, 2, 3, 5, 10, 20, 30, 50 and 60 ml).
- Tuberculin syringes (commonly used for intradermal injections) are 1-ml syringes marked to hundredths of a millilitre, allowing for accurate measurement of very small doses.
- Prefilled syringes – sterile syringes that contain a premeasured drug dose – require a special holder to release the drug from the cartridge.

Needle terminology

- Gauge: inside the diameter of the needle (the smaller the gauge, the larger the diameter)
- Bevel: angle at which the needle tip is open (may be short, medium or long)
- Length: distance from needle tip to hub: ranges from approximately 1 to approximately 7.5 cm

Important parts of a parenteral drug label

- Trade name
- Generic name
- Total volume of solution in the container
- Dose strength or concentration
- Approved routes of administration
- Expiration date
- Special instructions

Ratio solutions

- Solute is a drug in liquid or solid form that's added to a solvent (diluent) to make a solution.
- Solution is a liquid (usually sterile water) containing a dissolved solute.
- W:V solution: the first number represents the amount of drug in grams; the second number is the volume of finished solution in millilitres.
- V:V solution: the first number is the amount of drug in millilitres; the second number is the volume of finished solution in millilitres.

Insulin doses

- Measured in units
- Based on drug potency (not weight)
- Classified by origin (human or animal) and action time
- Most common (universal) concentration is U-100 insulin

Insulin action times

- Rapid-acting: regular, lispro
- Intermediate-acting: insuilin zinc suspension; NPH; isophane 70%/regular 30%; isophane 50%/regular 50%
- Long-acting: extended insulin zinc suspension, insulin glargine

Powders for reconstitution

- The fluid volume increases with the added diluent.
- Single-strength powders are reconstituted to one dose strength per administration route.
- Multiple-strength powders are reconstituted to appropriate strengths by adjusting the amount of diluent.

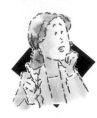

Quick quiz

1. To administer the medication in a prefilled syringe, you need:
   A. a specialised syringe system.
   B. a standard syringe.
   C. dead space.
   D. a tuberculin syringe.

Answer: A. Prefilled syringes come with a cartridge-needle unit and require a special holder to release the drug from the cartridge.

2. You need to purge a prefilled syringe before administering a drug because:
   A. the cartridge won't work otherwise.
   B. the syringe may contain air.
   C. doing so ensures needle patency.
   D. doing so ensures more accurate dosing.

Answer: B. You must purge the air from a prefilled syringe. Because a small amount of drug is wasted during purging, most manufacturers add a little extra drug to prefilled syringes.

3. The only insulin that can be given intravenously is:
   A. NPH.
   B. insulin zinc suspension.
   C. lispro.
   D. regular.

Answer: D. Regular insulin can be given intravenously. NPH, insulin zinc suspension and lispro insulin must be given subcutaneously.

4. The longest-acting insulin is:
   A. regular.
   B. insulin zinc suspension.
   C. extended insulin zinc suspension.
   D. NPH.

Answer: C. Extended insulin zinc insulin has a duration of 36 hours. Regular insulin lasts 6 to 8 hours, insulin zinc suspension lasts 18 to 24 hours, and NPH insulin lasts 18 to 24 hours.

5. The needle used for an intradermal injection is:
    A.   25 to 27G and approximately 1 to 1.75 cm long.
    B.   14 to 18G and approximately 2.5 to 3.75 cm long.
    C.   22G and approximately 2 cm long.
    D.   18 to 23G and approximately 2.5 to 7.5 cm long.

Answer: A. A 1-ml syringe, calibrated in 0.01-ml increments, is usually used with this needle for an intradermal injection.

6. In a subcutaneous injection, the drug is injected into the:
    A.   muscle.
    B.   tissue in the vastus lateralis.
    C.   tissue above the dermis.
    D.   tissue below the dermis.

Answer: D. A subcutaneous injection delivers the drug into the subcutaneous tissue, located below the dermis but above the muscle.

7. A percentage solution can be expressed in terms of:
    A.   weight/volume and volume/volume.
    B.   weight/weight and volume/volume.
    C.   weight/weight and strength/volume.
    D.   grams/weight and millilitres/volume.

Answer: A. Percentage solutions are expressed as weight/volume or volume/volume. These are the clearest and most common ways to label or describe solutions.

8. When a diluent is added to a powder for injection, the fluid volume:
    A.   increases.
    B.   decreases.
    C.   stays the same.
    D.   always doubles.

Answer: A. When a diluent is added to a powder, the fluid volume increases. That's why the label calls for less diluent than the total volume of the prepared solution.

9. If information about a drug's dose strength isn't on the label:
    A.   call the prescriber.
    B.   check the package insert.
    C.   mix it with 5 ml of normal saline solution.
    D.   ask your supervisor.

Answer: B. The package insert includes information about the drug's dose strength, the amount of diluent needed, the dose strength after reconstitution and any special instructions.

Scoring

☆☆☆ If you answered all nine items correctly, bravo! You've earned the right to say to anyone, 'This won't hurt a bit'.

☆☆ If you answered six to eight items correctly, you're almost a parenteral powerhouse!

☆ If you answered fewer than six items correctly, okay! Remember the golden rule of dosage calculations: keep things in proportion.

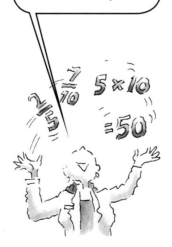

Wait until you see the dosage calculation feats you'll be able to accomplish after the next chapter!

⓵⓷ Calculating I.V. infusions

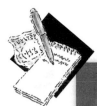

Just the facts

In this chapter, you'll learn:

♦ formulas for calculating drip rates and flow rates

♦ how to regulate an infusion manually and electronically

♦ how to calculate infusion time

♦ ways to calculate, monitor and regulate infusions of blood, total parenteral nutrition, heparin, insulin and electrolytes.

A look at I.V. infusions

Careful administration of I.V. fluids is critical, especially when dealing with patients who are susceptible to fluid volume changes. Rapid infusion of I.V. fluids or blood products may seriously threaten your patient's health.

Work from the outside in

To administer I.V. fluids safely, you need information specifying how much fluid to give, the correct length of time for administration, the type of fluid and what may be added to the fluid. Start by examining the outside of a full I.V. bag and learn to identify all its components. (See *Read the bag*.)

Next, you'll need to be able to select the proper tubing, calculate drip rates and flow rates, and become comfortable working with I.V. equipment such as electronic infusion devices. (See *Checking an I.V.*)

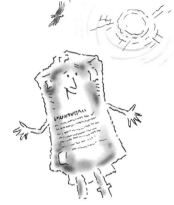

Getting to know me, getting to know all about me... (and my components!)

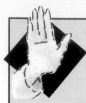

Before you give that drug!

Read the bag

The outside of an I.V. bag is an important source of information for calculating infusion rates and times. Read it carefully!

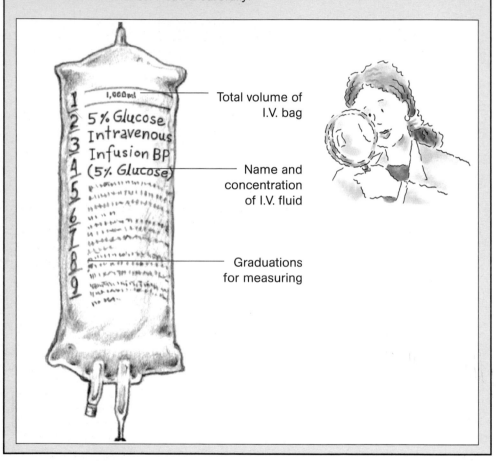

Total volume of I.V. bag

Name and concentration of I.V. fluid

Graduations for measuring

Administering I.V. fluids

To safely and accurately administer I.V. fluids to your patient, you must select the proper tubing. Selection of I.V. tubing plays an important role in calculating I.V. infusion rates.

Advice from the experts
Checking an I.V.

You can save time by assessing your patient's I.V. infusion at the beginning of every shift. Performing checks early on helps to avoid confusion when your ward gets busy.

- Are the time, volume and rate labelled correctly? If so, do they match the prescription?
- Check maintenance fluids and drug infusions, such as insulin, dopamine and morphine. Are the additives correct? Are they in the right solutions?
- After calculating the drug dosage, check the bag again to verify that the solution is labelled with the time, name and amount of drug added.
- If an electronic infusion device is being used, is it set correctly?
- Examine the tubing from the bag down to the patient to see whether the drug is infusing into the correct I.V. port. This is critical when a patient has multiple lines.

Most facilities stock I.V. tubing in two sizes: microdrip and macrodrip. Microdrip tubing, as its name implies, delivers smaller drops than macrodrip. Microdrip also delivers more drops per minute.

Targeting the right tube

To decide the right size of tubing for your patient, you should first understand the purpose of the infusion and the desired infusion rate. If the infusion rate for a solution is relatively fast – for example, 125 ml/hour – select macrodrip tubing. If the infusion rate is relatively slow – for example, 40 ml/hour – select microdrip tubing. If you use macrodrip tubing for a slow infusion, maintaining accurate I.V. flow may be difficult if not impossible. (See *Tube tips*.)

Calculating drip rates

Your next step is to determine the number of drops of solution you want to infuse per minute. In other words, you want to determine a drip rate.

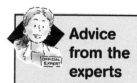

Advice from the experts
Tube tips

Follow these rules when selecting I.V. tubing:

- Use macrodrip tubing for infusions of at least 80 ml/hour.
- Use microdrip tubing for infusions of less than 80 ml/hour.
- With electronic infusion devices, select the tubing specifically made to work with those devices.

To calculate the drip rate, you need to know the calibration for the I.V. tubing you've selected. Different I.V. solution sets deliver fluids at varying amounts per drop. The drop factor refers to the number of drops per millilitre of solution calibrated for an administration set.

The drop factor is listed on the package containing the I.V. tubing administration set. For a standard (macrodrip) administration set, the drop factor is usually 15 or 20 gtt/ml (that's 'drops per millilitre'). For a microdrip (minidrip) set, it's 60 gtt/ml. (See *Quick drip rate guide*.)

A formula dripping with success

One way to calculate the drip rate is to use the formula below:

$$\frac{\text{drip rate}}{\text{in drops/minute}} = \frac{\text{total millilitres}}{\text{total minutes}} \times \frac{\text{drip factor}}{\text{in drops/ml}}$$

The following two examples show how to calculate the drip rate using this formula.

Getting to grips with glucose

Your patient needs an infusion of *glucose 5% in water at 125 ml/hour*. If the tubing set is calibrated at 15 gtt/ml, what's the drip rate?
- First, convert 1 hour to 60 minutes to fit the formula.
- Then set up a fraction. Place the volume of the infusion in the numerator. Place the number of minutes in which the volume is to be infused as the denominator:

$$\frac{125 \text{ ml}}{60 \text{ minutes}}$$

Before you give that drug!
Quick drip rate guide

When calculating the drip rate of I.V. solutions, for a given volume over time, remember that the number of drops required to deliver 1 ml varies with the type of administration set. To calculate the drip rate, you need to know the drop factor for each set. As a quick reference, consult the table below.

Drop factor	Drops/minute to infuse (drip rate)					
	500 ml/24 h	1000 ml/24 h	1000 ml/20 h	1000 ml/10 h	1000 ml/8 h	1000 ml/6 h
	21 ml/h	42 ml/h	50 ml/h	100 ml/h	125 ml/h	166 ml/h
15 gtt/ml	5 gtt	10 gtt	12 gtt	25 gtt	31 gtt	42 gtt
20 gtt/ml	7 gtt	14 gtt	17 gtt	34 gtt	42 gtt	56 gtt

- To determine X – or the number of drops per minute to be infused – multiply the fraction by the drop factor. Cancel units that appear in both the numerator and denominator:

$$X = \frac{125 \text{ ml}}{60 \text{ minutes}} \times \frac{15 \text{ gtt}}{\text{ml}}$$

- Solve for X by dividing the numerator by the denominator:

$$X = \frac{125 \times 15 \text{ gtt}}{60 \text{ minutes}}$$

$$X = \frac{1875 \text{ gtt}}{60 \text{ minutes}}$$

$$X = 31.25 \text{ gtt/minute}$$

The drip rate is 31.25 gtt/minute, rounded to 31 gtt/minute.

Pass the potassium, please!

You receive an prescription that reads *KCl 40 mmol in 100 ml normal saline over 40 minutes*. You decide to use a controller for the infusion, along with a tubing set calibrated at 20 gtt/ml. What's the drip rate? Here's how to solve this problem:
- Set up the fraction. Place the volume of the infusion in the numerator. Place the number of minutes for the infusion in the denominator:

$$\frac{100 \text{ ml}}{40 \text{ minutes}}$$

- To determine the number of drops per minute to be infused (solve for X), multiply the fraction by the drop factor. Cancel units that appear in both the numerator and denominator:

$$X = \frac{100 \text{ ml}}{40 \text{ minutes}} \times \frac{20 \text{ gtt}}{\text{ml}}$$

- To solve for X, divide the numerator by the denominator:

$$X = \frac{100 \times 20 \text{ gtt}}{40 \text{ minutes}}$$

$$X = \frac{2000 \text{ gtt}}{40 \text{ minutes}}$$

$$X = 50 \text{ gtt/minute}$$

The drip rate is 50 gtt/minute.

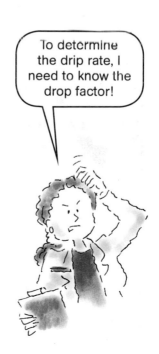

To determine the drip rate, I need to know the drop factor!

Calculating the flow rate

If your patient is receiving a large-volume infusion to maintain hydration or to replace fluids or electrolytes, you may need to calculate the flow rate. The flow rate is the number of millilitres of fluid to administer over 1 hour (it may also refer to the number of millilitres of fluid to administer per minute). To perform this calculation, you need to know the total volume to be infused in millilitres and the amount of time for the infusion.

Use this formula:

$$\text{flow rate} = \frac{\text{total volume ordered}}{\text{number of hours}}$$

The next two examples illustrate how to determine the correct flow rate.

So, how flows it?

Your patient needs 1000 ml of fluid over 8 hours. Find the flow rate by dividing the volume by the number of hours:

$$\text{flow rate} = \frac{1000 \text{ ml}}{8 \text{ hours}} = 125 \text{ ml/hour}$$

The flow rate is 125 ml/hour.

Salient saline solution

Your patient needs 250 ml of normal saline solution over 2 hours. What's the infusion rate?

To solve this problem, first set up the equation. Then divide 250 ml by 2 hours to find the flow rate in millilitres per hour:

$$\text{flow rate} = \frac{250 \text{ ml}}{2 \text{ hours}} = 125 \text{ ml/hour}$$

The flow rate is 125 ml/hour.

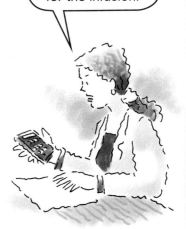

To determine the flow rate, I need to know the total volume and the amount of time for the infusion.

Quick calculation of drip rates

Here's a shortcut for calculating I.V. drip rates. It's based on the fact that all drop factors can be evenly divided into 60.

For macrodrip sets, use these rules to calculate drip rates:
* For sets that deliver 15 gtt/ml, divide the hourly flow rate by 4.
* For sets that deliver 20 gtt/ml, divide the hourly flow rate by 3.

With a microdrip set (drop factor of 60 gtt/ml), simply remember that the drip rate is the same as the flow rate.

Why the microdrip flow rate equals the drip rate

Here's the equation for determining the drip rate for a solution with a flow rate of 125 ml/hour (125 ml/60 minutes) when using a microdrip set (drop factor of 60 gtt/ml). Note that the number of minutes and the number of drops per millilitre cancel each other out.

$$\text{drip rate} = \frac{125 \ \cancel{ml}}{\cancel{60} \ \text{minutes}} \times \frac{\cancel{60} \ \text{gtt}}{1 \ \cancel{ml}}$$

The drip rate (125 gtt/minute) is the same as the number of millilitres of fluid per hour (flow rate).

Take the shortcut

A patient has been prescribed 1000 ml of normal saline to be infused over 12 hours. If your administration set delivers 20 gtt/ml, what's the drip rate?
- First, determine the flow rate (X) by dividing the number of millilitres to be delivered by the number of hours:

$$X = \frac{1000 \ \text{ml}}{12 \ \text{hours}} = 83.3 \ \text{ml/hour}$$

- Remember the rule: for sets that deliver 20 gtt/ml, divide the flow rate by 3 to determine the drip rate.
- Next, set up an equation to determine the drip rate, which now becomes X, and solve for X. Divide the flow rate by 3:

$$X = \frac{83.3}{3}$$

$$X = 27.7 \ \text{gtt/minute}$$

The drip rate is 27.7 gtt/minute, rounded up to 28 gtt/minute.

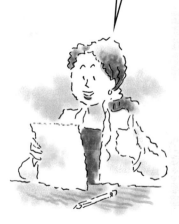

150 ml/hour equals 150 gtt/minute. Now that's the kind of maths I like!

Calculating infusion time

When you can calculate the flow rate and drip rate, you're ready to compute the time required for infusion of a specified volume of I.V. fluid. This calculation will help you keep the infusion on schedule and start the next infusion on time. It will also help you perform laboratory tests, such as the chemistry and electrolyte assessments that commonly accompany infusions, on time.

To calculate the infusion time, you must know the flow rate in millilitres per hour and the volume to be infused. Here's the formula:

$$\text{infusion time} = \frac{\text{volume to be infused}}{\text{flow rate}}$$

The following examples show how to use this formula to calculate infusion times.

Be back in _____ minutes!

If you plan to infuse 1 L of 5% glucose in water at 50 ml/hour, what's the infusion time?
• First, convert 1 L to 1000 ml to make units of measure that are equivalent.
• Then set up the fraction with the volume of the infusion as the numerator and the flow rate as the denominator:

$$\frac{1000\ ml}{50\ ml/hour}$$

• Next, solve for X by dividing 1000 by 50 and cancelling units that appear in both the numerator and denominator:

$$X = \frac{1000\ ml}{50\ ml/hour}$$

$$X = 20\ hours$$

The 5% glucose in water will infuse in 20 hours.

The bag will be empty at _____ o'clock

Your patient requires 500 ml of normal saline solution at 80 ml/hour. What's the infusion time? If the normal saline solution is hung at 5 a.m., what time will the infusion end?
• Set up a fraction. Place the volume of the infusion as the numerator and the flow rate as the denominator:

$$X = \frac{500\ ml}{80\ ml/hour}$$

• Solve for X by dividing 500 by 80 and canceling units that appear in both the numerator and denominator:

$$X = \frac{500\ ml}{80\ ml/hour}$$

$$X = 6.25\ hours$$

The normal saline solution will infuse in 6.25 hours (convert the decimal portion of this time to minutes by multiplying by 60 to get 15 minutes). This means that the bag will be empty at 11:15 a.m.

An alternative formula

Suppose all you know are the volume to be infused, the drip rate and the drop factor. Then you would use the alternative formula shown here to calculate the infusion time:

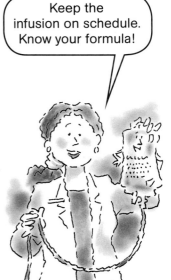

Keep the infusion on schedule. Know your formula!

$$\text{infusion time in hours} = \frac{\text{volume to be infused}}{(\text{drip rate} \div \text{drop factor}) \times 60 \text{ minutes}}$$

Another saline situation

A doctor prescribes *250 ml of normal saline I.V. at 32 gtt/minute*. The drop factor is 20 gtt/ml. What's the infusion time?
- Set up the formula with the known information:

$$\text{infusion time} = \frac{250 \text{ ml}}{(32 \text{ gtt/minute} \div 20 \text{ gtt/ml}) \times 60 \text{ minutes}}$$

- Divide the drip rate by the drop factor. (Remember, to divide a complex fraction, multiply the dividend by the reciprocal of the divisor.) Cancel units that appear in both the numerator and denominator:

$$\frac{32 \text{ gtt}}{1 \text{ min}} \times \frac{1 \text{ ml}}{20 \text{ gtt}} = \frac{32 \text{ ml}}{20 \text{ min}} = 1.6 \text{ ml/min}$$

- Rewrite the equation (solve for X) with the result (1.6 ml/minute) placed in the denominator. Cancel units that appear in both the numerator and denominator:

$$X = \frac{250 \text{ ml}}{\frac{1.6 \text{ ml}}{1 \text{ min}} \times \frac{60 \text{ min}}{1 \text{ hour}}}$$

- To find the infusion time, solve for X:

$$X = \frac{250}{1.6 \times 60 \text{ hours}}$$

$$X = \frac{250}{96 \text{ hours}}$$

$$X = 2.6 \text{ hours}$$

- The infusion time is 2.6 hours. Convert the decimal fraction portion of this time to minutes by multiplying by 60:

$$0.6 \text{ hours} \times 60 \text{ minutes} = 36 \text{ minutes}$$

The infusion time is 2 hours and 36 minutes.

> 2 hours and 36 minutes. Got the right time... just in time!

Heads-up! Here comes heta ...

If 500 ml of hetastarch are infusing at 40 gtt/minute with a set calibration of 20 gtt/ml, what's the infusion time?

- Use the information you know to set up a formula:

$$X = \frac{500 \text{ ml}}{(40 \text{ gtt/minute} \div 20 \text{ gtt/ml}) \times 60 \text{ minutes}}$$

- Divide the drip rate by the drop factor (remember to multiply the dividend by the reciprocal of the divisor). Cancel units that appear in both the numerator and denominator:

$$\frac{40 \text{ gtt}}{1 \text{ min}} \times \frac{1 \text{ ml}}{20 \text{ gtt}} = 2 \text{ ml/min}$$

- Rewrite the equation (solving for X) with the new denominator (2 ml/minute). Cancel units that appear in both the numerator and denominator:

$$X = \frac{500 \text{ ml}}{\dfrac{2 \text{ ml}}{1 \text{ min}} \times \dfrac{60 \text{ min}}{1 \text{ hour}}}$$

- To find the infusion time, solve for X:

$$X = \frac{500}{2 \times 60 \text{ hours}}$$

- Divide the numerator by the denominator:

$$X = \frac{500}{120 \text{ hours}}$$

- The infusion time is 4.166 hours, which rounds off to 4.17 hours. To convert the decimal fraction to minutes, multiply by 60 and then round off the number:

$$0.17 \text{ hour} \times 60 \text{ minutes} = 10.2 \text{ minutes} = 10 \text{ minutes}$$

The infusion time is 4 hours and 10 minutes.

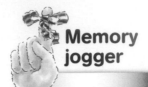

Memory jogger

When you need to divide a complex fraction, remember to multiply the dividend (the top number of the fraction) by the reciprocal (the inverse, or flipped, form) of the divisor (the bottom number).

In other words, change the division sign to a multiplication sign, and flip-flop the second fraction. Then proceed with the rest of the problem to solve for *X*.

Regulating infusions

After you start an infusion, you must be careful to regulate the I.V. flow. You can do this manually, using a pump, or using a patient-controlled analgesia (PCA) pump.

Regulating I.V. flow manually

To regulate the I.V. flow manually, count the number of drops going into the drip chamber. While counting the drops, adjust the flow with the roller clamp until the fluid is infusing at the appropriate number of drops per minute.

Fifteen seconds works fine

To save time, don't count for a full minute – calculate the drip rate for 15 seconds only. To do this, divide the prescribed drip rate by 4 (because 15 seconds is one quarter of a minute). For example, if the prescribed drip rate is 31 gtt/minute, divide 31 by 4 to get 8 (round 31 up to 32 first so it will divide evenly). Then adjust the roller clamp until the drip chamber shows 8 drops in 15 seconds.

Afterward, time-tape the I.V. bag to ensure that the solution is given at the prescribed rate and to make recording fluid intake easier. (See *Taped up and ready to drip*.)

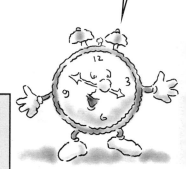

Save time. Calculate the drip rate for 15 seconds instead of a minute. Divide the prescribed rate by four.

Advice from the experts

Taped up and ready to drip

Time-taping an I.V. bag helps ensure that an I.V. solution is administered at the prescribed rate. It also helps facilitate recording of fluid intake.

To time-tape an I.V. bag, place a strip of adhesive tape from the top to the bottom of the bag, next to the fluid level markings. (This illustration shows a bag time-taped for a rate of 100 ml/hour beginning at 10 a.m.)

0 marks the spot

Next to the '0' marking, record the time that you hung the bag. Then, knowing the hourly rate, mark each hour on the tape next to the corresponding fluid marking. At the bottom of the tape, mark the time at which the solution will be completely infused.

Ink alert

Don't write directly on the bag with a felt tip marker because the ink may seep into the fluid. Some manufacturers provide printed time-tapes for use with their solutions.

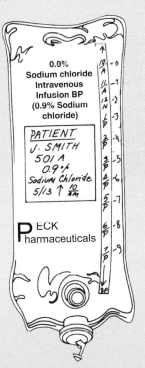

Electronic syringe drivers and infusion pumps

Electronic syringe drivers and infusion pumps facilitate I.V. administration. These specialised devices administer fluid under positive pressure and are calibrated by drip rate and volume.

Steady as she goes

When using a syringe driver or infusion pump, set the device to deliver a constant amount of solution per hour, following the manufacturer's directions.

The electronic edge

Electronic infusion pumps and syringe drivers offer many advantages, such as:
• allowing you easy control of the rate, or volume, by setting it on the machine
• shortening the time needed to calculate an infusion rate
• requiring less maintenance than standard devices that drip fluid by gravity
• providing greater accuracy than standard devices.

Special features

Most of these electronic devices keep track of the amount of fluid that has been infused, helping maintain accurate intake and output records. Many have alarms that signal when the fluid container is empty or when a mechanical problem occurs. Some devices have variable pressure limits that prevent them from pumping fluids into infiltrated sites.

Regulating I.V. flow with electronic devices

When using a syringe driver or infusion pump to regulate I.V. flow, programme the device based on your calculation of the infusion rate. Remember that these machines can make mistakes – they don't eliminate the need for careful calculations and assessment of infusion rates over time. So check the infusion by counting the drips in the chamber just as you would with manual regulation.

Programming the pump

To determine the pump settings, consider the volume of fluid to be given and the total infusion time. With most devices, you'll need to programme both the amount of fluid to be infused and the hourly flow rate. However, some devices require you to programme the flow rate per minute or the drip rate.

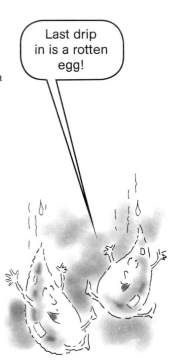

Last drip in is a rotten egg!

Patient-controlled analgesia apparatus

One popular infusion device is the computerised PCA pump, which allows a patient to self-administer an analgesic by pushing a button. You programme the pump to deliver a precise dose every time. The pump also can be programmed to deliver a basal dose of drug in addition to the patient-controlled dose. (See *Putting your patient in control*.)

No pain... all gains

The main advantage of using a PCA pump over the traditional approach – in which analgesics are injected intramuscularly every few hours – is that blood concentrations of analgesics remain consistent throughout the day. With the traditional approach,

Advice from the experts

Putting your patient in control

A computerised patient-controlled analgesia (PCA) pump, such as the one shown here, allows your patient to give themselves pain medication with the push of a button. With PCA pumps, patients tend to use less medication than they do with the traditional approach and also develop a greater feeling of control over their pain.

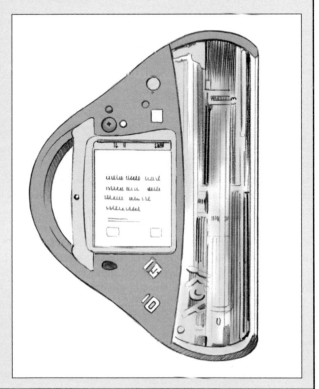

blood levels fluctuate, so patients have periods of heavy sedation alternating with periods of increasing pain.

Two added benefits of PCA pumps are that patients tend to take less medication than they do with the traditional approach and that they develop a greater feeling of control over their pain.

Pump-provided protection

Several safety features are built into PCA pumps. Drug dose and administration frequency are programmed, preventing the patient from medicating too often. If the patient tries to overmedicate, the machine simply ignores the request. Also, some pumps record the number of requests and the number of times the patient actually receives medication, which helps you evaluate whether the prescriber needs to increase or decrease the drug dose.

And the password is...

PCA pumps require you to use an access code or key before entering drug dose and frequency information into the system. This prevents unauthorised users from tampering with or accidentally resetting the pump. Some machines even record unauthorised entries.

I'll have another, but I think my friend has reached his limit!

PCA prep parameters

When preparing a PCA pump for a patient, follow these guidelines:
• Draw the correct amount and concentration of drug – usually morphine – and insert it into the PCA pump.
• Programme the pump according to the manufacturer's directions.
• Carefully read the PCA log, and then record the information based on your facility's policy. A typical prescription might state the following: *Start morphine sulphate PCA. Give 2 mg/hour basal rate and 1 mg every 15 minutes on demand, with a lock-out of 6 mg/4 hour.*

Recording drug dosage with a PCA

When interpreting the PCA log, note the strength (number of milligrams per millilitre) of drug solution in the syringe. You'll need this information to calculate the dose received by the patient.

Covering the basals

Also note the number of times the patient received the drug throughout the time covered by your assessment (usually over 4 hours). If your patient is receiving a basal dose, note that as well. By multiplying the number of injections by the volume of each injection and adding the basal dose, you can determine the amount of solution the patient received.

Multiply this amount by the solution strength to find the total amount of drug, as shown in this formula:

fluid volume $\times$ solution strength = total medication received

Record this amount in milligrams in the patient's medication administration record.

A double dose of accuracy

Most facilities require the nurse who prepares the syringe to record the amount of fluid and drug in the syringe. Each nurse who checks the PCA log double-checks and records this information. The record enables you to double-check the accuracy of everyone's calculations.

Adjusting the infusion rate

No matter how carefully you calculate the drip rate, and adjust the flow rate of an I.V. infusion, the rate still may change. Why? Perhaps the patient changed position, the I.V. tubing became kinked, or the drug infiltrated the patient's skin. Such factors cause the infusion to run ahead of or behind schedule.

Don't hesitate to recalculate

When problems occur, recalculate the drip rate, taking into account the remaining time and volume. If the fluid has infused too slowly, determine whether the patient can tolerate an increased rate by checking their cardiac and respiratory status. Look for a history of renal insufficiency, heart failure, pulmonary oedema or any other condition that increases the risk of fluid overload.

If I.V. fluid has infused too quickly, slow or stop the infusion and assess for signs of fluid overload, such as crackles and increased blood pressure. Call the prescriber if these occur.

Are you up for a fluid challenge?

You may also need to adjust the infusion rate to perform a fluid challenge – the protocol for monitoring how a patient tolerates increased fluids. The fastest way to do a fluid challenge is by increasing the I.V. flow rate for a specified time and then reducing it to a maintenance rate. However, be sure to use a fluid bolus cautiously in paediatric and elderly patients.

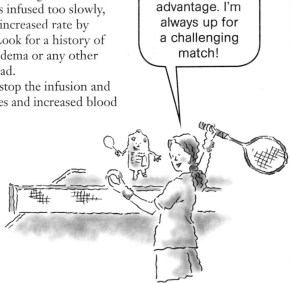

That's my advantage. I'm always up for a challenging match!

Heparin and insulin infusions

A doctor may prescribe heparin or insulin to be added to a large-volume I.V. infusion. These drugs are prescribed in units per hour. To administer them safely, you must calculate the drug dose so that it falls within therapeutic limits. (See Chapter 12, Calculating parenteral injections, for more information on heparin and insulin.)

Calculating heparin doses

A common anticoagulant, heparin prevents the formation of new clots and slows the development of pre-existing clots. Usually given by the I.V. route, it's prescribed in doses of units per hour or millilitres per hour. Each dose is individualised based on the patient's coagulation status, which is measured by the partial thromboplastin time.

Flow rate

Accurately calculating the flow rate ensures that the heparin dose falls within safe and therapeutic limits. This type of calculation differs from the flow-rate calculations discussed earlier because it's used to administer a drug, not just a fluid.

To calculate the hourly heparin flow rate, first determine the solution's concentration by dividing the units of drug added to the bag by the number of millilitres of solution. Then write a fraction stating the desired dose of heparin over the unknown flow rate. Then simply cross-multiply to find the unknown flow rate.

Here are some examples using simple proportions to find the solution.

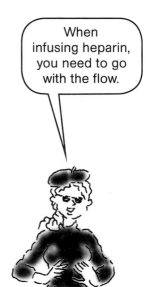

When infusing heparin, you need to go with the flow.

Go with the flow!

A prescription states *heparin 40 000 units in 1 L of 5% glucose in water I.V. Infuse at 1000 units/hour.* What's the flow rate in millilitres per hour?

• First, convert 1 L to 1000 ml. Then write a fraction to express the known solution strength (units of drug divided by millilitres of solution):

$$\frac{40\,000 \text{ units}}{1000 \text{ ml}}$$

• Write a second fraction with the desired dose of heparin in the numerator and the unknown flow rate in the denominator:

$$\frac{1000 \text{ units/hour}}{X}$$

- Put these fractions into a proportion:

$$\frac{40\,000\ \text{units}}{1000\ \text{ml}} = \frac{1000\ \text{units/hour}}{X}$$

- To find the flow rate, solve for X by cross-multiplying:

$$40\,000\ \text{units} \times X = 1000\ \text{units/hour} \times 1000\ \text{ml}$$

- Divide each side of the equation by 40 000 units and cancel units that appear in both the numerator and denominator:

$$\frac{40\,000\ \text{units} \times X}{40\,000\ \text{units}} = \frac{1000\ \text{units/hour} \times 1000\ \text{ml}}{40\,000\ \text{units}}$$

$$X = \frac{1\,000\,000\ \text{ml/hour}}{40\,000}$$

$$X = 25\ \text{ml/hour}$$

To administer heparin at 1000 units/hour, you should set the flow rate at 25 ml/hour.

Know this flow?

You're about to administer a continuous infusion of 25 000 units of heparin in 250 ml of 5% glucose in water. If the patient is to receive 600 units/hour, what's the flow rate?
- Write a ratio to express the known solution strength (units of drug to millilitres of solution):

$$25\,000\ \text{units} : 250\ \text{ml}$$

- Write a second ratio to describe the desired dose of heparin in relation to the unknown flow rate:

$$600\ \text{units/hour} : X$$

- Put these ratios into a proportion:

$$25\,000\ \text{units} : 250\ \text{ml} :: 600\ \text{units/hour} : X$$

- Solve for X by multiplying the extremes and the means:

$$25\,000\ \text{units} \times X = 600\ \text{units/hour} \times 250\ \text{ml}$$

- Divide each side of the equation by 25 000 units and cancel units that appear in both the numerator and denominator:

$$\frac{25\,000\ \text{units} \times X}{25\,000\ \text{units}} = \frac{600\ \text{units/hour} \times 250\ \text{ml}}{25\,000\ \text{units}}$$

$$X = \frac{600 \times 250 \text{ ml/hour}}{25\,000}$$

$$X = \frac{150\,000 \text{ ml/hour}}{25\,000}$$

$$X = 6 \text{ ml/hour}$$

To administer 600 units/hour, you should set the flow rate at 6 ml/hour.

Units per hour

If a heparin infusion is prescribed in millilitres per hour, you may want to calculate it in units per hour too. This determines the patient's drug dose so you can be sure it falls within a safe and therapeutic range.

Here's an example calculating units per hour.

Knowing your therapeutic range

A patient is receiving 20 000 units of heparin in 1000 ml of 5% glucose in water I.V. at 30 ml/hour. What heparin dose is he receiving?
• Write a fraction to describe the known solution strength (units of drug divided by millilitres of solution):

$$\frac{20\,000 \text{ units}}{1000 \text{ ml}}$$

• Set up the second fraction with the flow rate in the denominator and the unknown dose of heparin in the numerator:

$$\frac{X}{30 \text{ ml/hour}}$$

• Write these fractions into a proportion:

$$\frac{20\,000 \text{ units}}{1000 \text{ ml}} = \frac{X}{30 \text{ ml/hour}}$$

• Solve for X by cross-multiplying:

$$1000 \text{ ml} \times X = 30 \text{ ml/hour} \times 20\,000 \text{ units}$$

• Divide each side of the equation by 1000 ml and cancel units that appear in both the numerator and denominator:

$$\frac{\cancel{1000 \text{ ml}} \times X}{\cancel{1000 \text{ ml}}} = \frac{30 \cancel{\text{ ml}}/\text{hour} \times 20\,000 \text{ units}}{1000 \cancel{\text{ ml}}}$$

$$X = \frac{30 \times 20\,000 \text{ units/hour}}{1000}$$

$$X = \frac{600\,000 \text{ units/hour}}{1000}$$

$$X = 600 \text{ units/hour}$$

With the flow rate set at 30 ml/hour, the patient is receiving 600 units/hour of heparin.

Calculating continuous insulin infusions

An acutely ill diabetic patient may need to receive insulin by continuous infusion. Continuous infusion allows close control of insulin administration based on serial measurements of blood glucose levels.

You'll use an infusion pump to administer I.V. insulin. Regular insulin is the only type that can be administered by the I.V. route because it has a shorter duration of action than other insulins.

Insulin is usually prescribed in units per hour, but it may be prescribed in millilitres per hour. In either case, the infusion should be in a concentration of 1 unit/ml to avoid calculation errors that may have serious consequences. The examples here are based on common patient situations.

Insulin inquiry 1

Your patient needs a continuous infusion of 150 units of regular insulin in 150 ml of normal saline at 6 units/hour. What's the flow rate?

• Write a fraction to describe the known solution strength (units of drug over millilitres of solution):

$$\frac{150 \text{ units}}{150 \text{ ml}}$$

• Write a second fraction with the infusion rate in the numerator and the unknown flow rate in the denominator:

$$\frac{6 \text{ units/hour}}{X}$$

• Write the two fractions as a proportion:

$$\frac{150 \text{ units}}{150 \text{ ml}} = \frac{6 \text{ units/hour}}{X}$$

• Solve for X by cross-multiplying:

$$150 \text{ ml} \times X = 6 \text{ units/hour} \times 150 \text{ ml}$$

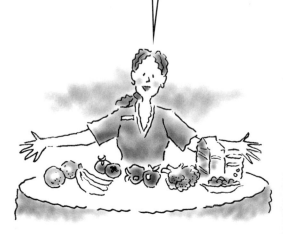

Doing all these calculations, you probably feel like you need an infusion of energy. Grab a bite to eat!

• Divide each side of the equation by 150 units and cancel units that appear in both the numerator and denominator:

$$\frac{\cancel{150 \text{ units}} \times X}{\cancel{150 \text{ units}}} = \frac{6 \text{ \cancel{units}/hour} \times 150 \text{ ml}}{150 \text{ \cancel{units}}}$$

$$X = 6 \text{ ml/hour}$$

To administer 6 units/hour of the prescribed insulin, you set the infusion pump's flow rate at 6 ml/hour.

Insulin inquiry 2

Your patient is receiving a continuous infusion of 100 units of regular insulin in 100 ml of normal saline at 10 ml/hour. How many units per hour is your patient receiving?
• Write a ratio to describe the known solution strength (units of insulin to millilitres of solution):

$$100 \text{ units} : 100 \text{ ml}$$

• Set up a second ratio comparing the unknown amount of insulin to the prescribed infusion rate:

$$X : 10 \text{ ml/hour}$$

• Put these ratios into a proportion:

$$100 \text{ units} : 100 \text{ ml} :: X : 10 \text{ ml/hour}$$

• Solve for X by multiplying the means and the extremes:

$$X \times 100 \text{ ml} = 100 \text{ units} \times 10 \text{ ml/hour}$$

• Divide each side of the equation by 100 ml and cancel units that appear in both the numerator and denominator:

$$\frac{X \times \cancel{100 \text{ ml}}}{\cancel{100 \text{ ml}}} = \frac{100 \text{ units} \times 10 \text{ \cancel{ml}/hour}}{\cancel{100 \text{ ml}}}$$

$$X = 10 \text{ units/hour}$$

When the insulin infusion runs at 10 ml/hour, the patient receives 10 units/hour.

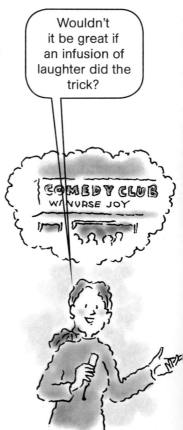

Wouldn't it be great if an infusion of laughter did the trick?

COMEDY CLUB W/ NURSE JOY

Electrolyte and nutrient infusions

I.V. fluids can be used to deliver electrolytes and nutrients directly into the patient's bloodstream.

Adding up the additives

Large-volume infusions with additives maintain or restore hydration or electrolyte status or supply additional electrolytes, vitamins or other nutrients. In such cases, you may have to calculate and prepare the correct amount and add it to the solution.

Common additives include potassium chloride, vitamins B and C, and trace elements. Electrolytes may also be given in small-volume, intermittent infusions piggybacked into existing I.V. lines. (See *Calculating piggyback infusions*.)

Sometimes, you may need to combine more than one additive into a solution. Before calculating the correct amounts of each substance to inject, check the compatibility chart or consult the pharmacist to make sure that the additives can be mixed safely.

> You have to prepare and serve the correct amount of I.V. fluids to your patient.

Prepare to prepare

If the additive isn't prepackaged in solution, either by the manufacturer or by the pharmacy, you must prepare the correct amount and add it to the solution. Then you must calculate the flow rate and the drip rate. To calculate the amount of additive, use the proportion method as you would for any prepared liquid drug. Here's an example.

Thinking about thiamine

Your patient requires 1000 ml of 5% glucose in water with 150 mg of thiamine/L over 12 hours. The thiamine is available in a prepared syringe of 25 mg/ml. How many millilitres of thiamine must be added to the solution? What's the flow rate?

- Write the first ratio to describe the known solution strength (amount of drug per 1 ml):

$$25\,\text{mg} : 1\,\text{ml}$$

- Set up the second ratio. Write the amount of thiamine prescribed on one side and the unknown amount to be added to the solution on the other side:

$$150\,\text{mg} : X$$

- Put these ratios into a proportion:

$$25\,\text{mg} : 1\,\text{ml} :: 150\,\text{mg} : X$$

Calculating piggyback infusions

An I.V. piggyback is a small-volume, intermittent infusion that's connected to an existing I.V. line containing maintenance fluid. Most piggybacks contain antibiotics or electrolytes. To calculate piggyback infusions, use proportions.

Piggyback problem

You receive an order for 500 mg of imipenem in 100 ml of normal saline solution, to be infused over 1 hour. The vial contains 1000 mg (1 g). The insert says to reconstitute the powder with 5 ml of normal saline solution. How much solution should you draw? What's the flow rate?

Solution solution

- Write the first ratio to describe the known solution strength (amount of drug compared with the known amount of solution):

$$1000\,mg : 5\,ml$$

- Write the second ratio, which compares the desired dose of imipenem and the unknown amount of solution:

$$500\,mg : X$$

- Put these ratios into a proportion:

$$1000\,mg : 5\,ml :: 500\,mg : X$$

- Multiply the extremes and the means:

$$1000\,mg \times X = 500\,mg \times 5\,ml$$

- Solve for X by dividing each side of the equation by 1000 mg and cancelling units that appear in both the numerator and denominator:

$$\frac{1000\,\cancel{mg} \times X}{1000\,\cancel{mg}} = \frac{500\,\cancel{mg} \times 5\,ml}{1000\,\cancel{mg}}$$

$$X = \frac{500 \times 5\,ml}{1000}$$

$$X = \frac{2500\,ml}{1000}$$

$$X = 2.5\,ml$$

You should draw 2.5 ml of solution to get 500 mg of imipenem.

Flow rate

Recall that the flow rate is the number of millilitres of fluid to administer over 1 hour. So, in this case, the flow rate is 100 ml/hour.

Compatibility counts

After you've calculated an I.V. piggyback dose, make sure that the drugs to be infused together are compatible. The same goes for drugs mixed in the same syringe or I.V. bag. Drug compatibility charts can be time-savers – you may have one hanging in your unit's medication room. If not, use a drug handbook that includes a compatibility chart.

- Solve for X by multiplying the extremes and the means:

$$X \times 25\,mg = 150\,mg \times 1\,ml$$

- Divide each side of the equation by 25 mg and cancel units that appear in both the numerator and denominator:

$$\frac{X \times 25\,\cancel{mg}}{25\,\cancel{mg}} = \frac{150\,\cancel{mg} \times 1\,ml}{25\,\cancel{mg}}$$

$$X = \frac{150 \text{ ml}}{25}$$

$$X = 6 \text{ ml}$$

- You must add 6 ml of thiamine to the solution. If the flow rate is 1000 ml over 12 hours, divide 1000 by 12 to find the flow rate for 1 hour:

$$\frac{1000 \text{ ml}}{12 \text{ hours}} = 83.3 \text{ ml/hours}$$

The flow rate is 83 ml/hour.

Blood and blood product infusions

The volume of fluid to be infused and the drop factor can be used to calculate transfusions of blood and blood products. During such transfusions, take care to prevent cell damage and ensure an adequate blood flow by using a special administration set that contains filters to remove agglutinated cells. The drop factor for these sets is usually 15 gtt/ml.

Generally, you'll use an 18G or larger I.V. catheter for administration. However, you may need a smaller catheter for elderly or paediatric patients, those with chronic illnesses who are hospitalised frequently, or severely dehydrated patients.

Written in blood

Your facility probably has specific protocols for infusing blood and blood products. For example, a unit of whole blood – about 500 ml – or packed red blood cells (PRBCs) – about 250 ml – should infuse for no longer than 4 hours because the blood can deteriorate and become contaminated with bacteria after this time. Many facilities recommend completing a transfusion in about 2 hours. However, this rate may be too fast for paediatric and elderly patients.

Product precautions

You'll also need to take special precautions when transfusing blood products, such as platelets, cryoprecipitate and granulocytes. Consult your facility's procedure manual to find out the type of tubing to use and the rate and duration of the transfusion.

In addition, some medical conditions require the use of special tubing. For example, cancer patients may need to use a leucocyte filter with blood products to prevent complications.

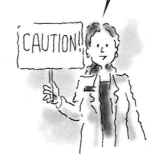

Be especially careful when infusing or transfusing blood. Use the right equipment, watch your time and always follow your facility's protocol.

CAUTION!

Blood cell brain teaser

Here's an example of a dosage calculation problem that involves PRBCs: your patient is to receive 250 ml of PRBCs over 4 hours. The drop factor of the tubing is 15 gtt/ml. What's the drip rate in drops per minute?

- First, find the flow rate in millilitres per minute:

$$\frac{250 \text{ ml PRCB}}{4 \text{ hours}} = \frac{62.5 \text{ ml}}{1 \text{ hour}}$$

> Use the flow rate in millilitres per hour …

$$\frac{62.5 \text{ ml}}{1 \text{ hour}} = \frac{1 \text{ hour}}{60 \text{minutes}} = 1.04 \text{ ml/minute} = \text{flow rate}$$

- Multiply the flow rate by the drop factor to find the drip rate in drops per minute:

$$\frac{1.04 \text{ ml}}{1 \text{ minute}} \times \frac{15 \text{ gtt}}{\text{ml}} = 15.6 \text{ gtt/minute}$$

> … to find the drip rate in drops per minute.

The drip rate is 15.6 gtt/minute, or approximately 16 gtt/minute.

Total parenteral nutrition

A patient receives parenteral nutrition when their nutritional needs can't be met enterally because of elevated requirements or impaired digestion or absorption in the GI tract. Total parenteral nutrition (TPN) refers to any nutrient solution, including lipids, given through a central venous line.

TPN can be administered through a central vein, such as the subclavian vein or internal jugular vein. Peripheral parenteral nutrition (PPN), which is administered through the veins of the arms, legs or scalp, supplies full caloric needs while avoiding the risks that accompany a central line. Most facilities have a written protocol regarding insertion sites and recommended solutions for both TPN and PPN.

TPN is available as commercially prepared products or individually formulated solutions from the pharmacy. Solutions are prepared under sterile conditions to guard against patient infection. Very rarely are nurses responsible for preparing TPN solutions on the unit.

> It's always good to brush up on your facility's protocol… no matter how busy you may be!

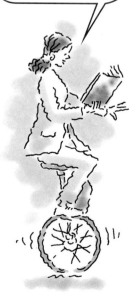

Added attractions

TPN solutions contain a 10% or greater glucose concentration. Amino acids are added to maintain or restore nitrogen balance, and vitamins, electrolytes and trace minerals are added to meet individual patient needs.

Lipids also may be added, but they're commonly given separately to prevent their destruction by the other nutrients. Remember that additives increase a solution's total volume, so they affect intake measurements.

For example, when assessing the amount of fluid remaining in the TPN bottle, don't be surprised to find 20 to 50 ml more than you expected. If this happens, find out whether the volume of additives explains the discrepancy.

What goes up... must come down

Initially, TPN is infused at a slow rate – usually 40 ml/hour – which is increased gradually to a maintenance level. The rate is decreased gradually before discontinuing TPN. Most solutions are administered through an infusion pump.

For example, a patient's TPN may be increased to a maintenance level of 2000 ml in 24 hours. To set the maintenance flow rate of the infusion pump, you need to find the hourly flow rate. To do this, simply divide the amount to be infused daily – 2000 ml – by 24 hours. You'll find that you should set the infusion pump at 83 ml/hour.

Infusion calculations

These problems are typical of the infusion calculations you're likely to encounter.

Real-world problems

Erythromycin drip rate drill

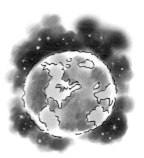

Your patient needs 15 ml of erythromycin, which is equal to 500 mg. The infusion is to be completed in 30 minutes using a tubing set calibrated to 20 gtt/ml. What's the drip rate?

Here's how to determine the answer:
• Set up a fraction. Place the volume of the infusion in the numerator. Place the number of minutes in which the volume is to be infused in the denominator:

$$\frac{15 \text{ ml}}{30 \text{ minutes}}$$

• Multiply the fraction by the drop factor to determine the number of drops per minute to be infused (solve for X). Cancel units that appear in both the numerator and denominator:

$$X = \frac{15 \text{ ml}}{30 \text{ minutes}} \times \frac{20 \text{ gtt}}{\text{ml}}$$

- Solve for X by dividing the numerator by the denominator:

$$X = \frac{15 \times 20 \text{ gtt}}{30 \text{ minutes}}$$

$$X = \frac{300 \text{ gtt}}{30 \text{ minutes}}$$

$$X = 10 \text{ gtt/minute}$$

The drip rate is 10 gtt/minute.

This should Ringer bell

If you infuse 1050 ml of Ringer-lactate solution at 25 gtt/minute using a set calibration of 15 gtt/ml, what's the infusion time?

- Use the information you know to set up the formula:

$$X = \frac{1050 \text{ ml}}{(25 \text{ gtt/minute} \div 15 \text{ gtt/ml}) \times 60 \text{ minutes}}$$

- Divide the drip rate by the drop factor. (Remember to multiply the dividend by the reciprocal of the divisor.) Cancel units that appear in both the numerator and denominator:

$$\frac{25 \text{ gtt}}{1 \text{ min}} \times \frac{1 \text{ ml}}{15 \text{ gtt}} = 1.67 \text{ ml/minute}$$

- Rewrite the equation (solving for X) using the result (1.67 ml/minute) in the denominator. Cancel units that appear in both the numerator and denominator:

$$X = \frac{1050 \text{ ml}}{\dfrac{1.67 \text{ ml}}{1 \text{ min}} \times \dfrac{60 \text{ min}}{1 \text{ hour}}}$$

- To find the infusion time, solve for X:

$$X = \frac{1050}{1.67 \times 60 \text{ hours}}$$

$$X = \frac{1050}{100.2 \text{ hours}}$$

- Divide the numerator by the denominator:

$$X = 10.47 \text{ hours}$$

The infusion time is 10.47 hours, which can be rounded to 10.5 hours. (This is equivalent to 10 hours 30 minutes.)

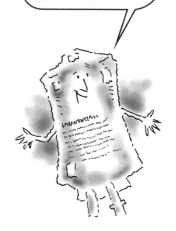

Let's see, 1050 ml of Ringer-lactate solution... well, I'll have to divide the drip rate by the drop factor.

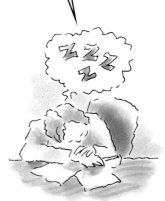

Okay, enough dosage calculations. Take a rest, and then give the Quick quiz a go!

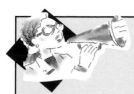

That's a wrap!

Calculating I.V. infusions review

Some important information about calculating I.V. infusions is highlighted below.

Drip rate

- Represents the number of drops infused per minute
- Formula to use:
total millilitres ÷ total minutes × drop factor in drops (gtt)/millilitre
- Drop factor represents the number of drops per millilitre of solution that the I.V. tubing is designed to deliver

Flow rate

- Represents the number of millilitres of fluid administered over 1 hour
- Formula to use:
total volume prescribed ÷ number of hours

Drip-rate shortcut

Macrodrips

- For 15 gtt/ml sets, divide hourly flow rate by 4
- For 20 gtt/ml sets, divide hourly flow rate by 3

Microdrips

- Drip rate = flow rate

Infusion time

- The amount of time required for infusion of a specified volume of I.V. fluid
- Method 1:
infusion time = infused volume ÷ flow rate

- Method 2:
infusion time = infused volume ÷ drip rate/drop factor × 60 minutes

Regulating I.V. flow manually

- Count the number of drops going into the drip chamber.
- Adjust the flow with the roller clamp to the appropriate drip rate.
- Time-tape the I.V. bag.

Regulating I.V. flow with electronic infusion pumps

- Programme the device based on the infusion rate.
- Count drips in the chamber to check the infusion.

PCA pump

- Allows the patient to self-administer an analgesic
- Also can be programmed to deliver a basal dose of drug
- Requires use of an access code or key to prevent unauthorised use of the device

Using a PCA pump

- Draw drug into a syringe and insert it into the PCA pump.
- Programme the pump according to the manufacturer's directions.
- Read the PCA log; then record information as per facility policy.

PCA log notes

- Strength of drug solution in syringe
- Number of drug administrations during assessment period

(continued)

Calculating I.V. infusions review (continued)

- Basal dose patient received, if any
- Amount of solution received (equals the number of injections × volume of injections + basal doses)
- Total amount of drug received (equals total amount of solution × solution strength)

Heparin flow-rate formula

- First determine the solution's concentration: divide units of drug added by the amount of solution in millilitres.
- Then state as a fraction (the desired dose over the unknown flow rate).
- Lastly, cross-multiply and solve for *X*.

Insulin infusions

- Regular insulin is the only type administered by I.V. route.
- Use an infusion pump.
- Use concentrations of 1 unit/ml.

Electrolyte and nutrient infusions

- Make sure that drugs to be infused together are compatible.
- Calculate the amount of additive using the proportion method as you would for any prepared liquid drug.
- Calculate the flow rate and the drip rate.

Blood infusions

- Filter out agglutinated cells with special administration sets.
- Drop factor is usually 15 gtt/ml.
- Use at least an 18G I.V. catheter.

TPN administration

- Can be given centrally or peripherally
- Initially infused at 40 ml/hour, then increased to maintenance
- Administered with an infusion pump

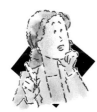

Quick quiz

1. To calculate the drip rate of an I.V. solution, you must first determine the:
    A. drop factor.
    B. flow rate.
    C. size of the tubing.
    D. total volume of the I.V. solution.

Answer: A. The drop factor, or number of drops/millilitre of solution, depends on the administration set you're using and is listed on the set's label.

2. The doctor prescribes 1000 ml of a drug to infuse over 10 hours at 25 gtt/minute. The set calibration is 15 gtt/ml. After 5 hours, 650 ml have infused instead of 500. To recalculate the drip rate for the remaining solution, you would:
    A. increase the rate to 18 gtt/minute.
    B. increase the rate to 35 gtt/minute.
    C. slow the rate to 10 gtt/minute.
    D. slow the rate to 18 gtt/minute.

Answer: D. To solve this problem, determine the amount of fluid remaining by subtracting 650 ml from 1000 ml. Convert the time remaining to minutes. Set up the equation using this formula:

$$\frac{\text{total ml}}{\text{total minutes}} \times \text{drop factor in gtt/minute} = \text{drip rate in gtt/minute}$$

3. Which test determines the therapeutic range for heparin?
   A. Activated partial thrombin test.
   B. Partial thromboplastin time (PTT).
   C. Partial thrombin activation test.
   D. Clotting test.

Answer: B. Heparin doses are individualised based on the patient's coagulation status, which is measured by PTT.

4. For a microdrip set with a drop factor of 60 gtt/ml, the drip rate is:
   A. half the hourly flow rate.
   B. 10 times greater than the hourly flow rate.
   C. the same as the hourly flow rate.
   D. 4 times greater than the hourly flow rate.

Answer: C. The drip rate is the same as the hourly flow rate because the number of minutes in an hour – 60 – is the same as the drop factor.

5. You start a continuous infusion of 150 units of regular insulin in 150 ml of normal saline solution. If the prescribed dose is 8 units/hour, what's the hourly flow rate?
   A. 8 ml/hour.
   B. 10 ml/hour.
   C. 18 ml/hour.
   D. 80 ml/hour.

Answer: A. Solve this problem by setting up the first fraction with the known solution strength and the second fraction with the desired dose and the unknown volume, putting these fractions into a proportion, cross-multiplying and then dividing and cancelling the units of measure that appear in both the numerator and denominator.

6. The PCA pump can provide a dose of medication on demand or at a:
   A. basil rate.
   B. basal rate.
   C. basic rate.
   D. base rate.

Answer: B. The basal rate is a continuous infusion administered by the PCA.

7. You need to infuse 1500 ml of 5% glucose in water over 10 hours. What's the flow rate?
   A.   50 ml/hour
   B.   100 ml/hour
   C.   150 ml/hour
   D.   250 ml/hour
Answer: C. Set up the equation using this formula:

$$\frac{\text{total volume prescribed}}{\text{number of hours}}$$

8. Your patient needs an infusion of 5% glucose in water at 75 ml/hour. If the tubing set is calibrated at 20 gtt/ml, what's the drip rate?
   A.   20 gtt/minute
   B.   25 gtt/minute
   C.   50 gtt/minute
   D.   75 gtt/minute
Answer: B. Set up the equation using this formula:

$$\frac{\text{total ml}}{\text{total minutes}} \times \text{drop factor in gtt/ml} = \text{drip rate in gtt/minute}$$

Scoring

☆☆☆   If you answered all eight items correctly, excellent! Enjoy every gtt of success.

☆☆   If you answered five to seven items correctly, great job! Your drop factor is beyond measure. (All right, if you insist, we'll give you 15 gtt/ml.)

☆   If you answered fewer than five items correctly, no problem! Go with the flow, keep calculating, and infuse in peace and joy.

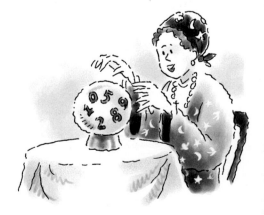

I see three more chapters of special calculations in your future …

Part VI

Special calculations

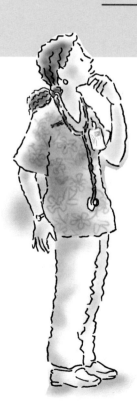

14 Calculating paediatric dosages

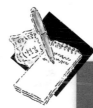

Just the facts

In this chapter, you'll learn:
- ♦ how to prepare drugs and administer them to infants and children by the four routes
- ♦ methods for calculating safe paediatric drug dosages according to body weight and body surface area
- ♦ recommended paediatric infusion guidelines and protocols
- ♦ how to calculate paediatric fluid needs based on body weight, calories of metabolism and body surface area.

A look at calculating paediatric dosages

When calculating drug dosages for paediatric patients, remember that children aren't just small adults. Because of their size, metabolism and other factors, children have special medication needs and require special care. Also, an incorrect dose is more likely to harm a child than an adult.

Same routes, different needs

Although children and adults both receive drugs by the oral, subcutaneous, intramuscular, intravenous and topical routes, the similarity ends there. The pharmacokinetics, pharmacodynamics and pharmacotherapeutics of drugs differ greatly between children and adults.

For example, a child's immature body systems may be unable to handle certain drugs. Also, a child's total volume of body water is much greater proportionally than an adult's, so drug distribution is altered. Because of these differences, you must be especially careful when calculating dosages for children. (See *A trio of time-saving tips*.)

Why is this chapter so important? Children have special dosage calculation needs.

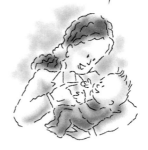

Administering paediatric drugs

The methods used to prepare drugs and administer them to paediatric patients also differ from the methods used for adults, depending on which route is used. There are specific administration guidelines and precautions for each route as well. (See *Giving medications to children*.)

Oral route

Infants and young children who can't swallow tablets or capsules are given oral drugs in liquid form. When a liquid preparation isn't available, you may generally crush a tablet and mix it with a small amount of liquid. Don't use essential fluids, such as breast milk and infant formula, because this could lead to feeding refusal. Additionally, mix it in only a small amount of liquid. If the medication is mixed in a large amount of liquid, such as a full bottle, the child won't receive the entire dose if the bottle isn't finished.

Remember: Never crush timed-release capsules or tablets or enteric-coated drugs. Crushing destroys the coating that causes drugs to release at the right time and prevent stomach irritation.

Measuring device advice

If a child can drink from a cup, measure and give liquid medications in one that's calibrated in metric units. If the child is very young or can't drink from a cup, use a medication dropper or syringe. These devices frequently come prepackaged with paediatric drugs.

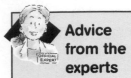

Advice from the experts

A trio of time-saving tips

When calculating safe paediatric dosages, save time and stop errors by following these suggestions:

- Carry a calculator for use when solving equations.
- Consult a formulary or drug handbook to verify a drug dose. When in doubt, call the pharmacist.
- Keep your patient's weight in kilograms at their bedside so you don't have to estimate it or weigh them in a hurry.

Advice from the experts

Giving medications to children

When giving oral and parenteral medications to children, safety is essential. Keep these points in mind:

- Check the child's mouth to make sure they have swallowed the oral drug.
- Carefully mix oral drugs that come in suspension form.
- Give intramuscular (I.M.) injections in the vastus lateralis muscle of infants who haven't started walking.
- Don't inject more than 1 ml into I.M. or subcutaneous sites.
- Rotate injection sites.

I.M. injections for infants

When giving intramuscular (I.M.) injections to infants, use the vastus lateralis muscle. Don't inject into the gluteus muscle until it's fully developed, which occurs when the child learns to walk. Use a 23 to 25G needle that's approximately 1.5 to 2.5 cm in length. These illustrations show how to give an I.M. injection using one- and two-person methods.

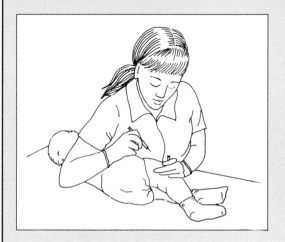
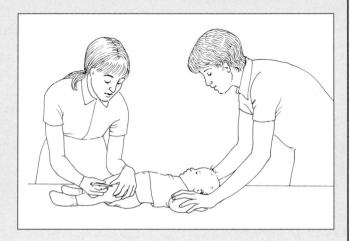

Mix it up

If the liquid drug is prepared as a suspension or as an insoluble drug in a liquid base, mix it thoroughly before you measure and administer it. This ensures that none of the drug remains settled out of the solution. Whenever you give an oral drug, check the child's mouth to make sure that all of the drug was swallowed.

Subcutaneous route

Paediatric patients also may receive childhood immunisations (such as the measles, mumps and rubella vaccine and other live-virus vaccines) and drugs such as insulin by the subcutaneous route. When giving subcutaneous injections, make sure each injection contains no more than 1 ml of solution. Any area with sufficient subcutaneous tissue may be used – the upper arm, abdomen and thigh are the most common.

Intramuscular route

Vaccines, such as that against diphtheria, pertussis and tetanus, are commonly administered by the I.M. route. (See *I.M. injections for infants*.) When giving I.M. injections, make sure each injection contains no more than 1 ml of solution. Give I.M. injections in the thighs of infants because their gluteal muscles don't develop until they learn to walk.

Finding the nerve

Be aware of the risk of nerve damage when selecting the site, needle length and injection technique.

Intravenous route

Fluids and drugs may also be administered by the I.V. route. I.V. site placement may be in a peripheral or central vein. Because paediatric patients can tolerate only a limited amount of fluid, dilute I.V. drugs and administer I.V. fluids cautiously. Always use an infusion pump with infants and small children.

Infiltration and inflammation alert!

Inspect I.V. sites frequently for signs of infiltration (cool, blanched and puffy skin) or inflammation (warm and reddened skin). Do this before, during and after the infusion because children's vessels are immature and damaged easily by drugs. If infiltration occurs, stop the infusion and consider placement for a new I.V. site.

Just passing through, making my I.V. inspection rounds... don't mind me!

Topical route

Medications may be administered topically in children as in adults. In infants and small children, the absorption of topical medications is greater because these children have:
- a thinner stratum corneum
- increased skin hydration
- a greater ratio of total body surface area to weight.

Also, the use of disposable nappies with a plastic-coated layer can increase topical drug absorption in the nappy area because the plastic coating can act like an occlusive dressing.

Baby wipes

When applying topical drugs on paediatric patients, wipe off any drug that remains on the skin from the previous application, and apply the new drug according to the prescription and the drug manufacturer's recommendations.

Calculation methods

To calculate and verify the safety of paediatric drug dosages, use the dosage-per-kilogram-of-body-weight method or the body surface area (BSA) method. Other methods, such as those based on age or the standard dosing used for adults, are less accurate and typically aren't used.

Whichever method you use, remember that you're professionally and legally responsible for checking the safety of a prescribed dose prior to administration.

Dosage per kilogram of body weight

Many pharmaceutical companies provide information about safe drug dosages for paediatric patients in milligrams per kilogram of body weight. This is the most accurate and common way to calculate paediatric dosages. Paediatric dosages are usually expressed as mg/kg/day or mg/kg/dose. Based on this information, you can determine the paediatric dose by multiplying the child's weight in kilograms by the required number of milligrams of drug per kilogram.

Shifting weight: from pounds to kilograms

While patients' weights should be measured using the metric system, they may sometimes be reported in pounds. In such cases, you must convert from pounds to kilograms before calculating the dosage per kilogram of body weight. Remember that 1 kg equals 2.2 lb.

Real-world problems

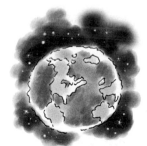

The following examples show how to use proportions to convert pounds to kilograms, how to calculate mg/kg/dose for one-time or as-needed (p.r.n.) medications, and how to calculate mg/kg/day for doses given around the clock to maintain a continuous drug effect.

A weighty problem

If your 6-year-old patient weighs 41.5 lb, how much does he weigh in kilograms?

Here's how to solve this problem using ratios:

- Set up the proportion, remembering that 2.2 lb equals 1 kg:

$$X : 41.5\,\text{lb} : : 1\,\text{kg} : 2.2\,\text{lb}$$

- Multiply the extremes and the means:

$$X \times 2.2\,\text{lb} = 1\,\text{kg} \times 41.5\,\text{lb}$$

- Solve for X by dividing each side of the equation by 2.2 lb and cancelling units that appear in both the numerator and denominator:

$$\frac{X \times 2.2 \,\text{lb}}{2.2 \,\text{lb}} = \frac{1 \,\text{kg} \times 41.5 \,\text{lb}}{2.2 \,\text{lb}}$$

$$X = \frac{41.5 \,\text{kg}}{2.2}$$

$$X = 18.9 \,\text{kg}$$

The child weighs 18.9 kg, rounded off to 19 kg.

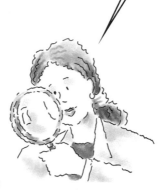

The real mystery is knowing what to put in the numerator and the denominator.

Milligram mystery

The nurse prescriber writes a prescription for a single dose of 20 mg/kg/dose of amoxicillin oral suspension for a toddler who weighs 9.1 kg. What's the dose in milligrams?

Here's how to solve this problem using fractions:

- Set up the proportion with the prescribed dosage in one fraction and the unknown dosage and the patient's weight in the other fraction:

$$\frac{20 \,\text{mg}}{1 \,\text{kg/dose}} = \frac{X}{9 \,\text{kg/dose}}$$

- Cross-multiply the fractions:

$$X \times 1 \,\text{kg/dose} = 20 \,\text{mg} \times 9 \,\text{kg/dose}$$

- Solve for X by dividing each side of the equation by 1 kg/dose and cancelling units that appear in both the numerator and denominator:

$$\frac{X \times 1 \,\text{kg/dose}}{1 \,\text{kg/dose}} = \frac{20 \,\text{mg} \times 9 \,\text{kg/dose}}{1 \,\text{kg/dose}}$$

$$X = 180 \,\text{mg}$$

The patient needs 180 mg of amoxicillin.

A perplexing penicillin problem

A child weighing 55 lb has been prescribed *phenoxymethylpenicillin oral suspension 56 mg/kg/day in four divided doses*. The suspension that is available is phenoxymethylpenicillin 125 mg/5 ml. What volume should you administer for each dose?

Here's how to solve this problem using ratios and fractions:

- First, convert the child's weight from pounds to kilograms by setting up the following proportion:

$$X : 55 \,\text{lb} : : 1 \,\text{kg} : 2.2 \,\text{lb}$$

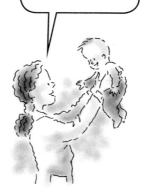

First, I need to figure out the child's weight in kilograms; then I can calculate the right dosage.

- Multiply the extremes and the means:

$$X \times 2.2 \text{ lb} = 1 \text{ kg} \times 55 \text{ lb}$$

- Solve for X by dividing each side of the equation by 2.2 lb and cancelling units that appear in both the numerator and denominator:

$$\frac{X \times 2.2\cancel{\text{ lb}}}{2.2\cancel{\text{ lb}}} = \frac{1 \text{ kg} \times 55\cancel{\text{ lb}}}{2.2\cancel{\text{ lb}}}$$

$$X = \frac{55 \text{ kg}}{2.2}$$

$$X = 25 \text{ kg}$$

- The child weighs 25 kg. Next, determine the total daily dosage by setting up a proportion with the patient's weight and the unknown dosage on one side and the prescribed dosage on the other side:

$$\frac{25 \text{ kg}}{X} = \frac{1 \text{ kg}}{56 \text{ mg}}$$

- Cross-multiply the fractions:

$$X \times 1 \text{ kg} = 56 \text{ mg} \times 25 \text{ kg}$$

- Solve for X by dividing each side of the equation by 1 kg and cancelling units that appear in both the numerator and denominator:

$$\frac{X \times 1\cancel{\text{ kg}}}{1\cancel{\text{ kg}}} = \frac{56 \text{ mg} \times 25 \cancel{\text{ kg}}}{1 \cancel{\text{ kg}}}$$

$$X = \frac{56 \text{ mg} \times 25}{1}$$

$$X = 1400 \text{ mg}$$

- The child's daily dosage is 1400 mg. Now, divide the daily dosage by 4 doses to determine the dose to administer every 6 hours:

$$X = \frac{1400 \text{ mg}}{4 \text{ doses}}$$

$$X = 350 \text{ mg/dose}$$

The child should receive 350 mg every 6 hours.
- Lastly, calculate the volume to give for each dose by setting up a proportion with the unknown volume and the amount in one dose on one side and the available dose on the other side:

$$\frac{X}{350 \text{ mg}} = \frac{5 \text{ ml}}{125 \text{ mg}}$$

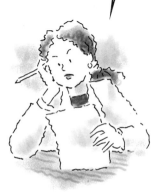

Next, I determine the dose to administer every 6 hours.

- Cross-multiply the fractions:

$$X \times 125 \text{ mg} = 5 \text{ ml} \times 350 \text{ mg}$$

- Solve for X by dividing each side of the equation by 125 mg and cancelling units that appear in both the numerator and denominator:

$$\frac{X \times \cancel{125 \text{ mg}}}{\cancel{125 \text{ mg}}} = \frac{5 \text{ ml} \times 350 \cancel{\text{ mg}}}{125 \cancel{\text{ mg}}}$$

$$X = \frac{5 \text{ ml} \times 350}{125}$$

$$X = \frac{1700 \text{ ml}}{125}$$

$$X = 14 \text{ ml}$$

You should administer 14 ml of the drug at each dose.

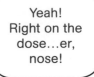

Yeah! Right on the dose...er, nose!

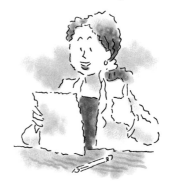

Dosage by BSA

The body surface area (BSA) method is used to calculate safe paediatric dosages for a limited number of drugs, such as anti-neoplastic or chemotherapeutic agents. (It's also used to calculate safe dosages for adult patients receiving these extremely potent drugs or drugs requiring great precision.)

BSA plot thickens

Calculating dosages by BSA involves two steps:

Plot the patient's height and weight on a chart called a nomogram to determine the BSA in square metres (m²). (See *What's in a nomogram?*)

Multiply the BSA by the prescribed paediatric dose in mg/m²/day.
Here's the formula:

$$\text{child's dose in mg} = \text{child's BSA in m}^2 \times \frac{\text{paediatric dose in mg}}{\text{m}^2/\text{day}}$$

What's in a nomogram?

Body surface area (BSA) is critical when calculating dosages for paediatric patients or for drugs that are extremely potent and need to be given in precise amounts. The nomogram shown here lets you plot the patient's height and weight to determine the BSA. Here's how it works:

- Locate the patient's height in the left column of the nomogram and weight in the right column.
- Use a ruler to draw a straight line connecting the two points. The point where the line intersects the surface area column indicates the patient's BSA in square metres.
- For an average-sized child, use the simplified nomogram in the box. Just find the child's weight in pounds on the left side of the scale, and then read the corresponding BSA on the right side.

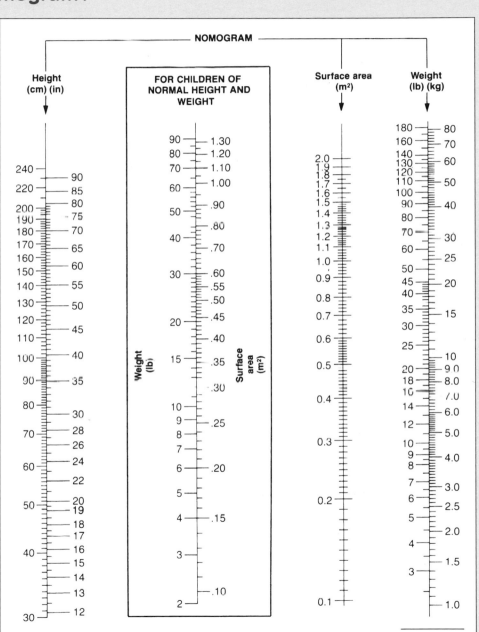

More real-world problems

The following problems show how this formula is used in the BSA method of dosage calculation.

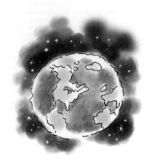

An engrossing etoposide equation

Etoposide 100 mg/m²/day has been prescribed for a child who's 40″ tall and weighs 64 lb. How much etoposide should the child receive daily?

- Use the nomogram to determine that the child's BSA is 0.96 m².
- Using the appropriate formula, determine the daily dosage:

$$X = 0.96 \text{ m}^2 \times \frac{100 \text{ mg}}{1 \text{ m}^2/\text{day}}$$

- Solve for X:

$$X = 0.96 \text{ m}^2 \times \frac{100 \text{ mg}}{1 \text{ m}^2/\text{day}}$$

The child needs 96 mg of etoposide per day.

A captivating chemotherapy question

A child prescribed *chemotherapy (120 mg/m²/day)* is 90 cm tall and weighs 18.2 kg. How much chemotherapeutic agent should the child receive each day?

- Use the nomogram to determine that the child's BSA is 0.72 m².
- Then, using the appropriate formula, determine the daily dose:
- Solve for X by cancelling units that appear in both the numerator and denominator, multiplying the child's BSA by the average adult dose, and dividing the result by the average adult BSA:

$$X = 0.72 \text{ m}^2 \times \frac{120 \text{ mg}}{1 \text{ m}^2/\text{day}}$$

- Solve for X:

$$X = 0.72 \text{ m}^2 \times \frac{120 \text{ mg}}{1 \text{ m}^2/\text{day}}$$

A dose of 86.4 mg should be administered daily.

Verifying calculations

Although the prescriber determines the medication dosage, the nurse is an important 'last line of defence' who verifies that the prescribed dosage is safe. Depending on your facility, you may have access to several reliable sources of information, including online computer services, drug references and other staff.

Look it up

Some nursing drug handbooks contain usual (recommended) paediatric dosages for commonly prescribed drugs (paediatric drug handbooks specifically developed for the special needs of infants and children are also available). The pharmacist is another excellent resource for verifying drug safety. And remember, you should always double-check complex calculations with another nurse.

Yet more real-world problems

Here are some real-world examples of verifying calculations.

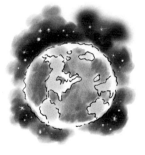

Clearing the way for chloral hydrate

Chloral hydrate 75 mg by mouth has been prescribed to sedate a 3-kg neonate for an electroencephalogram. The drug resource states that the usual (recommended) dosage of chloral hydrate for a neonate is 25 mg/kg/dose for sedation prior to a procedure. Was the correct dosage prescribed? Here's how to solve this problem using fractions:

• Set up the proportion with the usual dosage in one fraction and the unknown dosage and the patient's weight in the other fraction:

$$\frac{25 \text{ mg}}{1 \text{ kg/dose}} = \frac{X}{3 \text{ kg/dose}}$$

• Cross-multiply the fractions:

$$X \times 1 \text{ kg/dose} = 25 \text{ mg} \times 3 \text{ kg/dose}$$

• Solve for X by dividing each side of the equation by 1 kg/dose and cancelling units that appear in both the numerator and denominator:

$$\frac{X \times 1 \text{ kg/dose}}{1 \text{ kg/dose}} = \frac{25 \text{ mg} \times 3 \text{ kg/dose}}{1 \text{ kg/dose}}$$

The patient needs 75 mg of chloral hydrate. That's what was stated on the prescription and, therefore, the dose is safe to administer.

Penicillin puzzler

Phenoxymethylpenicillin oral suspension 250 mg, every 6 hours, has been prescribed for a patient who weighs 55 lb. Is the dose safe? The suspension that's available is phenoxymethylpenicillin 125 mg/5 ml. What volume should you administer for each dose?

Here's how to answer these questions using ratios and fractions:
• First, convert the child's weight from pounds to kilograms by setting up the following proportion:

$$X : 55 \text{ lb} :: 1 \text{ kg} : 2.2 \text{ lb}$$

• Multiply the extremes and the means:

$$X \times 2.2 \text{ lb} = 1 \text{ kg} \times 55 \text{ lb}$$

• Solve for X by dividing each side of the equation by 2.2. lb and cancelling units that appear in both the numerator and denominator:

$$\frac{X \times 2.2 \text{ lb}}{2.2 \text{ lb}} = \frac{1 \text{ kg} \times 55 \text{ lb}}{2.2 \text{ lb}}$$

$$X = \frac{55 \text{ kg}}{2.2}$$

$$X = 25 \text{ kg}$$

The child weighs 25 kg.
• Now verify the usual (recommended) dosage. The drug reference states to give phenoxymethylpenicillin 25 to 50 mg/kg/day orally in divided doses every 6 to 8 hours. This indicates a safe daily dosage range – a low dosage (25 mg/kg/day) and a high dosage (50 mg/kg/day). These are also the minimum (low dosage) and the maximum (high dosage) dosages for the day.
• Next, determine the usual total daily dosage range by setting up two proportions with the patient's weight on one side and the usual dosage (either the low dosage or the high dosage) on the other side. Let's look at the high dose first:

$$\frac{25 \text{ kg}}{X} = \frac{1 \text{ kg}}{50 \text{ mg}}$$

• Cross-multiply the fractions:

$$X \times 1 \text{ kg} = 50 \text{ mg} \times 25 \text{ kg}$$

• Solve for X by dividing each side of the equation by 1 kg and cancelling units that appear in both the numerator and denominator:

$$\frac{X \times 1 \text{ kg}}{1 \text{ kg}} = \frac{50 \text{ mg} \times 25 \text{ kg}}{1 \text{ kg}}$$

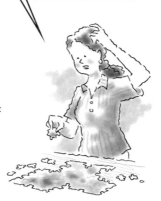

Let's see... I need to determine whether the dose is safe and what volume to give for each dose. Hmm... this really is a puzzle!

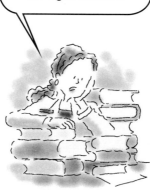

The first step is to see whether the prescribed dose is safe, based on the usual or recommended dosage listed in these drug references. So, let's get started.

$$X = \frac{50 \text{ mg} \times 25}{1}$$

$$X = 1250 \text{ mg}$$

• The child's maximum daily dosage is 1250 mg. Now divide the daily dosage by four doses to determine the maximum safe dose to administer every 6 hours:

$$X = \frac{1250 \text{ mg}}{4 \text{ doses}}$$

• Now repeat the same steps to determine the low or minimum dose:

$$\frac{25 \text{ kg}}{X} = \frac{1 \text{ kg}}{25 \text{ mg}}$$

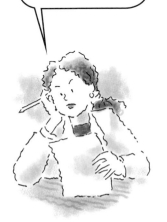

And now on to the minimum daily dosage and minimum safe dose to give every 6 hours.

• Cross-multiply the fractions:

$$X \times 1 \text{ kg} = 25 \text{ mg} \times 25 \text{ kg}$$

• Solve for X by dividing each side of the equation by 1 kg and cancelling like units:

$$\frac{X \times \cancel{1 \text{ kg}}}{\cancel{1 \text{ kg}}} = \frac{25 \text{ mg} \times 25 \cancel{\text{ kg}}}{1 \cancel{\text{ kg}}}$$

$$X = \frac{25 \text{ mg} \times 25}{1}$$

$$X = 625 \text{ mg}$$

• The child's minimum daily dosage is 625 mg. Now divide the daily dosage by four doses to determine the minimum safe dose to administer every 6 hours:

$$X = \frac{625 \text{ mg}}{4 \text{ doses}}$$

$$X = 156.25 \text{ mg or } 156 \text{ mg/dose}$$

The safe daily dosage range is 625 to 1250 mg per day for this child. In this case, 250 mg every 6 hours (or four doses per day) or a total dosage of 1000 mg (250 mg/dose × four doses) was prescribed. This falls within the safe daily range.

• The child can safely receive 250 mg every 6 hours. Lastly, calculate the volume to give for each dose by setting up a proportion with the unknown volume and the amount in one dose on one side and the available dose on the other side:

$$\frac{X}{250 \text{ mg}} = \frac{5 \text{ ml}}{125 \text{ mg}}$$

$$X \times 125 \text{ mg} = 5 \text{ ml} \times 250 \text{ mg}$$

- Solve for X by dividing each side of the equation by 125 mg and cancelling units that appear in both the numerator and denominator:

$$\frac{X \times \cancel{125 \text{ mg}}}{\cancel{125 \text{ mg}}} = \frac{5 \text{ ml} \times 250 \cancel{\text{mg}}}{125 \cancel{\text{mg}}}$$

$$X = \frac{5 \text{ ml} \times 250}{125}$$

$$X = \frac{1250 \text{ ml}}{125}$$

$$X = 10 \text{ ml}$$

You should administer 10 ml of the drug at each dose.

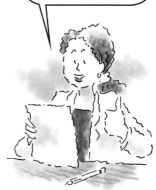

So, if my calculations are correct, the prescribed dose is safe to give, and the patient should receive 10 ml at each dose.

I.V. guidelines

I.V. fluids and drugs are administered by continuous or intermittent infusion. Because paediatric I.V. drug administration is so complex, be sure to follow all written guidelines and protocols about dosages, fluid volumes for dilution and administration rates when giving the drug.

Continuous infusions

A continuous infusion is used when the paediatric patient requires around-the-clock fluids, drug therapy or both. Fluids may be infused to maintain volume or to correct an existing fluid or electrolyte imbalance.

To prepare for a continuous drug infusion, add the drug to a small-volume bag of I.V. fluid or a volume-control device. Be sure to follow the manufacturer's guidelines for mixing the solution carefully. Remember that paediatric patients can tolerate only small amounts of fluid.

Usually, a volume-control device such as the Buretrol set, which maintains flow rate by using a positive-pressure pumping mechanism, is used for continuous as well as intermittent infusion. (See *I.V. infusion control*.)

Infusion basics: 5 steps

Follow these steps to start a continuous infusion:

✋ Calculate the dosage.

✌ Draw up the drug in a syringe; then add the drug to the I.V. bag or fluid chamber through the drug additive port, using aseptic technique.

🤟 Mix the drug thoroughly.

🖐 Label the I.V. bag or fluid chamber with the drug's name, the dosage, the time and date it was mixed, and your initials.

🖐 Hang the solution and administer the drug by infusion pump at the prescribed flow rate.

Intermittent infusions

Intermittent infusion is used commonly in acute and home care settings. If the paediatric patient is capable of normal enteral fluid intake, I.V. fluids or drug infusions may be necessary only at periodic intervals. A vascular access device can be kept in place, eliminating the need for continuous fluid infusion. The child can remain mobile, minimising the potential for volume overload.

Adjusting the volume

Volume-control devices have 100- to 150-ml fluid chambers, which are calibrated in 1-ml increments to allow accurate fluid administration. Medication-filled syringes with microtubing can also be used to infuse small volumes via syringe pumps. Accuracy is especially important with paediatric patients because children can't tolerate as much fluid as adults and are more prone to fluid and electrolyte imbalances. The rate of I.V. infusion must be carefully controlled to ensure proper absorption and to prevent or minimise toxicity associated with rapid infusion.

Starting an infusion: 10 steps

If you're using a volume-control device, follow these steps to start an intermittent infusion:
• Carefully calculate the prescribed volume of drug. Some facilities consider the drug volume as part of the diluent volume. For example, if 100 mg of a drug is contained in 5 ml of fluid and the total fluid volume should be 50 ml, add 45 ml of diluent because

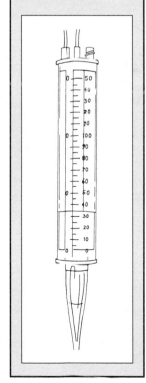

I.V. infusion control

Accurate fluid administration is extremely important for paediatric patients. So syringes, infusion pumps and other volume-control devices are used extensively to regulate continuous and intermittent I.V. infusions. One typical device, the Buretrol set, is shown below.

45 ml of diluent plus 5 ml of fluid drug volume equals a total of 50 ml.
- After careful calculation, draw up the prescribed volume of drug into a syringe.
- Add the drug to the fluid chamber through the drug additive port, using aseptic technique.
- Mix the drug thoroughly.
- Attach the volume-control device to an electronic infusion pump to control the infusion rate.
- Calculate the appropriate flow rate and infuse the drug.
- Label the volume-control device with the name of the drug.
- When the infusion is complete, flush the line to clear the tubing of the drug. A specific flush volume may be requested by the prescriber or a standard volume protocol may be followed based on the tubing volume, the patient's condition or both. Administer the flush at the same rate as the drug. Label the volume-control device to indicate that the flush is infusing.
- With an intermittent infusion, disconnect the device when the flush is complete.
- During the infusion, check the I.V. site frequently for infiltration because children's veins are more prone to this problem.

Calculating paediatric fluid needs

Children's fluid needs are proportionally greater than those of adults, so children are more vulnerable to changes in fluid and electrolyte balance. Because their extracellular fluid has a higher percentage of water, children's fluid exchange rates are two to three times greater than those of adults, leaving them more susceptible to dehydration.

Three ways to figure fluids

Determining and meeting the fluid needs of children are important nursing responsibilities. You can calculate the number of millilitres of fluid a child needs based on:
- weight in kilograms
- metabolism (calories required)
- BSA in square metres.
    Although results may vary slightly, all three methods are appropriate. Keep in mind that fluid replacement can also be affected by clinical conditions that cause fluid retention or loss. Children with these conditions should receive fluids based on their individual needs.

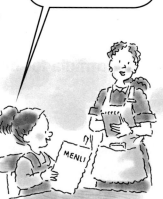

...and I'd like the apple juice, the milk and the fruit smoothie.... You know how I need my fluids!

Fluid needs based on weight

You may use three different formulas to calculate a child's fluid needs based on their weight.

Fluid formula for tiny tots

A child who weighs less than 10 kg requires 100 ml of fluid per kilogram of body weight. To determine this child's fluid needs, first convert the weight (if required) from pounds to kilograms. Then multiply the results by 100 ml/kg/day.

Here's the formula:

weight in kg × 100 ml/kg/day = fluid needs in ml/day

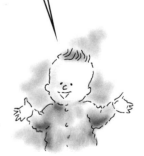

As you've probably guessed, my fluid needs keep changing as I grow.... Think I'm due for a change now!

Fluid formula for middleweights

A child weighing 10 to 20 kg requires 1000 ml of fluid per day for the first 10 kg plus 50 ml for every kilogram over 10. To determine this child's fluid needs, follow these steps:
• Convert the weight (again, if necessary) from pounds to kilograms.
• Subtract 10 kg from the child's total weight, and then multiply the result by 50 ml/kg/day to find the child's additional fluid needs.

Here's the formula:

(total kg − 10 kg) × 50 ml/kg/day = additional fluid need in ml/day

• Add the additional daily fluid need to the 1000 ml/day required for the first 10 kg. The total is the child's daily fluid requirement:

1000 ml/day + additional fluid need = fluid needs in ml/day

Fluid formula for bigger kids

A child weighing more than 20 kg requires 1500 ml of fluid for the first 20 kg plus 20 ml for each additional kilogram. To determine this child's fluid needs, follow these steps:
• Convert the child's weight from pounds to kilograms (if given in pounds).
• Subtract 20 kg from the child's total weight, and then multiply the result by 20 ml/kg to find the child's additional fluid need.

Here's the formula:

(total kg − 20 kg) × 20 ml/kg/day = additional fluid need in ml/day

- Because the child needs 1500 ml of fluid per day for the first 20 kg, add the additional fluid need to 1500 ml. The total is the child's daily fluid requirement:

    1500 ml/day + additional fluid need = fluid needs in ml/day

    Use this information to solve the following problem.

Finding a fluid solution

How much fluid should you give a 44-lb patient over 24 hours to meet her maintenance needs?

- First, convert 44 lb to kilograms by setting up a proportion with fractions. (Remember that 1 kg equals 2.2 lb.)

$$\frac{44 \text{ lb}}{X} = \frac{2.2 \text{ lb}}{1 \text{kg}}$$

- Cross-multiply the fractions, and then solve for X by dividing both sides of the equation by 2.2 lb and cancelling units that appear in both the numerator and denominator:

$$X \times 2.2 \text{ lb} = 44 \text{ lb} \times 1 \text{kg}$$

$$\frac{X \times 2.2 \text{ lb}}{2.2 \text{ lb}} = \frac{44 \text{ lb} \times 1 \text{ kg}}{2.2 \text{ lb}}$$

$$X = \frac{44 \text{ kg}}{2.2}$$

$$X = 20 \text{ kg}$$

- The child weighs 20 kg. Now, subtract 10 kg from the child's weight, and multiply the result by 50 ml/kg/day to find the child's additional fluid need:

$$X = (20 \text{ kg} - 10 \text{ kg}) \times 50 \text{ ml/kg/day}$$

$$X = 10 \text{ kg} \times 50 \text{ ml/kg/day}$$

$$X = 500 \text{ ml/day additional fluid need}$$

- Next, add the additional fluid need to the 1000 ml/day required for the first 10 kg (because the child weighs between 10 and 20 kg).

$$X = 1000 \text{ ml/day} + 500 \text{ ml/day}$$

$$X = 1500 \text{ ml/day}$$

The child should receive 1500 ml of fluid in 24 hours to meet her fluid maintenance needs.

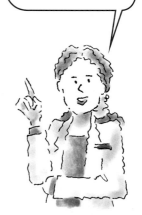

Look closely! I can cancel kilograms in this equation to find the child's additional fluid need in ml/day.

Fluid needs based on calories

You can calculate fluid needs based on calories because water is necessary for metabolism. A child should receive 120 ml of fluid for every 100 kilocalories (kcal) of metabolism, also commonly called calories.

Fluids help burn calories

To calculate fluid requirements based on calorie requirements, follow these steps:
• Find the child's calorie requirements. You can take this information from a table of recommended dietary allowances for children, or you can have a dietitian calculate it.
• Divide the calorie requirements by 100 kcal because fluid requirements are determined for every 100 calories.
• Multiply the results by 120 ml – the amount of fluid required for every 100 kcal. Here's the formula:

$$\text{fluid requirements in ml/day} = \frac{\text{calorie requirements}}{100 \text{ kcal}} \times 120 \text{ ml}$$

Use the information above to solve the following problem.

Calorie-conscious problem

Your paediatric patient uses 900 calories/day. What are his daily fluid requirements?
• Set up the formula, inserting the appropriate numbers and substituting X for the unknown amount of fluid:

$$X = \frac{900 \text{ kcal}}{100 \text{ kcal}} \times 120 \text{ ml}$$

$$X = 9 \times 120 \text{ ml}$$

$$X = 1080 \text{ ml}$$

The patient needs 1080 ml of fluid per day.

Fluid needs based on BSA

Another method for determining paediatric maintenance fluid requirements is based on the child's BSA. To calculate the daily fluid needs of a child who isn't dehydrated, multiply the BSA by 1500, as shown in this formula:

$$\text{fluid maintenance needs in ml/day} = \text{BSA in m}^2 \times 1500 \text{ ml/day/m}^2$$

Use this formula to solve the following problem.

BSA-based problem

Your patient is 90 cm tall and weighs 18.2 kg. If his BSA is 0.72 m², how much fluid does he need each day?
• Set up the equation, inserting the appropriate numbers and substituting X for the unknown amount of fluid. Then solve for X:

$$X = 0.72 \text{ m}^2 \times 1500 \text{ ml/day/m}^2$$

$$X = 1080 \text{ ml/day/ m}^2$$

The child needs 1080 ml of fluid per day.

A final real-world problem

Use your calculation skills to solve the following paediatric dosage problem.

An ampicillin answer

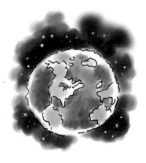

A single dose of *360 mg of ampicillin* has been prescribed for an infant who weighs 8 lb. Your paediatric drug handbook states that the usual (recommended) ampicillin dose as 100 mg/kg/dose. After reconstituting with sterile water, the ampicillin is available in a concentration of 500 mg/5 ml. Is the dose prescribed correct for the patient? What volume of ampicillin should you administer to the infant?

First, you'll need to determine whether the dose prescribed is correct.
• Set up the proportion to determine the child's weight in kilograms. Remember that 1 kg = 2.2 lb:

$$\frac{X}{8 \text{ lb}} = \frac{1 \text{ kg}}{2.2 \text{ lb}}$$

• Cross-multiply the fractions:

$$X \times 2.2 \text{ lb} = 8 \text{ lb} \times 1 \text{ kg}$$

• Solve for X by dividing both sides of the equation by 2.2 lb and cancelling units that appear in both the numerator and denominator:

$$\frac{X \times 2.2 \text{ lb}}{2.2 \text{ lb}} = \frac{8 \text{ lb} \times 1 \text{ kg}}{2.2 \text{ lb}}$$

$$X = \frac{8 \times 1 \text{ kg}}{2.2}$$

$$X = 3.63 \text{ kg}$$

The infant weighs 3.63 kg, rounded off to 3.6 kg.

- Next, set up a proportion with the recommended dosage (from the paediatric drug reference) in one fraction and the unknown dosage and the patient's weight in the other fraction:

$$\frac{100 \text{ mg}}{1 \text{ kg/dose}} = \frac{X}{3.6 \text{ kg/dose}}$$

- Cross-multiply the fractions:

$$X \times 1 \text{ kg/dose} = 100 \text{ mg} \times 3.6 \text{ kg/dose}$$

- Solve for X by dividing each side of the equation by 1 kg/dose and cancelling units that appear in both the numerator and denominator:

$$\frac{X \times 1 \text{ kg/dose}}{1 \text{ kg/dose}} = \frac{100 \text{ mg} \times 3.6 \text{ kg/dose}}{1 \text{ kg/dose}}$$

$$X = \frac{100 \text{ mg} \times 3.6}{1}$$

$$X = 360 \text{ mg}$$

So, the prescription was correct: 100 mg/kg/dose for a child who weighs 3.6 kg is 360 mg.

Next, determine the volume of drug you should administer to the infant.

- Set up a proportion with the known concentration in one fraction and the desired dose and unknown volume in the other fraction:

$$\frac{500 \text{ mg}}{5 \text{ ml}} = \frac{360 \text{ mg}}{X}$$

- Cross-multiply the fractions:

$$500 \text{ mg} \times X = 360 \text{ mg} \times 5 \text{ ml}$$

- Solve for X by dividing both sides of the equation by 500 mg and cancelling units that appear in both the numerator and denominator:

$$\frac{500 \text{ mg} \times X}{500 \text{ mg}} = \frac{360 \text{ mg} \times 5 \text{ ml}}{500 \text{ mg}}$$

$$X = \frac{360 \times 5 \text{ ml}}{500 \text{ mg}}$$

$$X = 3.6 \text{ ml}$$

You should administer 3.6 ml of reconstituted ampicillin to give the patient 360 mg.

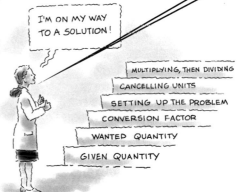

Now that you know the dose is correct, you need to determine how much medication to administer. Just follow the steps you've been using all along.

I'M ON MY WAY TO A SOLUTION!

MULTIPLYING, THEN DIVIDING

CANCELLING UNITS

SETTING UP THE PROBLEM

CONVERSION FACTOR

WANTED QUANTITY

GIVEN QUANTITY

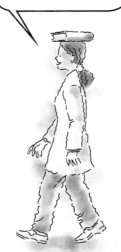

See, taking the right steps will lead you to the correct solution every time.

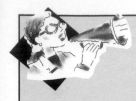

That's a wrap!

Calculating paediatric dosages review

When determining paediatric dosage calculations, be sure to keep these points in mind.

Route guidelines

- Oral medications may be given as liquid suspensions
  - Mix drug before measuring out dose
  - Never crush timed-release capsules or tablets or enteric-coated drugs
- Subcutaneous routes are commonly used for childhood immunisations and insulin injections
  - Make sure injection contains no more than 1 ml of solution
  - Administer in any area with sufficient subcutaneous tissue
- I.M. injection routes are commonly used for vaccines
  - Never inject more than 1 ml of solution
  - Administer in the thigh of infants
- I.V. drugs should be diluted carefully and administered cautiously
  - Use an infusion pump used with infants and small children
- For topical route, absorption is greater in infants and small children
  - Wipe off any remaining drug after application
  - Apply according to doctor's prescription and drug manufacturer's recommendations

Dosage per kilogram

- Dosages are expressed as mg/kg/day or mg/kg/dose.

- Multiply the child's weight in kilograms by the required milligrams of drug per kilogram.

BSA

- Measured in m^2
- Determined through intersection of height and weight on a nomogram
- Multiplied by the prescribed dose in $mg/m^2/day$ to calculate safe paediatric dosages

Weight-based formulas for fluid needs

- A child weighing less than 10 kg: weight in kg $\times$ 100 ml = fluid needs in ml/day
- A child weighing 10 to 20 kg: (total kg − 10 kg) $\times$ 50 ml = additional fluid need in ml/day; 1000 ml/day + additional fluid need = fluid needs in ml/day
- A child weighing more than 20 kg: (total kg − 20 kg) = 20 ml $\times$ additional fluid need in ml/day; 1500 ml/day + additional fluid need = fluid needs in ml/day

Calorie-based formula for fluid needs

- Fluid-to-calorie ratio: 120 ml per 100 kcal
- Fluid requirements in ml/day = (calorie requirements ÷ 100 kcal) $\times$ 120 ml

BSA-based formula for fluid needs

- For a nondehydrated child: fluid maintenance needs in ml/day = BSA in m^2 $\times$ 1500 ml/day/m^2

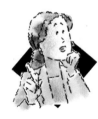

Quick quiz

1. If the suggested paediatric dosage for a drug is 35 mg/kg/day, the amount to give an infant weighing 5 kg is:
 A. 250 mg
 B. 175 mg
 C. 75 mg
 D. 50 mg

Answer: B. To solve this problem, set up a proportion with the suggested dosage in one ratio and the unknown quantity in the other. Multiply the means and extremes, and then divide each side of the equation by the value that appears on the X side of the equation. Cancel units that appear in the numerator and denominator.

2. A child who uses 1000 calories per day has a daily fluid requirement of:
 A. 1200 ml
 B. 1000 ml
 C. 500 ml
 D. 200 ml

Answer: A. Use the equation for calculating fluid needs based on kilocalories, inserting the appropriate numbers. Then solve for X.

3. If a patient is 100 cm tall, weighs 29 kg, and has a BSA of $0.96 \, m^2$, how much fluid does he require per day?
 A. 140 ml
 B. 1040 ml
 C. 1400 ml
 D. 1440 ml

Answer: D. Use the equation for calculating fluid needs based on BSA, inserting the appropriate numbers. Then solve for X.

4. Your patient weighs 8 kg. What are her daily fluid needs?
 A. 1000 ml/day
 B. 900 ml/day
 C. 800 ml/day
 D. 600 ml/day

Answer: C. Set up the equation using the formula weight in kilograms multiplied by 100 ml/kg/day. Cancel like units:

$$8 \, \cancel{kg} \times 100 \, ml/\cancel{kg}/day$$

$$800 \, ml/day$$

5.   The chart used to determine BSA is the:
     A.   monogram.
     B.   nomogram.
     C.   paediagram.
     D.   infogram.
Answer: B. A nomogram lets you plot the patient's height and weight to determine BSA.

Scoring

☆☆☆   If you answered all five items correctly, way to go! You're the pride and joy of precise paediatric dosages.

☆☆   If you answered four items correctly, we're impressed! There's nothing infantile about your abilities.

☆   If you answered fewer than four items correctly, review and try again! You'll be a specialist in special calculations before you know it.

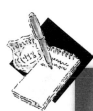

15 Calculating obstetric drug dosages

Just the facts

In this chapter, you'll learn:

♦ how to assess the mother and foetus during medication administration
♦ common obstetric drugs and their adverse effects
♦ how to calculate obstetric dosages.

A look at obstetric drug administration

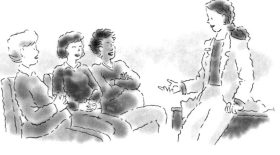

Drugs have multiple uses during labour and delivery.

During pregnancy, labour and delivery, and the postpartum period, drugs are commonly given to the mother for four reasons:

- to control pregnancy-induced hypertension

- to inhibit preterm labour

- to induce labour

- to prevent postpartum haemorrhage.

Drugs administered to the mother before delivery can also affect the foetus, so both mother and foetus require meticulous monitoring. *Remember:* you're caring for two patients at once, so there's a narrow margin for error.

Assessing the mother and foetus

When administering medications, frequently check the mother's vital signs, urine output, uterine contractions and deep tendon

Assessing the mother's body systems

Assessment is a critical part of obstetric nursing. Here's what to assess in each of the mother's body systems.

Neurological system

- Deep tendon reflexes when magnesium sulphate is infusing
- Pain
- Orientation (because disorientation can indicate hypoxaemia or water intoxication)

Cardiovascular system

- Vital signs
- Extremities for peripheral oedema with large-volume infusions
- Pulses and skin temperature in the lower extremities for evidence of deep-vein thrombosis; also for Homans' sign by dorsiflexing the foot while supporting the leg (deep calf pain may indicate thrombophlebitis)
- I.V. site to prevent infiltration

Respiratory system

- Breath sounds
- Need for oxygen
- Lungs for pulmonary oedema with large-volume infusions

GI system

- Abdomen for contractions when oxytocin is infusing
- Abdomen for bowel sounds after delivery
- Ability to pass flatus or move bowels before discharge

Genitourinary system

- Urine output
- Fluid balance to check for decreased renal function

reflexes. Carefully assess fluid intake and output along with breath sounds to reduce the mother's risk of fluid overload, which can lead to acute pulmonary oedema. (See *Assessing the mother's body systems*.)

Fluid monitoring is especially critical in women with pregnancy-induced hypertension, which can cause decreased renal function. It's also important with drugs given to inhibit preterm labour because of their anti-diuretic effect.

The foetus is also the focus

While you're evaluating the mother, be sure to evaluate the foetus's response to drug therapy. Constantly assess foetal heart tones and heart rate by connecting the mother to an electronic foetal monitor. This monitor records the heart rate and also provides a tracing of it.

Be alert for a sudden increase or decrease in foetal heart rate, which may signal an adverse reaction to treatment. If either occurs, discontinue the drug immediately. (See *It's got a good beat: contractions and foetal heart rate*.)

Continuous monitoring of foetal heart tones and heart rate is necessary during drug therapy.

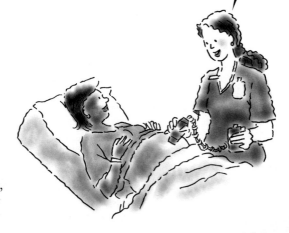

Advice from the experts

It's got a good beat: contractions and foetal heart rate

Electronic foetal monitoring allows you to assess the mother's contractions as well as the foetal heart rate. Follow these steps.

1. Evaluate the mother's contraction pattern.

2. Note the characteristics of the contractions.
   • What's the frequency?
   • What's the duration?
   • What's the intensity?

3. Evaluate the foetal heart rate after establishing a baseline.
   • Is the rate within normal range?
   • Is tachycardia present?
   • Is bradycardia present?

4. Determine the foetal heart rate variability.
   • What's the short-term variability (only with internal foetal monitoring)?
   • What's the long-term variability?

5. Assess for changes in foetal heart rate characteristics.
   • Is acceleration or increased heart rate present with contractions?
   • Is deceleration or decreased heart rate present with contractions?
   • Is the heart rate waveform regular and uniform in shape?
   • Is the heart rate waveform irregular in shape?

Common obstetric drugs

Drugs used during pregnancy, labour and delivery, and the postpartum period include:
• terbutaline
• magnesium sulphate
• dinoprostone
• oxytocin. (See *The lowdown on four obstetric drugs*.)

Terbutaline

Terbutaline is used to inhibit preterm labour. It stimulates the beta$_2$-adrenergic receptors in the uterine smooth muscle and inhibits contractility.

A preterm proposition

To administer terbutaline, mix it in a compatible I.V. solution and administer it through an infusion pump. Then titrate the dose every 10 minutes until the contractions subside, the maximum dose is reached, or the patient is unable to tolerate the drug because of its adverse effects.

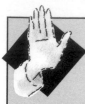

Before you give that drug!

The lowdown on four obstetric drugs

This table lists some common drugs used in the obstetric setting along with their actions, adverse reactions and nursing considerations.

Drug	Action	Adverse reactions	Nursing considerations
Terbutaline	Relaxes uterine muscle by acting on beta$_2$-adrenergic receptors; inhibits uterine contractions	**Maternal** • Blood: increased liver enzymes • Central nervous system (CNS): seizures, nervousness, tremour, headache, drowsiness, flushing, sweating • Cardiovascular (CV): increased heart rate, changes in blood pressure, palpitations, chest discomfort • Eye, ear, nose and throat (EENT): tinnitus • GI: nausea, vomiting, altered taste • Respiratory: dyspnea, wheezing	• Use cautiously in patients with diabetes, hypertension, hyperthyroidism, severe cardiac disease and arrhythmias. • Protect from light. Don't use if discoloured. • Explain the need for the drug to the patient and family. • Give subcutaneous injection in lateral deltoid area. • Warn the patient about the possibility of paradoxical bronchospasm. • Tell the patient she may use tablets and aerosol concomitantly. • Tell the patient how to administer a metered dose. • Monitor the neonate for hypoglycaemia. • Monitor the patient's blood glucose level with long-term use.
Magnesium sulphate	May decrease acetylcholine released by nerve impulse, but anti-convulsant mechanisms unknown	**Maternal** • CNS: sweating, drowsiness, depressed reflexes, flaccid paralysis, hypothermia, flushing, blurred vision • CV: hypotension, circulatory collapse, depressed cardiac function, heart block • Other: fatal respiratory paralysis, hypocalcaemia with tetany	• Use cautiously in labour and in those with impaired renal function, myocardial damage or heart block. • This drug may be used as a tocolytic agent to inhibit premature labour; it can decrease the frequency and force of uterine contractions. • Keep calcium gluconate available to reverse magnesium sulphate intoxication. • Use cautiously in patients undergoing digitalisation because arrhythmias may occur. • Watch for respiratory depression. • Monitor intake and output. • Monitor deep tendon reflexes. • Maximum infusion is 150 mg/minute. • Signs of hypermagnesaemia begin to appear at blood levels of 4 mmol/L. • This drug should be stopped at least 2 hours before delivery to avoid foetal respiratory depression. • Monitor the neonate for magnesium sulphate toxicity.

The lowdown on four obstetric drugs (continued)

Drug	Action	Adverse reactions	Nursing considerations
Dinoprostone	A prostaglandin that produces strong, prompt contractions of uterine smooth muscle; facilitates cervical dilations by directly softening the cervix	*Maternal* • CNS: fever, headache, dizziness, anxiety, paresthesia, weakness, syncope • CV: chest pain, arrhythmias • EENT: blurred vision, eye pain • GI: nausea, vomiting, diarrhoea • Genitourinary: vaginal pain, vaginitis, endometritis *Foetal* • CNS: hypotonia, hyperstimulation • Respiratory: respiratory depression • CV: bradycardia • Other: intrauterine foetal sepsis	• Use only with the patient in or near a delivery suite. Critical care facilities should be available. • After administration of the gel form of the drug, the patient should remain supine for 10 minutes. • Have the patient remain supine for 2 hours after insertion of the vaginal insert form of the drug. • Remove the vaginal insert with onset of active labour or 12 hours after insertion. • Monitor the foetus accordingly. • If hyperstimulation of the uterus occurs, gently flush the vagina with sterile saline solution. • Treat dinoprostone-induced fever (usually self-limiting and transient) with water sponging and increased fluid intake, not with aspirin.
Oxytocin	Causes potent and selective stimulation of uterine and mammary gland smooth muscle	*Maternal* • Blood: afibrinogenaemia (may be from postpartum bleeding) • CNS: subarachnoid haemorrhage resulting from hypertension; seizures or coma resulting from water intoxication • CV: hypotension, increased heart rate, systemic venous return, increased cardiac output, arrhythmias • Other: hypersensitivity, tetanic uterine contractions, abruptio placentae, impaired uterine blood flow, increased uterine motility, uterine rupture *Foetal* • Blood: hyperbilirubinaemia, hypercapnia • CV: bradycardia, tachycardia, premature ventricular contractions, variable deceleration of heart rate • Respiratory: hypoxia, asphyxia, death • CNS: brain damage, seizures • EENT: retinal haemorrhage • GI: hepatic necrosis	• Oxytocin is contraindicated in cephalopelvic disproportion; where delivery requires conversion, as in transverse lie; in foetal distress; when delivery isn't imminent; and in other obstetric emergencies. • Administer by piggyback infusion so the drug can be discontinued without interrupting the I.V. line. Don't give by I.V. bolus injection. • Don't infuse in more than one site. • Monitor and record uterine contractions, heart rate, blood pressure, intrauterine pressure, foetal heart rate and character of blood loss every 15 minutes. • Have magnesium sulphate (20% solution) available for relaxation of myometrium. • Monitor fluid intake and output. Anti-diuretic effect may lead to fluid overload, seizures and coma.

Magnesium sulphate

Another drug used during labour and delivery is magnesium sulphate, which prevents or controls seizures that may be caused by pregnancy-induced hypertension. The drug may decrease acetylcholine levels, but its exact anti-convulsant mechanism is unknown.

Control those seizures

To administer magnesium sulphate, first give a loading dose (a high dose given over a short time to rapidly reach a therapeutic drug level). This should be followed by an infusion at a lower dose, as prescribed.

During the infusion, closely assess knee jerk and patellar reflexes; loss of these signals drug toxicity. If toxicity is suspected, immediately stop the infusion and notify the prescriber. Calcium gluconate may be prescribed as an antidote.

Dinoprostone

Dinoprostone – a drug used to induce labour – is used to open the cervix in pregnant patients at or near term.

Scope it out

Dinoprostone is available as an endocervical gel, a vaginal insert or a vaginal suppository.

Warm and... gel-like

For administration of dinoprostone, have the patient lie on her back; the cervix will then be examined using a speculum. Then assist with insertion of the gel, using aseptic technique. A catheter provided with the drug is used to administer the gel into the cervical canal just below the level of the internal os. Warm the gel to room temperature before using. It isn't necessary to warm the vaginal inserts before giving; however, a minimal amount of water-soluble jelly may be used to aid insertion.

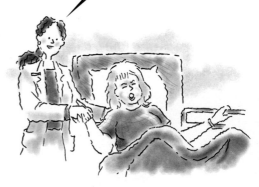

Okay, Mrs Brown. We'll be inducing labour very soon now. Just try to hang in there!

Oxytocin

Oxytocin – the drug most commonly used to induce labour – selectively stimulates uterine smooth muscle.

Compelling contractions

After mixing oxytocin with a compatible solution, administer it by piggyback with an I.V. infusion pump and titrate until a normal contraction pattern occurs. When labour is firmly established, a decrease in the infusion rate may be prescribed. Carefully monitor contraction strength because the drug can cause severe contractions that can lead to uterine rupture as well as foetal and maternal death.

Bleeding blockade

Oxytocin may also be used to control bleeding after delivery of the placenta. To control bleeding, add the drug to 1 L of I.V. fluid, and then infuse it at a rate that controls bleeding but doesn't exceed 20 milliunits (mU) per minute. Don't administer oxytocin by I.V. push.

Dosage calculations

In the labour and delivery unit, you must be especially careful to calculate and administer drugs accurately. For one thing, you may be dealing with life-threatening problems, such as haemorrhage and seizures caused by pregnancy-induced hypertension.

Administering accurate dosages to the mother helps avoid foetal complications. Be sure to examine drug labels closely. They contain valuable information for calculating dosages.

Real-world problems

These examples show how to calculate obstetric drugs using proportions.

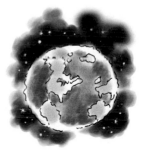

Overdue? Order oxytocin

Your patient is 10 days overdue, so oxytocin has been prescribed to stimulate labour. The prescription reads *1 ml (10 units) oxytocin in 1 L (1000 ml) in normal saline; infuse via pump at 2 mU/minute for 20 minutes and then increase flow rate to 3 mU/minute*. What's the solution's concentration? What's the flow rate needed to deliver 2 mU/minute for 20 minutes? What's the flow rate needed to deliver 3 mU/minute thereafter?

• Determine the concentration of the solution by setting up a proportion with the prescribed concentration in one fraction and the unknown concentration in the other fraction:

$$\frac{10 \text{ units}}{1000 \text{ ml}} = \frac{X}{1 \text{ ml}}$$

• Cross-multiply the fractions:

$$X \times 1000 \text{ ml} = 10 \text{ units} \times 1 \text{ ml}$$

- Solve for X by dividing both sides of the equation by 1000 ml and cancelling units that appear in both the numerator and denominator:

$$\frac{X \times \cancel{1000\ ml}}{\cancel{1000\ ml}} = \frac{10\ units \times 1\ \cancel{ml}}{1000\ \cancel{ml}}$$

$$X = \frac{10\ units}{1000}$$

$$X = 0.01\ unit$$

- The amount 0.01 unit can be written in milliunits (mU): 1 mU is $\frac{1}{1000}$ of a unit; 1000 mU is 1 unit. Therefore, 0.01 unit times 1000 equals 10 mU. So the concentration is 10 mU/ml.
- Next, determine the flow rate. If the prescribed dosage of oxytocin is 2 mU/minute for 20 minutes, the patient receives a total of 40 mU. To calculate the rate needed to provide that dose, set up a proportion with the known concentration in one fraction and the total oxytocin dose and unknown flow rate in the other:

$$\frac{10\ mU}{1\ ml} = \frac{40\ mU}{X}$$

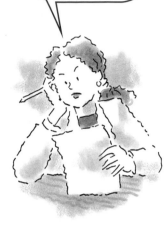

I need to determine the flow rate for the first 20 minutes.

- Cross-multiply the fractions:

$$X \times 10\ mU = 1\ ml \times 40\ mU$$

- Solve for X by dividing both sides of the equation by 10 mU and cancelling units that appear in both the numerator and denominator:

$$\frac{X \times \cancel{10\ mU}}{\cancel{10\ mU}} = \frac{1\ ml \times 40\ \cancel{mU}}{10\ \cancel{mU}}$$

$$X = \frac{40\ ml}{10}$$

$$X = 4\ ml$$

- The flow rate is 4 ml/20 minutes. Because this drug must be delivered by infusion pump, compute the hourly flow rate by multiplying the 20-minute rate by 3:

$$4\ ml/20\ minutes \times 3 = 12\ ml/hour$$

- The hourly flow rate is 12 ml/hour. Lastly, calculate the flow rate to be used after the first 20 minutes, resulting in 3 mU/minute (180 mU/hour). Having calculated the solution's concentration as 10 mU/ml, set up a proportion with the known concentration in one fraction and the increased oxytocin dose and the unknown flow rate in the other fraction:

$$\frac{10\ mU}{1\ ml} = \frac{180\ mU}{X}$$

- Cross-multiply the fractions:

$$X \times 10\ mU = 1\ ml \times 180\ mU$$

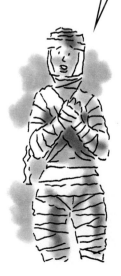

I think we'll have a new 'mummy' on the unit by the time this problem is finished!

- Solve for X by dividing both sides of the equation by 10 mU and cancelling units that appear in both the numerator and denominator:

$$\frac{X \times \cancel{10\,mU}}{10\,mU} = \frac{1\;ml \times 180\,\cancel{mU}}{10\,\cancel{mU}}$$

$$X = \frac{180\;ml}{10}$$

$$X = 18\,ml$$

- After 20 minutes, reset the pump to deliver 18 ml/hour. That's 18 ml/60 minutes, or 0.3 ml/minute. Because there are 10 mU/ml, multiply 10 by 0.3 ml/minute to verify that this flow rate does provide 3 mU/minute.

Seizure? Stop it with magnesium sulphate

Your patient is at risk from a seizure due to pregnancy-induced hypertension. The doctor prescribes *4 g (4000 mg) magnesium sulphate in 250 ml 5% glucose in water, to be infused at 2 g/hour*. What's the flow rate in millilitres per hour?

Here's one approach to solving this problem:
- Set up a proportion with the known concentration in one fraction and the flow rate in grams and the unknown flow rate in millilitres in the other fraction:

$$\frac{4\;g}{250\;ml} = \frac{2\;g}{X}$$

- Cross-multiply the fractions:

$$X \times 4\,g = 250\,ml \times 2\,g$$

- Solve for X by dividing each side of the equation by 4 g and cancelling units that appear in both the numerator and denominator:

$$\frac{X \times \cancel{4\,g}}{\cancel{4\,g}} = \frac{250\;ml \times 2\,\cancel{g}}{4\,\cancel{g}}$$

$$X = \frac{250\;ml \times 2}{4}$$

$$X = \frac{500\;ml}{4}$$

$$X = 125\,ml$$

The magnesium sulphate solution should be infused at 125 ml/hour.

Let's seize that problem again

Here's another approach to solving the same problem:

- First, calculate the strength of the solution by setting up a proportion with the known strength in one fraction and the unknown strength in the other fraction:

$$\frac{4\,g}{250\,ml} = \frac{X}{1\,ml}$$

- Cross-multiply the fractions:

$$X \times 250\,ml = 4\,g \times 1\,ml$$

- Solve for X by dividing each side of the equation by 250 ml and cancelling units that appear in both the numerator and denominator:

$$\frac{X \times 250\,\cancel{ml}}{250\,\cancel{ml}} = \frac{4\,g \times 1\,\cancel{ml}}{250\,\cancel{ml}}$$

$$X = \frac{4\,g}{250}$$

$$X = 0.016\,g$$

- The solution's strength is 0.016 g/ml. Next, calculate the flow rate by setting up another proportion with the solution concentration in one fraction and the unknown flow rate in the other fraction:

$$\frac{1\,ml}{0.016\,g} = \frac{X}{2\,g}$$

- Cross-multiply the fractions:

$$X \times 0.016\,g = 1\,ml \times 2\,g$$

- Solve for X by dividing each side of the equation by 0.016 g and cancelling units that appear in both the numerator and denominator:

$$\frac{X \times \cancel{0.016\,g}}{\cancel{0.016\,g}} = \frac{1\,ml \times 2\,\cancel{g}}{0.016\,\cancel{g}}$$

$$X = \frac{2\,ml}{0.016}$$

$$X = 125\,ml$$

The same flow rate of 125 ml per hour is obtained using this method.

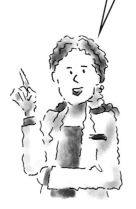

Let's try to solve the same problem using another method.

Preterm labour? Try terbutaline

Your patient is in preterm labour. The prescriber decides that *10 mg terbutaline sulphate in 250 ml 5% glucose in water should be administered, to infuse at 5 mcg/minute*. What's the flow rate for this solution?

- First, find the solution's strength. Set up a proportion with the known strength in one fraction and the unknown strength in the other fraction:

$$\frac{10 \text{ mg}}{250 \text{ ml}} = \frac{X}{1 \text{ ml}}$$

- Cross-multiply the fractions:

$$X \times 250 \text{ ml} = 10 \text{ mg} \times 1 \text{ ml}$$

- Solve for X by dividing each side of the equation by 250 ml and cancelling units that appear in both the numerator and denominator:

$$\frac{X \times \cancel{250 \text{ ml}}}{\cancel{250 \text{ ml}}} = \frac{10 \text{ mg} \times 1 \cancel{\text{ ml}}}{250 \cancel{\text{ ml}}}$$

$$X = \frac{10 \text{ mg}}{250}$$

$$X = 0.04 \text{ mg}$$

- The strength of the solution is 0.04 mg/ml. Next, convert to micrograms (mcg) by multiplying by 1000 (0.04 mg/ml × 1000 = 40 mcg/ml). Then calculate the flow rate needed to deliver the prescribed dose of 5 mcg/minute. To do this, set up a proportion with the known solution strength in one fraction and the unknown flow rate in the other:

$$\frac{1 \text{ ml}}{40 \text{ mcg}} = \frac{X}{5 \text{ mcg}}$$

- Cross-multiply the fractions:

$$X \times 40 \text{ mcg} = 1 \text{ ml} \times 5 \text{ mcg}$$

- Solve for X by dividing each side of the equation by 40 mcg and cancelling units that appear in both the numerator and denominator:

$$\frac{X \times \cancel{40 \text{ mcg}}}{\cancel{40 \text{ mcg}}} = \frac{1 \text{ ml} \times 5 \cancel{\text{ mcg}}}{40 \cancel{\text{ mcg}}}$$

$$X = \frac{5 \text{ mcg}}{40}$$

$$X = 0.125 \text{ ml}$$

- The flow rate is 0.125 ml/minute. Because the infusion must be administered with a pump, compute the hourly flow rate by setting up a proportion with the known flow rate per minute in one fraction and the unknown flow rate per hour in the other fraction:

$$\frac{0.125 \text{ ml}}{1 \text{ minute}} = \frac{X}{60 \text{ minutes}}$$

- Cross-multiply the fractions:

$$X \times 1 \text{ minute} = 0.125 \text{ ml} \times 60 \text{ minutes}$$

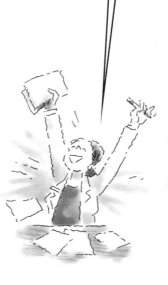

Nothing feels better than getting the right answer twice!

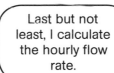

Last but not least, I calculate the hourly flow rate.

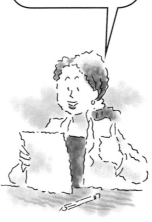

- Solve for X by dividing each side of the equation by 1 minute and cancelling units that appear in both the numerator and denominator:

$$\frac{X \times \cancel{1\ minute}}{1\ minute} = \frac{0.125\ ml \times 60\ \cancel{minutes}}{1\ \cancel{minute}}$$

$$X = 7.5\ ml$$

Round off the answer of 7.5 ml to the nearest millilitre, and set the infusion pump to deliver 8 ml/hour.

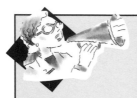

That's a wrap!

Calculating obstetric drug dosages review

Here are some important facts about obstetric drug dosages to keep in mind.

Assessing the mother during drug administration

- Frequently check vital signs, urine output, uterine contractions and deep tendon reflexes.
- Monitor and record fluid intake and output.
- Assess breath sounds.

Evaluating foetal response to drug therapy

- Monitor foetal heart rate during mother's drug therapy.
- If a sudden increase or decrease occurs, immediately discontinue the drug.

Common obstetric drugs
Terbutaline

- Inhibits preterm labour
- Administered via an infusion pump and titrated every 10 minutes as needed

Magnesium sulphate

- Prevents or controls seizures caused by pregnancy-induced hypertension

- Given as a loading dose first, then followed with infusion at a lower dose
- Suspected toxicity requires stopping infusion immediately and notifying doctor

Oxytocin

- Selectively stimulates uterine smooth muscle to induce labour
- May also be used to control bleeding after delivery of the placenta
- Administered I.V. piggyback with an infusion pump and titrated until normal contraction pattern occurs
- Requires careful monitoring of contraction strength

Dinoprostone

- Ripens the cervix (to induce labour) in pregnant patients at or near term
- Available as endocervical gel, vaginal inserts or vaginal suppositories

Dosage calculations

- Accurate dosages of drugs given to the mother help avoid foetal complications.
- Proportions can be used to solve obstetric dosage calculations.

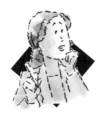

Quick quiz

1. If the prescription reads *20 units oxytocin in 1000 ml of Ringer-lactate solution*, the solution's concentration is:
   A. 20 units/ml
   B. 2 units/ml
   C. 0.2 unit/ml
   D. 0.02 unit/ml

Answer: D. To solve this problem, set up a proportion with the known concentration in one fraction and the unknown concentration in the other fraction. Then solve for *X*.

2. A sudden increase or decrease in the foetal heart rate after drug treatment is a:
   A. sign that the infant is about to be delivered.
   B. sign of an adverse reaction to the drug.
   C. temporary reaction to many obstetric drugs.
   D. sign indicating that the drug has reached its peak level.

Answer: B. Changes in the foetal heart rate may signal an adverse reaction to the drug; therefore, discontinue the drug immediately.

3. Which drug should be kept readily available to reverse magnesium sulphate intoxication?
   A. Potassium chloride
   B. Atropine
   C. Calcium gluconate
   D. Sodium chloride

Answer: C. During magnesium sulphate infusion, calcium gluconate should be readily available to reverse magnesium intoxication should it occur.

4. If a prescription reads *infuse 20 mg terbutaline sulphate in 1000 ml 5% glucose in water, at 0.01 mg/minute for 20 minutes*, the flow rate should be:
   A. 1 ml
   B. 10 ml
   C. 100 ml
   D. 200 ml

Answer: B. First, calculate the concentration, which is 0.02 mg/ml. Then determine the amount of drug provided in 20 minutes by multiplying 0.01 by 20 minutes to get 0.2 mg. Lastly, set up a proportion with the concentration in one fraction and the total amount of medication and the unknown flow rate in the other fraction. Solve for *X*.

5. If 5 g of magnesium sulphate are added to 1 L of normal saline solution, the concentration of magnesium sulphate is:
    A. 0.05 mg/ml
    B. 0.5 mg/ml
    C. 5 mg/ml
    D. 50 mg/ml

Answer: C. First, convert 5 g to 5000 mg and 1 L to 1000 ml. Then divide the 1000 into 5000 to obtain the concentration: 5 mg/ml.

6. If a patient is prescribed *20 g magnesium sulphate in 1000 ml 5% glucose in water, to be infused at 5 g/hour*, the flow rate in millilitres per hour should be:
    A. 2 ml/hour
    B. 25 ml/hour
    C. 250 ml/hour
    D. 300 ml/hour

Answer: C. To solve this problem, set up a proportion with the prescribed concentration in one fraction and the flow rate in grams and the unknown flow rate in millilitres in the other. Solve for X.

7. The best way to administer oxytocin is by:
    A. I.V. piggyback infusion.
    B. I.V. bolus injection.
    C. direct I.V. infusion.
    D. I.M. injection.

Answer: A. Administer oxytocin by I.V. piggyback infusion using an infusion pump so that the drug can be discontinued without interrupting the I.V. line.

Scoring

✩✩✩ If you answered all seven items correctly, fantastic! Your labours have helped you become a confident calculator.

✩✩ If you answered five or six items correctly, keep at it! You'll soon be able to deftly deliver drugs in any delivery unit.

✩ If you answered fewer than five items correctly, chin up! You still have one chapter left to conquer the Quick quiz.

16 Calculating critical care dosages

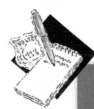

Just the facts

In this chapter, you'll learn:

♦ special points to consider when giving critical care drugs

♦ how to calculate dosages for I.V. push drugs

♦ how to calculate I.V. flow rates for critical care drugs

♦ how to calculate drugs not prescribed at a specific flow rate or dosage.

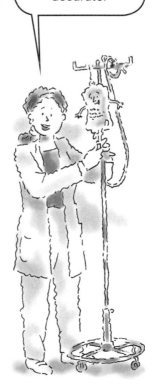

In the critical care unit, dosage calculations need to be quick and accurate.

A look at critical care dosages

If you work on a critical care unit, not only do you need to perform dosage calculations accurately, you also need to perform them quickly because of the patient's life-threatening condition. (See *Quick list of critical care meds and measurements*.)

Many I.V. drugs – such as the anti-arrhythmics lidocaine and procainamide, the vasodilators sodium nitroprusside and glyceryl trinitrate, and the adrenergics noradrenaline (norepinephrine) and dopamine – are administered in life-threatening situations. The nurse's job is to prepare the drug for infusion, give it to the patient and then observe to evaluate the drug's effectiveness.

Administering I.V. injections

Many drugs administered on critical care units are given by direct injection, also called I.V. push. These potent, fast-acting drugs rapidly control heart rate, respiration, blood pressure, cardiac output or kidney function. They usually have a short duration of action, so you can evaluate their effectiveness immediately and begin other treatment promptly if they aren't working.

One critical difference

Generally, I.V. push drugs are prescribed by dosage, which can sometimes include the specific unit of measure to administer over a short time (such as mg/minute or mcg/kg/minute). Calculate dosages on the critical care unit the same as you would on other units. However, take extra care because drugs used on critical care units are extremely potent and have serious adverse effects, which can include death.

Be prepared to be under stress

You're responsible for calculating and administering the dose accurately, following any special instructions. Many drugs used on critical care units come in small vials, so double-check the label to make sure you're giving the right dose or concentration. Giving the wrong concentration could be fatal.

Because calculating dosages during an emergency is stressful, and stress makes you more error-prone, do everything you can to be prepared. (See *Stress busters*.)

Calculating dosages

The following examples demonstrate how to use proportions to calculate I.V. push drugs. Note that the calculations are very similar to those for I.M. drugs.

Also note how the administration times vary. If you aren't sure how slowly or quickly to push a drug, look it up or call the pharmacist. It's better to be safe than sorry with rapid-acting drugs.

Are you label able?

Your patient is admitted with frequent ventricular arrhythmias. They are prescribed *procainamide 200 mg every 5 min by slow I.V. push (no faster than 25 to 50 mg/minute) until arrhythmias disappear*. If the drug label says the dose strength is 100 mg/ml, how many millilitres of procainamide should you give to the patient every 5 minutes?

• Set up a proportion with the prescribed dose and the unknown volume in one fraction and the dose strength in milligrams per millilitre in the other fraction:

$$\frac{200 \text{ mg}}{X} = \frac{100 \text{ mg}}{1 \text{ ml}}$$

• Cross-multiply the fractions:

$$X \times 100 \text{ mg} = 1 \text{ ml} \times 200 \text{ mg}$$

Quick list of critical care meds and measurements

The lists below show some of the common critical care drugs and associated units of measure. Memorising these units of measure will help speed up your calculations.

mg/minute

• lidocaine
• glyceryl trinitrate
• procainamide

mcg/minute

• adrenaline (epinephrine)
• noradrenaline (norepinephrine)
• phenylephrine

mcg/kg/minute

• dobutamine
• dopamine
• nitroprusside

- Solve for X by dividing each side of the equation by 100 mg and cancelling the units that appear in both the numerator and denominator:

$$\frac{X \times \cancel{100\ mg}}{\cancel{100\ mg}} = \frac{1\ ml \times 200\ \cancel{mg}}{100\ \cancel{mg}}$$

$$X = \frac{200\ ml}{100}$$

$$X = 2\ ml$$

You should administer 2 ml, or one-fifth of the contents of the procainamide vial. According to the package insert, you should administer the drug only intramuscularly or intravenously. Also, note that when giving I.V. procainamide, the drug must be diluted.

Rapid heartbeat riddle

Your patient suddenly develops supraventricular tachycardia and is prescribed *6 mg adenosine by rapid I.V. push*. If the only vial available contains 3 mg/ml, how many millilitres should you give?
- Set up a proportion with the available solution in one ratio and the prescribed dose and the unknown volume in the other ratio:

$$3\ mg : 1\ ml :: 6\ mg : X$$

- Multiply the means and the extremes:

$$X \times 3\ mg = 1\ ml \times 6\ mg$$

- Solve for X by dividing both sides of the equation by 3 mg and cancelling units that appear in both the numerator and denominator:

$$\frac{X \times 3\ \cancel{mg}}{3\ \cancel{mg}} = \frac{1\ ml \times 6\ \cancel{mg}}{3\ \cancel{mg}}$$

$$X = \frac{6\ ml}{3}$$

$$X = 2\ ml$$

You should administer 2 ml of the solution. According to the package insert, this drug should be administered by rapid I.V. push because of its very short half-life. It also should be administered directly into the vein or in the most proximal port, followed by a rapid saline flush.

Digoxin difficulty

Your patient has a history of rapid atrial fibrillation and takes digoxin at home. When his digoxin level is found to be sub-therapeutic, the

Advice from the experts

Stress busters

Here are four hot tips to help reduce your stress level when calculating drugs during an emergency:

Carry a list of all the drug-calculation formulas.

Carry a calculator for quick use (know how to operate it correctly!).

Keep patients' weights in kilograms, with other relevant information, at their bedsides.

Become familiar with the different critical care drugs given intravenously as well as your unit's medication protocols.

doctor prescribes *0.125 mg I.V. digoxin* as a single dose to control his heart rate. The only available digoxin vial contains 0.25 mg/ml. How many millilitres should you give?

• Set up a proportion with the available solution in one ratio and the prescribed dose and the unknown volume in the other ratio:

$$0.25 \text{ mg} : 1 \text{ ml} :: 0.125 \text{ mg} : X$$

• Multiply the means and the extremes:

$$X \times 0.25 \text{ mg} = 1 \text{ ml} \times 0.125 \text{ mg}$$

• Solve for X by dividing both sides of the equation by 0.25 mg and cancelling units that appear in both the numerator and denominator:

$$\frac{X \times 0.25 \text{ mg}}{0.25 \text{ mg}} = \frac{1 \text{ ml} \times 0.125 \text{ mg}}{0.25 \text{ mg}}$$

$$X = \frac{0.125 \text{ ml}}{0.25}$$

$$X = 0.5 \text{ ml}$$

You should administer 0.5 ml of digoxin. According to the package insert, the drug should be given by I.V. push over 5 minutes (not 1 minute, as with some other critical care drugs).

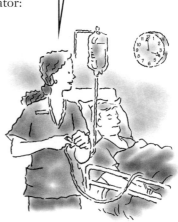

When giving an injection by I.V. push, it's very important to note how long to push the drug... too fast or too slow can have serious consequences.

Calculating I.V. flow rates

Because many drugs given on the critical care unit are used to treat life-threatening problems, you can't waste any time when calculating I.V. flow rates. You must swiftly do the calculations, prepare the drug for infusion, administer it and then observe the patient closely to evaluate the drug's effectiveness.

Three critical calculations

You may need to perform three calculations before administering critical care drugs:

concentration of the drug in the I.V. solution

flow rate required to deliver the desired dose

number of micrograms needed, based on the patient's weight in kilograms. You may need to perform this calculation if the drug is prescribed in micrograms per kilogram of body weight per minute. *Remember:* if you need to convert milligrams to micrograms, multiply by 1000.

Concentrate on this formula

To calculate the drug's concentration, use this formula:

$$\text{concentration in mg/ml} = \frac{\text{mg of drug}}{\text{ml of fluid}}$$

- If you need to express the concentration in mcg/ml, multiply the answer by 1000.

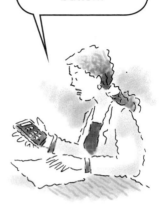

I wish there were some way to perform all three calculations with one push of a button!

Figure the flow rate

You can determine the I.V. flow rate per minute using this formula:

$$\frac{\text{dose/minute}}{X} = \frac{\text{concentration of solution}}{1 \text{ ml of fluid}}$$

- To calculate the hourly flow rate, first multiply the prescribed dose, given in milligrams or micrograms per minute, by 60 minutes to determine the hourly dose. Then use this proportion to compute the hourly flow rate:

$$\frac{\text{hourly dose}}{X} = \frac{\text{concentration of solution}}{1 \text{ ml of fluid}}$$

Determine the dosage

To determine the dosage in milligrams per kilogram of body weight per minute, perform the following steps:
- First, determine the concentration of the solution in milligrams per millilitre. To determine the dose in milligrams per hour, multiply the hourly flow rate by the concentration using this formula:

$$\text{dose in mg/hour} = \text{hourly flow rate} \times \text{concentration}$$

- To calculate the dose in milligrams per minute, first divide the hourly dose by 60 minutes. Here's the formula:

$$\text{dose in mg/minute} = \frac{\text{dose in mg/hour}}{60 \text{ minutes}}$$

- Then divide the dose per minute by the patient's weight, using this formula:

$$\text{mg/kg/minute} = \frac{\text{mg/minute}}{\text{patient's weight in kg}}$$

No time for books?

Suppose you don't have time to refer to your dosage calculation book in a critical situation. Keep these formulas on a card with your calculator for quick reference. They're foolproof!

- To find out how many micrograms per kilogram per minute your patient is receiving, use this formula:

$$\frac{mg}{\text{volume of bag}} \times 1000 \div 60 \div kg \times \text{infusion rate} = mcg/kg/min$$

- To find out how many millilitres per hour you should give, use this formula:

$$\frac{\text{weight in kg} \times \text{dose in mcg/kg/min} \times 60}{\text{concentration in 1 L}} = ml/hour$$

- After you've performed these calculations, make sure that the drug is being given within a safe and therapeutic range. Compare the amount in milligrams per kilogram per minute with the safe range shown in a drug reference book. (See *No time for books?*)

Real-world problems

The following examples show how to calculate an I.V. flow rate using the different formulas.

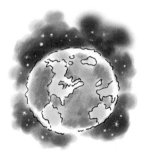

A lidocaine lifeline

Your patient is having frequent runs of ventricular tachycardia that subside after 10 to 12 beats. The doctor prescribes *2 g (2000 mg) lidocaine in 500 ml 5% glucose in water, to infuse at 2 mg/minute.* What's the flow rate in millilitres per minute? In millilitres per hour?
- First, find the solution's concentration by setting up a proportion with the unknown concentration in one fraction and the prescribed dose in the other fraction:

$$\frac{X}{1\ ml} = \frac{2000\ mg}{500\ ml}$$

- Cross-multiply the fractions:

$$X \times 500\ ml = 2000\ mg \times 1\ ml$$

- Solve for X by dividing each side of the equation by 500 ml and cancelling units that appear in both the numerator and denominator:

$$\frac{X \times 500\ \cancel{ml}}{500\ \cancel{ml}} = \frac{2000\ mg \times 1\ \cancel{ml}}{500\ \cancel{ml}}$$

$$X = \frac{2000 \text{ mg}}{500}$$

$$X = 4 \text{ mg}$$

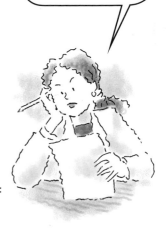

Next, I calculate the flow rate per minute.

• The solution's concentration is 4 mg/ml. Next, calculate the flow rate per minute needed to deliver the prescribed dose of 2 mg/minute. To do this, set up a proportion with the unknown flow rate per minute in one fraction and the solution's concentration in the other fraction:

$$\frac{2 \text{ mg}}{X} = \frac{4 \text{ mg}}{1 \text{ ml}}$$

• Cross-multiply the fractions:

$$X \times 4 \text{ mg} = 1 \text{ ml} \times 2 \text{ mg}$$

• Solve for X by dividing each side of the equation by 4 mg and cancelling units that appear in both the numerator and denominator:

$$\frac{X \times \cancel{4 \text{ mg}}}{\cancel{4 \text{ mg}}} = \frac{1 \text{ ml} \times 2 \cancel{\text{mg}}}{4 \cancel{\text{mg}}}$$

$$X = \frac{2 \text{ ml}}{4}$$

$$X = 0.5 \text{ ml}$$

• The patient should receive 0.5 ml/minute of lidocaine. Because lidocaine must be infused through an infusion pump, compute the hourly flow rate. Do this by setting up a proportion with the unknown flow rate per hour in one fraction and the flow rate per minute in the other fraction:

$$\frac{X}{60 \text{ minutes}} = \frac{0.5 \text{ ml}}{1 \text{ minute}}$$

• Cross-multiply the fractions:

$$X \times 1 \text{ minute} = 0.5 \text{ ml} \times 60 \text{ minutes}$$

• Solve for X by dividing each side of the equation by 1 minute and cancelling units that appear in both the numerator and denominator:

$$\frac{X \times \cancel{1 \text{ minute}}}{\cancel{1 \text{ minute}}} = \frac{0.5 \text{ ml} \times 60 \cancel{\text{minutes}}}{\cancel{1 \text{ minute}}}$$

$$X = 30 \text{ ml}$$

Set the infusion pump to deliver 30 ml/hour.

Don't doubt dobutamine

A 200-lb patient is to receive an *I.V. infusion of dobutamine at 10 mcg/ kg/minute*. The label instructs to check the package insert. There it says to dilute 250 mg of the drug in 50 ml of 5% glucose in water.

Because the drug vial contains 20 ml of solution, the total to be infused is 70 ml (50 ml of 5% glucose in water + 20 ml of solution). How many millilitres of the drug should the patient receive each minute? Each hour?

- First, compute the patient's weight in kilograms. To do this, set up a proportion with the weight in pounds and the unknown weight in kilograms in one fraction and the number of pounds per kilogram in the other fraction:

$$\frac{200 \text{ lb}}{X} = \frac{2.2 \text{ lb}}{1 \text{ kg}}$$

- Cross-multiply the fractions:

$$X \times 2.2 \text{ lb} = 1 \text{ kg} \times 200 \text{ lb}$$

- Solve for X by dividing each side of the equation by 2.2 lb and cancelling units that appear in both the numerator and denominator:

$$\frac{X \times 2.2 \text{ lb}}{2.2 \text{ lb}} = \frac{1 \text{ kg} \times 200 \text{ lb}}{2.2 \text{ lb}}$$

$$X = \frac{200 \text{ kg}}{2.2}$$

$$X = 90.9 \text{ kg}$$

- The patient weighs 90.9 kg. Next, determine the dose in millilitres per minute by setting up a proportion with the patient's weight in kilograms and the unknown dose in micrograms per minute in one fraction and the known dose in micrograms per kilogram per minute in the other fraction:

$$\frac{90.9 \text{ kg}}{X} = \frac{1 \text{ kg}}{10 \text{ mcg/minute}}$$

- Cross-multiply the fractions:

$$X \times 1 \text{ kg} = 10 \text{ mcg/minute} \times 90.9 \text{ kg}$$

- Solve for X by dividing each side of the equation by 1 kg and cancelling units that appear in both the numerator and denominator:

$$\frac{X \times 1 \text{ kg}}{1 \text{ kg}} = \frac{10 \text{ mcg/minute} \times 90.9 \text{ kg}}{1 \text{ kg}}$$

$$X = 909 \text{ mcg/minute}$$

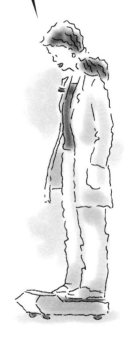

First, compute the patient's weight in kilograms. Hmm... don't like the looks of this!

- The patient should receive 909 mcg, or 0.909 mg, of dobutamine every minute. To determine the flow rate in millilitres per minute, set up a proportion using the solution's concentration and solve for X:

$$\frac{0.909 \text{ mg}}{X} = \frac{250 \text{ mg}}{70 \text{ ml}}$$

$$\frac{\cancel{250 \text{ mg}} \times X}{\cancel{250 \text{ mg}}} = \frac{0.909 \cancel{\text{mg}} \times 70 \text{ ml}}{250 \cancel{\text{mg}}}$$

$$X = \frac{63.63 \text{ ml}}{250}$$

$$X = 0.25 \text{ ml/minute}$$

- To find the flow rate in millilitres per hour, multiply by 60.

$$0.25 \text{ ml/minute} \times 60 \text{ minutes/hour} = 15 \text{ ml/hour}$$

The patient should receive dobutamine at a rate of 15 ml/hour.

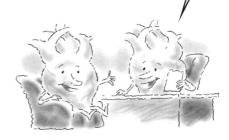

Here we go, folks… just in from the home office: the top 10 reasons why dobutamine is so effective…

Special cases

Critical care drugs aren't always prescribed at a specific flow rate or dosage. Sometimes, they're prescribed according to the patient's heart rate, blood pressure or other parameters.

In some cases, a starting dose and a maximum dose to which the drug can be titrated may be prescribed. To deliver the correct amount of drug, you must calculate the starting dose and the maximum dose.

Here are some examples of drug calculations that you may use in special cases.

Nitroprusside number cruncher

A patient with severe hypertension weighs 85 kg. Their prescription reads *nitroprusside 50 mg in 250 ml 5% glucose in water. Start at 0.5 mcg/kg/minute. Titrate to keep systolic BP <170 mmHg. Maximum dose is 10 mcg/kg/minute.* At what rate should you start the infusion?

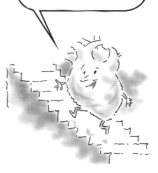

Sometimes drugs are prescribed according to heart rate. Only one more flight to go!

- First, find the concentration of the infusion. Start by converting 50 mg to 50 000 mcg.

$$\frac{50\ 000\ \text{mcg}}{250\ \text{ml}} = 200\ \text{mcg/ml}$$

- Then set up the following equation:

$$X = \frac{85\ \text{kg} \times 0.5\ \text{mcg/kg/min} \times 60}{200\ \text{mcg/ml}}$$

$$X = 12.75\ \text{ml/hour}$$

The starting dose is 13 ml/hour.

Keep the phenylephrine flowing

A patient with terminal Hodgkin's disease who weighs 41 kg has been hypotensive for several hours despite receiving I.V. fluid boluses. A prescription is given for *100 mg phenylephrine in 250 ml of normal saline solution*. The drug is to start at 30 mcg/minute and then be titrated to keep the systolic blood pressure at 90 mmHg. What's the flow rate in millilitres per minute?
- First, determine the solution's concentration by dividing the prescribed dose of phenylephrine by the amount of normal saline solution:

$$X = \frac{100\ \text{mg}}{250\ \text{ml}}$$

$$X = 0.4\ \text{mg/ml}$$

- The concentration is 0.4 mg/ml. Next, convert milligrams to micrograms by multiplying by 1000:

$$0.4\ \text{mg/ml} \times 1000 = 400\ \text{mcg/ml}$$

- The concentration is 400 mcg/ml. Now calculate the flow rate by setting up a proportion with the starting flow rate and the unknown flow rate in one fraction and the concentration in the other fraction:

$$\frac{30\ \text{mcg/minute}}{X\ \text{ml/minute}} = \frac{400\ \text{mcg}}{1\ \text{ml}}$$

- Cross-multiply the fractions:

$$X\ \text{ml/minute} \times 400\ \text{mcg} = 30\ \text{mcg/minute} \times 1\ \text{ml}$$

- Solve for X by dividing each side of the equation by 400 mcg and cancelling units that appear in both the numerator and denominator:

$$\frac{X \text{ ml/minute} \times \cancel{400 \text{ mcg}}}{\cancel{400 \text{ mcg}}} = \frac{30 \cancel{\text{ mcg}}/\text{minute} \times 1 \text{ ml}}{400 \cancel{\text{ mcg}}}$$

$$X = \frac{30 \text{ ml/minute}}{400}$$

$$X = 0.075 \text{ ml/minute}$$

- The flow rate is 0.075 ml/minute. To calculate the hourly flow rate, multiply 0.075 ml by 60:

$$0.075 \text{ ml} \times 60 = 4.5 \text{ ml}$$

The hourly flow rate is 4.5 ml, which can be rounded off to 5 ml/hour.

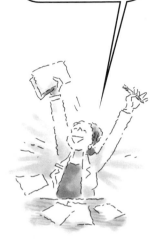

Finally, I know the hourly flow rate!

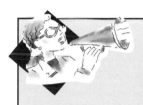

That's a wrap!

Calculating critical care dosages review

When working with critical care dosages, keep in mind these important facts.

Calculating I.V. push dosages

- Use proportions to calculate dosages.
- Determine administration time.

Calculating a drug's concentration

$$\text{concentration in mg/ml} = \frac{\text{mg of drug}}{\text{ml of fluid}}$$

- Remember to multiply the answer by 1000 if you need to express concentration in mcg/ml.

Calculating the flow rate

- Per minute:

$$\frac{\text{dose/minute}}{X} = \frac{\text{concentration of solution}}{1 \text{ ml of fluid}}$$

- Per hour:

$$\frac{\text{hourly dose}}{X} = \frac{\text{concentration of solution}}{1 \text{ ml of fluid}}$$

Calculating a dosage in mg/kg of body weight/minute

- Determine the dose in milligrams per hour:
  hourly flow rate × concentration
- Calculate the dose in milligrams per minute:
  dose in mg/hour ÷ 60 minutes
- Solve for mg/kg/minute:
  mg/minute ÷ patient's weight in kg

More formulas!

- To determine how many micrograms per kilogram per minute a patient is receiving:

$$\frac{\text{mg}}{\text{volume of bag}} \times 1000 \div 60 \div \text{kg} \times \text{infusion rate} = \text{mcg/kg/minute}$$

- To determine how many millilitres per hour to give:

$$\frac{\text{weight in kg} \times \text{dose in mcg/kg/min} \times 60}{\text{concentration in 1L}} = \text{ml/hr}$$

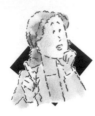

Quick quiz

1. If a patient has a dopamine drip of 800 mg in 500 ml 5% glucose in water, the concentration is:
   A. 0.16 mg/ml
   B. 1.6 mg/ml
   C. 16 mg/ml
   D. 160 mg/ml

Answer: B. Concentration is determined by dividing the total in milligrams (800 mg) by the volume (500 ml).

2. Procainamide is measured in:
   A. mg/minute
   B. mcg/kg/minute
   C. mg/hour
   D. mcg/minute

Answer: A. This information is necessary before you can calculate dosages of procainamide.

3. To convert milligrams to micrograms, multiply by:
   A. 10
   B. 60
   C. 100
   D. 1000

Answer: D. When converting a number from milligrams to micrograms, move the decimal three spaces to the right.

4. How many kilograms does a 250-lb man weigh?
   A. 11.4 kg
   B. 114 kg
   C. 550 kg
   D. 125 kg

Answer: B. To convert pounds to kilograms, divide by 2.2 and round off the number.

5. A prescription reads *furosemide 80 mg I.V. as a single dose*. The available vial contains 100 mg in 10 ml of normal saline solution. What volume should you give to administer this dose?
   A. 0.08 ml
   B. 0.8 ml
   C. 1.8 ml
   D. 8 ml

Answer: D. Set up a proportion with the available solution in one ratio and the prescribed dose and the unknown volume in the other ratio. Solve for *X*.

6.   If a patient weighs 50 kg, his weight in pounds is:
    A.   28 lb
    B.   100 lb
    C.   110 lb
    D.   200 lb

Answer: C. To convert kilograms to pounds, multiply by 2.2.

7.   A patient requires nitroprusside to lower her blood pressure. This dose should be prescribed in:
    A.   mcg/hour
    B.   mcg/minute
    C.   mg/minute
    D.   mcg/kg/minute

Answer: D. Nitroprusside should be prescribed in doses of mcg/kg/minute.

Scoring

☆☆☆   If you answered all seven items correctly, fantastic! You can calculate confidently in critical cases.

☆☆   If you answered five or six items correctly, that isn't bad! You're a cool, calm and collected calculator.

☆   If you answered fewer than five items correctly, keep at it! You have the best dosage calc book ever. Keep it with you always and refer to it frequently.

Appendices and index

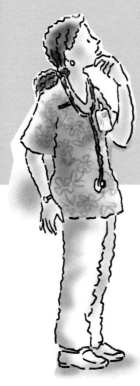

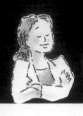

Practice makes perfect

1. The improper fraction $^{11}\!/_2$ converted into a mixed number is:
   A. $^2\!/_{11}$
   B. $5\frac{1}{11}$
   C. $5\frac{1}{2}$
   D. $^{22}\!/_{11}$

2. The sum of $\frac{1}{2} + \frac{3}{4} + \frac{6}{10}$ is:
   A. $1\frac{8}{10}$
   B. $1\frac{17}{20}$
   C. $2\frac{1}{4}$
   D. $^{10}\!/_{16}$

3. The complex fraction $^1\!/_{75}$ divided by the complex fraction $^1\!/_{25}$ equals:
   A. $\frac{1}{3}$
   B. 3
   C. $^1\!/_{100}$
   D. $\frac{2}{3}$

4. The decimal fraction 4.3 divided by 8.6 yields:
   A. 0.5
   B. 2
   C. 20
   D. 50

5. When 21.3478 is rounded off to the nearest hundredth, it becomes:
   A. 21.34
   B. 21.3
   C. 21.348
   D. 21.35

6. 31% of 105 is:
   A. 3.15
   B. 31.5
   C. 32.55
   D. 33.3

7. When 20% is converted to a decimal fraction, it becomes:
   A. 0.02
   B. 2.0
   C. 0.2
   D. 2.2

8. In fraction form, the proportion 1 : 4 :: 4 : 16 is:
    A. $\frac{4}{1} = \frac{4}{16}$
    B. $\frac{1}{4} = \frac{4}{16}$
    C. $\frac{4}{4} = \frac{1}{16}$
    D. $\frac{4}{1} = \frac{16}{4}$

9. If a vial has 20 mg of drug in 50 ml of solution, the amount of drug in 10 ml of solution is:
    A. 15 mg
    B. 10 mg
    C. 5 mg
    D. 4 mg

10. In the proportion 3 : 9 :: 9 : X, X equals:
    A. 81
    B. 3
    C. 27
    D. 18

11. How much chlorine bleach should you add to 500 ml of water to make a solution that contains 10 ml of chlorine bleach for every 100 ml of water?
    A. 5 ml
    B. 50 ml
    C. 10 ml
    D. 100 ml

12. A patient tells you that he weighs 154 lbs. How many kilograms is this?
    A. 63 kg
    B. 70 kg
    C. 49 kg
    D. 89 kg

13. A patient has been prescribed *ampicillin 250 mg*. The medication is supplied as an oral suspension, 125 mg per 5 ml. How many millilitres should the patient receive?
    A. 10 ml
    B. 5 ml
    C. 25 ml
    D. 1 ml

14. Your patient has been prescribed *pethidine 25 mg*. The pharmacy stocks a multidose vial containing 50 mg/ml. How many millilitres should you administer?
    A. 7.5 ml
    B. 5 ml
    C. 1.5 ml
    D. 0.5 ml

15. Convert 0.025 litres to mililitres.
    A. 250 ml
    B. 2.5 ml
    C. 0.25 ml
    D. 25 ml

16. During a 24-hour period, a patient received 600 ml, 1.25 L and 2.5 L of I.V. fluid. How many millilitres did the patient receive altogether?
    A. 43 500 ml
    B. 43.5 ml
    C. 4350 ml
    D. 435 ml

17. The weight in kilograms of an infant who weighs 8300 g is:
    A. 8300 kg
    B. 8.3 kg
    C. 83.0 kg
    D. 830 kg

18. A patient receives 250 mcg of digoxin. How many milligrams did they receive?
    A. 25 mg
    B. 2.5 mg
    C. 0.25 mg
    D. 0.00025 mg

19. A patient's fingerstick glucose level was 19.5 mmol/l. The doctor has prescribed *10 units of regular insulin* for the patient. The bottle is labelled 100 units/ml. The volume of insulin you'll administer is:
    A. 0.01 ml
    B. 0.1 ml
    C. 1 ml
    D. 10 ml

20. A patient needs 20 mmol of potassium chloride oral solution. The solution contains 60 mmol in every 15 ml. How many millilitres of solution should you give the patient?
    A. 5 ml
    B. 2.5 ml
    C. 7.5 ml
    D. 3 ml

21. A doctor prescribes *digoxin 0.125 mg, by mouth, 0900 daily* for a patient with heart failure. How should you interpret this order?
    A. Give 125 grams of digoxin orally at 9 a.m. every other day.
    B. Give 0.125 milligrams of digoxin orally every day at 9 p.m.
    C. Give 0.125 milligrams of digoxin orally every day at 9 a.m.
    D. Give 0.125 micrograms of digoxin orally at 9 a.m. every other day.

22. Which prescription is incomplete?
    A. Indometacin 100 mg P.O. stat
    B. Aspirin 325 P.O. every a.m.
    C. Seconal 100 mg P.O. at bedtime, p.r.n.
    D. Rocephin 1 g I.V. daily

23. The doctor prescribes *nifedipine 300 mg SL every 4 h* for a patient with hypertension. You should understand that this drug is to be given:
    A. four times per day.
    B. in a suspension.
    C. as needed.
    D. under the tongue.

24. You're administering medication to a 58-year-old patient who was admitted with heart failure. In giving a regularly scheduled drug, you must:
    A. give the drug half an hour before or after the prescribed time.
    B. give the drug 1 hour before or after the prescribed time.
    C. give the drug 15 minutes before or after the prescribed time.
    D. give the drug exactly at the prescribed time.

25. You need to administer morphine to a patient who just returned from the post-anaesthesia care unit after undergoing surgery. The information recorded on the controlled inventory record when you remove a controlled substance from a locked storage site should include:
    A. date and time of removal, patient's name, drug dose and your initials.
    B. date and time of removal, patient's name, drug dose and your signature.
    C. date and time of removal, patient's name, prescriber's name, drug dose and your signature.
    D. date and time of removal, patient's initials, prescriber's name and your initials.

26. You're caring for a 49-year-old patient with metastatic breast cancer. You need to administer the patient's 9 a.m. medications. When administering regularly scheduled drugs, you should:
    A. document the time of administration before giving the drug to the patient.
    B. document the time of administration after giving the drug to the patient.
    C. document the time of administration for all regularly scheduled drugs on your shift at the beginning of the shift.
    D. document the time of administration at the end of your shift.

27. A patient tells you that she typically takes two ibuprofen tablets for menstrual cramps. If one tablet of ibuprofen contains 200 mg, how many milligrams does the patient usually take?
    A. 500 mg
    B. 600 mg
    C. 400 mg
    D. 300 mg

28. Before administering a patient's medication, you should compare the drug prescribed with the drug's label. The non-proprietary name on a drug label is the drug's:
    A. trade name.
    B. generic name.
    C. manufacturer name.
    D. chemical name.

29. A patient is prescribed *minoxidil 5 mg, by mouth, daily*, for treatment of hypertension. The medication is supplied as 2.5 mg per tablet. How many tablets should be administered?
    A. ½ tablet
    B. 1 tablets
    C. 1½ tablets
    D. 2 tablets

30. A patient is prescribed *paracetamol 250 mg supp per rectum* to treat post-operative pain. You have paracetamol 125 mg supp available. What should be prepared?
    A. 1½ suppositories
    B. 1 suppository
    C. 2 suppositories
    D. ½ suppository

31. A paediatric patient is prescribed *domperidone 15 mg supp per rectum, stat*, for treatment of post-operative nausea. Domperidone 30 mg per supp is available. How much should be given?
    A. 2 suppositories
    B. 1½ suppositories
    C. 1 suppository
    D. ½ suppository

32. A patient is prescribed bacitracin for treatment of a wound he received in a road traffic accident. Before giving the patient a topical preparation, it's important to read the label first because:
    A. you want to know the manufacturer's name.
    B. the patient may be allergic to the ingredients.
    C. you like to read small print.
    D. there's probably no package insert.

33. A 52-year-old patient requires transdermal glyceryl trinitrate to control angina. You know that these transdermal patches should be removed 12 to 14 hours after application to:
    A. prevent it from falling off while the patient sleeps.
    B. prevent it from irritating the patient's skin.
    C. prevent the patient from developing a tolerance to the drug.
    D. prevent toxicity.

34. A patient returns from the post-anaesthesia care unit after undergoing an exploratory laparotomy and a lysis of adhesions. The patient is prescribed *morphine sulphate 10 mg I.M. every 4 h p.r.n.* for pain. The medication is available in a vial containing 20 mg/ml of morphine sulphate. How many millilitres of the drug should you administer?
   A. 1 ml
   B. 0.75 ml
   C. 0.5 ml
   D. 0.25 ml

35. A patient is prescribed *heparin 8000 units, by subcutaneous injection, every 8 hours* for a deep-vein thrombosis. The heparin available is 20 000 units per 1 ml. How many millilitres of heparin should you give?
   A. 0.2 ml
   B. 0.3 ml
   C. 0.4 ml
   D. 0.5 ml

36. A patient with type 1 diabetes mellitus is prescribed *45 units of NPH insulin subcutaneously in the morning daily.* You have NPH insulin 100 units/ml available. Using a U-100 syringe, how many millilitres will be in the syringe?
   A. 0.045 ml
   B. 0.45 ml
   C. 4.5 ml
   D. 5 ml

37. A patient needs an infusion of 5% glucose in water, at 100 ml/hour. If the tubing set is calibrated at 15 gtt/ml, what's the drip rate?
   A. 31 gtt/minute
   B. 33 gtt/minute
   C. 25 gtt/minute
   D. 30 gtt/minute

38. A patient diagnosed with pneumonia needs 2000 ml of fluid over 24 hours. What's the flow rate?
   A. 150 ml/hour
   B. 125 ml/hour
   C. 110 ml/hour
   D. 83 ml/hour

39. You're about to administer a continuous infusion of 25 000 units of heparin in 500 ml of half-normal saline solution. If the patient is to receive 750 units/hour, what's the flow rate?
   A. 25 ml/hour
   B. 15 ml/hour
   C. 10 ml/hour
   D. 5 ml/hour

40. A 4-year-old patient weighs 46 lb. How many kilograms is this?
    A. 21 kg
    B. 20 kg
    C. 23 kg
    D. 12 kg

41. The doctor prescribes a *single dose of paracetamol 10 mg/kg/dose oral suspension* for a child with a fever who weighs 6 kg. What's the dose in milligrams?
    A. 1.6 mg
    B. 16 mg
    C. 60 mg
    D. 80 mg

42. A child weighing 66 lb is admitted with appendicitis. How much maintenance I.V. fluid should the child receive in 24 hours?
    A. 1500 ml/day
    B. 1700 ml/day
    C. 1800 ml/day
    D. 1900 ml/day

43. A 25-year-old primagravida has been in labour for 20 hours with little progress. The doctor prescribes oxytocin. The prescription reads *10 units oxytocin in 1000 ml normal saline, to infuse via pump at 1 mU/minute for 15 minutes; then increase flow rate to 2 mU/minute*. What's the flow rate needed to deliver 1 mU/minute for 15 minutes?
    A. 4 ml/hour
    B. 6 ml/hour
    C. 8 ml/hour
    D. 12 ml/hour

44. Use the calculations in the previous problem. After 15 minutes, the pump needs to be reset to deliver 2 mU/minute. What's the flow rate?
    A. 10 ml/hour
    B. 20 ml/hour
    C. 12 ml/hour
    D. 15 ml/hour

45. A patient is prescribed *4 g magnesium sulphate in 250 ml 5% glucose in water, infused at 1 g/hour for pre-eclampsia*. What's the flow rate?
    A. 125 ml/hour
    B. 250 ml/hour
    C. 25 ml/hour
    D. 63 ml/hour

46. A patient is prescribed *150 mg of ritodrine in 500 ml 5% glucose in water, to infuse at 0.15 mg/minute* following admission for pre-term labour. What's the flow rate?
    A. 30 ml/hour
    B. 15 ml/hour
    C. 10 ml/hour
    D. 5 ml/hour

47. A patient experiencing an acute myocardial infarction is to receive *glyceryl trinitrate 10 mcg/minute I.V.* The I.V. solution contains 250 ml 5% glucose in water, with 25 mg glyceryl trinitrate. How many millilitres should the patient receive each hour?
   A.   16 ml
   B.   10 ml
   C.   6 ml
   D.   4 ml

48. A patient experienced a sustained ventricular tachycardia that required cardioversion. They are prescribed *1 g lidocaine in 250 ml 5% glucose in water, to infuse at 3 mg/minute* to help maintain a normal sinus rhythm. What's the flow rate?
   A.   30 ml/hour
   B.   45 ml/hour
   C.   60 ml/hour
   D.   70 ml/hour

49. The doctor writes a prescription for *2 L of Ringer-lactate solution to be infused over 16 hours.* The drop factor of the administration set is 20 gtt/ml. What should the drip rate be?
   A.   25 gtt/minute
   B.   33 gtt/minute
   C.   20 gtt/minute
   D.   42 gtt/minute

50. The nurse is to administer *ceftriaxone 2 g in 500 ml over 10 hours.* What hourly flow rate should the nurse set the infusion pump to deliver?
   A.   50 ml/hour
   B.   65 ml/hour
   C.   35 ml/hour
   D.   15 ml/hour

51. A nurse receives a prescription to administer *4000 ml of normal saline solution I.V. over 12 hours.* What should the drip rate be if the drop factor of the tubing is 15 gtt/ml?
   A.   46 gtt/min
   B.   91 gtt/min
   C.   166 gtt/min
   D.   83 gtt/min

52. A 68-kg patient is to receive *gentamicin 3 mg/kg daily in 3 divided doses.* Gentamicin is available to the nurse in 80 mg/2 ml. How many millilitres should the nurse administer every 8 hours?
   A.   1.7 ml
   B.   4 ml
   C.   2.7 ml
   D.   1.3 ml

53. The doctor prescribes *digoxin 250 mcg by mouth every day*. The pharmacy stocks digoxin 0.5-mg scored tablets. How many tablets should the nurse administer?
    A. ¼ tablet
    B. 1 tablet
    C. ½ tablet
    D. 2 tablets

54. A patient is prescribed *co-amoxiclav suspension 250 mg by mouth, 3 times, every day*. Co-amoxiclav is available to the nurse in a suspension of 125 mg/5 ml. How many millilitres should the nurse administer per dose?
    A. 5 ml
    B. 10 ml
    C. 12.5 ml
    D. 25 ml

55. The doctor prescribes *azathioprine 75 mg by mouth every day*. The drug is available to the nurse in 50-mg unscored tablets. How should the nurse administer the dose?
    A. Administer 2 tablets.
    B. Administer 1½ tablets.
    C. Administer 1 tablet.
    D. Withhold the dose until the pharmacy sends a 75-mg tablet.

56. An infant weighing 2.3 kg is ordered to receive *gentamicin 2.5 mg/kg/dose I.V. every 4 hours*. The pharmacy stocks gentamicin in a solution of 2 mg/ml. How many millilitres of the solution should the nurse administer for each dose?
    A. 3.2 ml
    B. 2.6 ml
    C. 1.9 ml
    D. 2.9 ml

57. An infant weighing 3.6 kg is about to receive a blood transfusion of *15 ml/kg of packed red blood cells over 4 hours*. What hourly flow rate should the nurse set the infusion pump to deliver?
    A. 8 ml/hour
    B. 10.6 ml/hour
    C. 13.5 ml/hour
    D. 15.2 ml/hour

58. Your patient is prescribed *ceftriaxone 1 g in 10 ml of 5% glucose in water, to be given at a dose of 250 mg I.V. every 12 h*. How many millilitres should the nurse administer for each dose?

59. The doctor prescribes *morphine sulphate 60 mg I.M. stat*. The drug is available in a 1-ml vial containing 100 mg/ml. How many millilitres are discarded after the nurse has administered the prescribed dose?

60. Which conversion factors are correct? Select all that apply.
    A. 2.2 kilograms = 1 pound
    B. 1000 milligrams = 1 gram
    C. 1 kilogram = 2.2 pounds
    D. 1 litre = 1000 millilitres

Answers

1. C. Divide the numerator (11) by the denominator (2). The calculation looks like this:

$$^{11}\!/_2 = 11 \div 2 = 5\tfrac{1}{2}$$

   You get 5 with 1 left over. The 1 becomes the new numerator and the denominator stays the same.

2. B. Determine the lowest common denominator (20). Then convert each to the lowest common denominator: $\tfrac{1}{2} = {}^{10}\!/_{20}$, $\tfrac{3}{4} = {}^{15}\!/_{20}$, $^{6}\!/_{10} = {}^{12}\!/_{20}$. Add all the numerators and place over the denominators: $^{10}\!/_{20} + {}^{15}\!/_{20} + {}^{12}\!/_{20} = {}^{37}\!/_{20}$. Reduce to lowest terms: $1^{17}\!/_{20}$.

3. A. Divide the dividend $^{1}\!/_{75}$ by the divisor $^{1}\!/_{25}$. Invert the divisor ($^{1}\!/_{25}$) and multiply $^{1}\!/_{75} \times {}^{25}\!/_1 = {}^{25}\!/_{75}$. Reduce to lowest terms: $\tfrac{1}{3}$.

4. A. Move the decimal points of both the divisor and the dividend one place to the right before dividing. Place the quotient's decimal point over the new decimal point in the dividend.

5. D. The number 4 is in the hundredth place. Look at the number to the right of it, which is 7. Seven is greater than 5 so add 1 to 4 to round off the number.

6. C. To solve this, restate the question as a decimal fraction by removing the per cent sign and moving the decimal point two places to the left. (The decimal fraction 0.31 is obtained.) Then multiply 0.31 by 105.

7. C. Remove the per cent sign and move the decimal point two places to the left.

8. B. Make the ratio on both sides into fractions by substituting slashes for colons; replace the double colon in the centre with an equals sign.

9. D. Substitute X for the amount of drug in 10 ml of solution; then set up a proportion with ratios or fractions and solve for X:

$$X : 10\,\text{ml} :: 20\,\text{mg} : 50\,\text{mg} \ \ or \ \ \frac{X}{10\ \text{ml}} = \frac{20\ \text{mg}}{50\ \text{ml}}$$

10. C. Multiply the means and the extremes. Put the products of the means and extremes into an equation. Solve for X by dividing both sides by 3. The calculation looks like this:

$$9 \times 9 = 3 \times X$$

$$81 = 3X$$

$$X = 27$$

11. B. Substitute X for the amount of chlorine bleach in 500 ml of water. Then set up a proportion with ratios or fractions and solve for X. The set up looks like this:

$$X \text{ ml bleach}/500 \text{ ml of water} = 10 \text{ ml bleach}/100 \text{ ml water}$$

or

$$X \text{ ml bleach} : 500 \text{ ml water} :: 10 \text{ ml bleach} : 100 \text{ ml water}$$

12. B. Use the conversion factor 2.2 lb equals 1 kg to find that 154 lb equals 70 kg.

13. A. Use the conversion factor 125 mg equals 5 ml to find that the patient should receive 10 ml.

14. D. Set up the following equation and solve for X (X represents the millilitres needed to administer 25 mg):

$$\frac{50 \text{ mg}}{1 \text{ ml}} = \frac{25 \text{ mg}}{X}$$

15. D. Using the *Amazing metric decimal place finder*, count the number of places to the right or left of litres to reach millilitres. In this case, it's three places to the right, so move the decimal point three places to the right.

16. C. Knowing that there are 1000 ml in 1 L, convert all the measurements to millilitres and add all the numbers together.

17. B. Knowing that 1 kg equals 1000 g, set up an equation with X as the unknown quantity:

$$\frac{1 \text{ kg}}{1000 \text{ kg}} = \frac{X}{8300 \text{ g}}$$

Cross-multiply and then divide both sides of the equation by 1000 g to isolate X, cancelling like units. Finish solving for X.

18. C. Using the *Insta-metric conversion table*, you'll see that 1 mg is equal to 1000 mcg. Set up the equation with X as the unknown quantity:

$$\frac{X}{250 \text{ mcg}} = \frac{1 \text{ mg}}{1000 \text{ mcg}}$$

Cross-multiply and then divide both sides of the equation by 1000 mg to isolate X, cancelling like units. Finish the calculation.

19. B. Set up the equation with X as the unknown quantity:

$$\frac{X}{10 \text{ units}} = \frac{1 \text{ ml}}{100 \text{ units}}$$

Cross-multiply both sides of the equation. To isolate X, divide both sides by 100 units. Finish the calculation.

20. A. Set up the equation using X as the unknown quantity:

$$\frac{X}{20 \text{ mmol}} = \frac{15 \text{ ml}}{60 \text{ mmol}}$$

Cross-multiply the fractions. Then find X by dividing both sides by 60 mmol to isolate X and cancel like units. Finish the calculation.

21. C. In the correct answer, daily is interpreted as 'every day' and 0900 represents 9 a.m. when using the 24-hour clock. Also, mg stands for milligrams not grams or micrograms.

22. B. This answer is incomplete because the unit of measure for the dose is missing.

23. D. SL is the abbreviation for sublingual, which means 'under the tongue'.

24. A. Scheduled drugs are considered on time if they're given half an hour before or after the prescribed time.

25. C. When a controlled substance is removed from the locked storage site, the date and time the dose is removed, the patient's full name, the prescriber's name, the drug dose and your signature must be recorded on the controlled inventory record. You may also be required to note the amount of the controlled substance remaining in the locked storage site.

26. B. Document the time of administration of a drug immediately after giving the drug to the patient to keep from mistakenly giving the drug again.

27. C. Set up the equation with 200 mg per 1 tablet as the known amount and X as the unknown factor:

$$\frac{200 \text{ mg}}{1 \text{ tablet}} = \frac{X}{2 \text{ tablets}}$$

Solve for X.

28. B. The generic name is the accepted non-proprietary name, which is a simplified form of the drug's chemical name.

29. D. Set up the equation with 2.5 mg equals 1 tablet as the known factor and X as the unknown factor:

$$\frac{2.5 \text{ mg}}{1 \text{ tablet}} = \frac{5 \text{ mg}}{X}$$

Solve for X.

30. C. Set up the equation with 125 mg per 1 supp as the known factor and X as the unknown factor:

$$125 \text{ mg} : 1 \text{ supp} :: 250 \text{ mg} : X$$

Solve for X.

31. D. Set up the equation with 30 mg equals 1 supp as the known factor and X as the unknown factor:

$$30\,\text{mg} : 1\,\text{supp} : : 15\,\text{mg} : X$$

Solve for X.

32. B. Topical preparations may contain one or more ingredients and you need to make sure the patient isn't allergic to any of them.

33. C. A new patch is applied daily (usually in the morning) and removed after 12 to 14 hours to prevent the patient from developing a tolerance to the drug.

34. C. Set up the equation with the known factor 20 mg/1 ml and X as the unknown factor:

$$\frac{20\,\text{mg}}{1\,\text{ml}} = \frac{10\,\text{mg}}{X}$$

Solve for X.

35. C. Set up the equation with 20 000 units/1 ml as the known factor and X as the unknown factor:

$$\frac{20\,000\,\text{units}}{1\,\text{ml}} = \frac{8000\,\text{units}}{X}$$

Solve for X.

36 B. Set up the equation with 100 units/1 ml as the known factor and X as the unknown factor:

$$\frac{100\,\text{units}}{1\,\text{ml}} = \frac{45\,\text{units}}{X}$$

Solve for X. Cross-multiply the fractions. Then find X by dividing both sides by 100 units to isolate X and cancel like units. Finish the calculation.

37. C. Convert hours to minutes. Then set up the equation using this formula to find drops/minute: total ml/total minutes × drop factor in drops/ml:

$$X = \frac{100\,\text{ml}}{60\,\text{min}} \times \frac{15\,\text{gtt}}{1\,\text{ml}}$$

Multiply the fraction by the drop factor and cancel like units. Solve for X by dividing the numerator by the demoninator.

38. D. Set up the equation using the formula: total volume ordered divided by the number of hours.

39. B. Set up the equation using 25 000 units/500 ml as the known factor and X ml as the unknown factor:

$$\frac{25\,000 \text{ units}}{500 \text{ ml}} = \frac{750 \text{ units}}{X}$$

Solve for X.

40. A. Divide the weight in pounds by 2.2 kg (1 kg = 2.2 lb), and round off the answer (20.9) to 21.

41. C. Set up the proportion with the ordered dosage in one fraction and the unknown dosage and the patient's weight in the other fraction:

$$\frac{10 \text{ mg}}{1 \text{ kg}} = \frac{X}{6 \text{ kg}}$$

Cross-multiply and solve for X.

42. B. First, convert the child's weight to kilograms by dividing by 2.2. Then calculate the dosage, remembering that the first 20 kg of a child's weight requires 1500 ml and each additional kilogram of weight requires 20 ml/kg. Because the child weighs 30 kg, he needs 1500 ml for the first 20 kg and 200 ml for the additional 10 kg of weight.

43. B. First determine the concentration of the solution by setting up the equation with 10 units/1000 ml as the known factor and X as the unknown factor:

$$\frac{10 \text{ units}}{1000 \text{ ml}} = \frac{X}{1 \text{ ml}}$$

Cross-multiply and solve for X. Then convert to milliunits by multiplying by 1000. Next, determine the flow rate by setting up the equation with 10 mU/1 ml as the known factor and 15 mU/X as the unknown factor:

$$\frac{10 \text{ mU}}{1 \text{ ml}} = \frac{15 \text{ mU}}{X}$$

Cross-multiply and solve for X. Convert to an hourly rate by multiplying by 4 (60 minutes/15 minutes = 4).

44. C. Using the calculation for the solution above, 10 mU/1 ml, determine that the patient needs 120 mU in 1 hour (2 mU/minute × 60 minutes). Set up the equation with 10 mU/1 ml as the known factor and 120 mU/X as the unknown factor:

$$\frac{10 \text{ mU}}{1 \text{ ml}} = \frac{120 \text{ mU}}{X}$$

Cross-multiply and solve for X.

45. D. Set up the equation with 4 g/250 ml as the known factor and 1 g/X as the unknown factor:

$$\frac{4\text{ g}}{250\text{ ml}} = \frac{1\text{ g}}{X}$$

Cross-multiply and solve for X. Round off the answer.

46. A. First find the fluid's strength by setting up the equation 150 mg/500 ml as the known factor and X/1 ml as the unknown factor:

$$\frac{150\text{ mg}}{500\text{ ml}} = \frac{X}{1\text{ ml}}$$

Cross-multiply and solve for X to determine 0.3 mg/ml of magnesium sulphate. Next, set up the equation with 1 ml/0.3 mg as the known factor and X/0.15 mg as the unknown factor:

$$\frac{1\text{ ml}}{0.3\text{ mg}} = \frac{X}{0.15\text{ mg}}$$

Cross-multiply and solve for X. Convert to hourly flow rate by multiplying by 60.

47. C. First, determine the concentration. It's easier to do this if you first convert the 25 mg of glyceryl trinitrate to micrograms by multiplying by 1000. Then divide this by the number of millilitres to determine the concentration of the solution. Then determine ml/hour by multiplying the ordered dose by 60 minutes and dividing by the concentration.

48. B. Multiply 1 g by 1000 to convert to milligrams. Then set up the equation with 1000 mg/250 ml as the known factor and X as the unknown factor to determine the concentration in 1 ml:

$$\frac{1000\text{ mg}}{250\text{ ml}} = \frac{X}{1\text{ ml}}$$

Cross-multiply and solve for X. Using this information, set up an equation with the concentration per millilitre as the known factor and 3 mg/X as the unknown factor:

$$\frac{4\text{ mg}}{1\text{ ml}} = \frac{3\text{ mg}}{X}$$

Cross-multiply and solve for X. You find 0.75 ml for 3 mg of lidocaine. Now set up the final equation to determine hourly flow rate with 0.75 ml/1 minute and X/60 minutes. Cross-multiply and solve for X.

49. D. First, convert 2 L to millilitres by setting up an equation with the conversion of 1000 ml/1 L:

$$\frac{1\ L}{1000\ ml} = \frac{2\ L}{X}$$

The total to be infused is 2000 ml.

Next, convert 16 hours to minutes by multiplying by 60 to determine that the solution needs to be infused over 960 minutes. Then determine the drip rate using the formula: total ml/total minutes × drop factor in drops/ml:

$$\text{Drip rate} = \frac{2000\ ml}{960\ min} \times \frac{20\ gtt}{ml}$$

Multiply the fraction by the drip rate and cancel like units. Then divide the numerator by the denominator, and round off the answer.

50. A. Use the formula: total volume ordered ÷ number of hours. In this case, it would be 500 ml ÷ 10 hours.

51. D. First, convert 12 hours to minutes by multiplying by 60 to determine that the fluid must be infused over 720 minutes. Then determine the drip rate using the formula: total ml/total minutes × drop factor in drops/ml.

$$\frac{4000\ ml}{720\ min} \times \frac{15\ gtt}{ml}$$

Multiply the fraction by the drip rate and cancel like units. Then divide the numerator by the denominator, and round off the answer.

52. A. First, determine the number of milligrams the patient is to receive per day by multiplying the desired dose per day (3 mg) by the weight in kilograms (68 kg). Then determine the number of milligrams to administer every 8 hours by dividing the total number of milligrams per day (204 mg) by 3. Lastly, determine the number of millilitres to administer every 8 hours by cross-multiplying the drug's available concentration (80 mg/2 ml) and the unknown factor (68 mg/X) and solving for X.

53. C. Convert the dose in micrograms to milligrams by dividing by 1000 (1 mg = 1000 mcg). Then set up an equation using 0.5 mg/tablet as the known factor, and 0.25 mg/X as the unknown factor:

$$\frac{0.5\ mg}{1\ tab} = \frac{0.25\ mg}{X}$$

Solve for X by cross-multiplying, dividing both sides by 0.5 mg, and cancelling units that appear in both the numerator and denominator. Because the tablet is scored, the nurse may administer ½ of a tablet.

54. B. Set up an equation using the drug's available concentration as the known factor, and the desired dose as the unknown factor:

$$\frac{125 \text{ mg}}{5 \text{ ml}} = \frac{250 \text{ mg}}{X}$$

Cross-multiply and solve for X, cancelling units that appear in both the numerator and denominator.

55. D. Determine the number of tablets to administer by setting up an equation using 50 mg/tablet as the known factor and 75 mg/X as the unknown factor, and solve for X. Because the tablet is unscored, the nurse shouldn't break it in half to administer the necessary 1½ tablet dose. The nurse must call the pharmacy to have the dose sent as a single tablet or, if this is unavailable, the pharmacist should crush and measure out the tablet so that the nurse may administer the most accurate dosage.

56. D. First, determine the number of milligrams per dose by multiplying the infant's weight in kg (2.3 kg) by the ordered dose (2.5 mg/kg). Then cross-multiply the known drug concentration (2 mg/1 ml) by the unknown factor (5.75 mg/X) and solve for X to calculate the number of millilitres to administer for each dose.

57. C. Multiply the child's weight in kilograms (3.6 kg) by 15 ml/kg to determine the total volume of the blood transfusion. Calculate the hourly flow rate by dividing the total volume of the transfusion (54 ml) by the number of hours (4).

58. 2.5 ml. Determine the concentration of the solution in milligrams using the conversion factor 1 g = 1000 mg. Calculate the final concentration of the solution by cross-multiplying the known factor of 1000 mg/10 ml and the unknown factor of X/1 ml, to get the final concentration of 100 mg/1 ml. Then calculate the dose in millilitres:

$$\frac{100 \text{ mg}}{1 \text{ ml}} = \frac{250 \text{ mg}}{X}$$

Cross-multiply, and solve for X by dividing both sides of the equation by 100 mg and cancelling units that appear in the numerator and denominator.

59. 0.4 ml. First, determine the required dose in millilitres using 100 mg/1 ml as the known factor and 60 mg/X as the unknown factor. The patient should receive 0.6 ml of morphine sulphate. Subtract the volume of the dose (0.6 ml) from the total volume of the vial (1 ml) to determine the volume to be discarded.

60. B, C, D. Commit frequently used conversion factors to memory to administer dosages quickly and accurately.

Drug therapy conversions

Metric weight	
1 kilogram (kg)	= 1000 grams (g)
1 g	= 1000 milligrams (mg)
1 mg	= 1000 micrograms (mcg)
0.6 g	= 600 mg
0.3 g	= 300 mg
0.1 g	= 100 mg
0.06 g	= 60 mg
0.03 g	= 30 mg
0.015 g	= 15 mg
0.001 g	= 1 mg

Metric volume	
1 litre (L)	= 1000 millilitres (ml)
1 ml	= 1000 microlitres (µl)

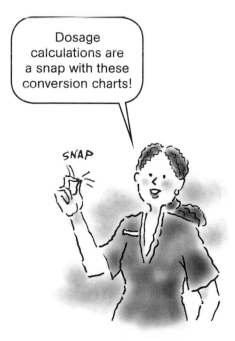

Dosage calculations are a snap with these conversion charts!

SNAP

Weight conversion

To convert a patient's weight in pounds to kilograms, divide the number of pounds by 2.2 kg.

Pounds	Kilograms
10	4.5
20	9.1
30	13.6
40	18.2
50	22.7
60	27.3
70	31.8
80	36.4
90	40.9
100	45.5
110	50
120	54.5
130	59.1
140	63.6
150	68.2
160	72.7
170	77.3
180	81.8
190	86.4
200	90.9

Temperature conversion

To convert Fahrenheit to Celsius, subtract 32 from the temperature in Fahrenheit and then divide by 1.8.

$$(F - 32) \div 1.8 = \text{degrees Celsius}$$

Degrees Fahrenheit (°F)	Degrees Celsius (°C)	Degrees Fahrenheit (°F)	Degrees Celsius (°C)
89.6	32	101	38.3
91.4	33	101.2	38.4
93.2	34	101.4	38.6
94.3	34.6	101.8	38.8
95	35	102	38.9
95.4	35.2	102.2	39
96.2	35.7	102.6	39.2
96.8	36	102.8	39.3
97.2	36.2	103	39.4
97.6	36.4	103.2	39.6
98	36.7	103.4	39.7
98.6	37	103.6	39.8
99	37.2	104	40
99.3	37.4	104.4	40.2
99.7	37.6	104.6	40.3
100	37.8	104.8	40.4
100.4	38	105	40.6
100.8	38.2		

Dosage calculation formulas

Calculating drip rates

When calculating the flow rate of I.V. solutions, remember that the number of drops required to deliver 1 ml varies with the type of administration set you're using. To calculate the drip rate, you must know the calibration of the drip rate for each specific manufacturer's product. As a quick guide, refer to the chart below. Use this formula to calculate specific drip rates:

$$\frac{\text{volume of infusion (in ml)}}{\text{time of infusion (in minutes)}} \times \text{drip factor (in drops/ml)} = \text{drops/minute}$$

	Prescribed volume					
	500 ml/24 hour or 21 ml/hour	1000 ml/24 hour or 42 ml/hour	1000/20 hour or 50 ml/hour	1000/10 hour or 100 ml/hour	1000 ml/8 hour or 125 ml/hour	1000 ml/6 hour or 166 ml/hour
Drops/ml	Drops/minute to infuse					
Macrodrip						
15	5	11	13	25	31	42
20	7	14	17	33	42	55
Microdrip						
60	21	42	50	100	125	166

Common calculation formulas

$$\text{body surface area in m}^2 = \sqrt{\frac{\text{height in cm} \times \text{weight in kg}}{3600}}$$

$$\text{mcg/ml} = \text{mg/ml} \times 1000$$

$$\text{ml/minute} = \frac{\text{ml/hour}}{60}$$

$$\text{gtt/minute} = \frac{\text{volume in ml to be infused}}{\text{time in minutes}} \times \text{drip factor in gtt/ml}$$

$$\text{mg/minute} = \frac{\text{mg in bag}}{\text{ml in bag}} \times \text{flow rate} \div 60$$

$$\text{mcg/minute} = \frac{\text{mg in bag}}{\text{ml in bag}} \div 0.06 \times \text{flow rate}$$

$$\text{mcg/kg/minute} = \frac{\text{mcg/ml} \times \text{ml/minute}}{\text{weight in kilograms}}$$

Glossary

body surface area (BSA): The area covered by a person's external skin calculated in square metres (m²) according to height and weight; used to calculate safe paediatric dosages for all drugs and safe dosages for adult patients receiving extremely potent drugs or drugs requiring great precision, such as anti-neoplastic and chemotherapeutic agents.

common factor: A number that's a factor of two different numbers (for example, 2 is a common factor of 4 and 6).

common fraction: A fraction with a whole number in both the numerator and denominator (such as ⁷⁄₁₂).

complex fraction: A fraction in which the numerator and the denominator are fractions, such as:

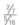

concentration: A ratio that expresses the amount of a drug in a solution; sometimes called *drug strength*.

denominator: The bottom number in a fraction, which represents the total number of equal parts of a whole (for example, in the fraction ⁷⁄₁₀, the denominator is 10).

dividend: In division, the number to be divided (for example, in the problem 33 ÷ 7, 33 is the dividend).

divisor: In division, the number by which the dividend is divided (for example, in the problem 33 ÷ 7, 7 is the divisor).

dosage: The amount, frequency and number of doses of a drug.

dose: The amount of a drug to be given at one time.

drip rate: The number of drops of I.V. solution to be infused per minute; based on the drop factor (number of drops delivered per millilitre) and calibrated for the selected I.V. tubing.

drop factor: The number of drops to be delivered per millilitre of solution in an I.V. administration set; measured in gtt/ml (drops per millilitre); listed on the package containing the I.V. tubing administration set.

enteral: Within or by way of the small intestine.

equianalgesic dose: Amount of an opioid analgesic that provides the same pain relief as 10 mg of I.M. morphine; used to recalculate the necessary dose when substituting one analgesic for another.

flow rate: The number of millilitres of I.V. fluid to administer over 1 hour; based on the total volume to be infused in millilitres and the amount of time for the infusion.

fraction: A representation of the division of one number by another number; mathematical expression for parts of a whole, with the bottom number (denominator) describing the total number of parts and the top number (numerator) describing the parts of the whole being considered (for example, ½, ⅓, ⁷⁄₁₈).

generic name: The accepted non-proprietary name, which is a simplified form of the drug's chemical name.

glucometer: A device used to calculate blood glucose levels – and, thereby, insulin levels – from one drop of blood.

gram (g): The basic unit of weight in the metric system; represents the weight of one cubic centimetre of water at 4°C.

improper fraction: A fraction in which the numerator is larger than or equal to the denominator, such as ³⁄₂, ¹⁰⁄₇, and ⁵⁄₅.

International System of Units: (abbreviated **SI** from the French-*Système International d'Unités*) system adopted in 1960 by the International Bureau of Weights and Measures to promote the use of standard metric abbreviations to prevent drug transcription errors.

intradermal route: Drug administration into the dermis of the skin.

intramuscular (I.M.) route: Drug administration into a muscle.

intravenous (I.V.) route: Drug administration into a vein.

largest common divisor: In a fraction, the largest whole number that can be divided into both the numerator and denominator of a fraction (for example, in the fraction ⁸⁄₁₀, the largest common divisor is 2).

litre (L): A basic unit of fluid volume in the metric system; equivalent to the volume of 1 kg of water at 4°C and standard temperature and pressure.

lowest common denominator: The smallest number that's a multiple of all denominators in a set of fractions; also called least common multiple (for example, for the fractions, ¹⁄₁₀₀ and ³⁄₁₅₀, the lowest common denominator is 300).

lowest terms: In a fraction, the smallest numbers possible in the numerator and denominator. (Reduce a fraction to its lowest terms by dividing the numerator and denominator by the largest common divisor. For example, in the fraction $\frac{3}{15}$, divide both the numerator and denominator by 3, the largest common divisor, to find $\frac{1}{5}$, the lowest terms of this fraction.)

metre (m): The basic unit of length in the metric system; equivalent to 39.37 inches.

metric system: A decimal-based measurement system that uses the units metre (for length), litre (for volume) and gram (for weight); the most widely used system for measuring amounts of drugs.

millimole (mmol): A measurement of concentration defined as one thousandth of a gram molecule; used to measure electrolytes.

mixed number: A number that consists of a whole number and a fraction (such as $1\frac{1}{2}$).

multiplied common denominator: For a set of fractions, the product of all the denominators, which is found by multiplying all the denominators together (for example, for the fractions, $\frac{1}{2}$, $\frac{2}{3}$ and $\frac{3}{5}$, multiply the denominators together to find the multiplied common denominator, which is 30 [$2 \times 3 \times 5 = 30$]).

non-parenteral drugs: Drugs administered by the oral, topical or rectal route, as opposed to drugs administered by the parenteral route.

nomogram: A chart used to determine body surface area in square metres, based on the patient's height and weight.

numerator: The top number in a fraction, which represents the number of parts being considered (for example, in the fraction $\frac{7}{10}$, the numerator is 7).

oral route (P.O.): Drug administration through the mouth.

parenteral route: Drug administration through a route other than the digestive tract, such as I.V., I.M. and subcutaneous means.

percentage: A quantity stated as a part per hundred; written with a per cent sign (%), which means 'for every hundred' (for example, 50% represents 50 parts out of 100 total parts).

prime factor: Prime numbers that can be divided into some part of a mathematical expression such as the denominators in a set of fractions; used to find the lowest common denominator for a set of fractions (for example, the prime factors for the denominators in the fractions $\frac{1}{10}$ and $\frac{2}{3}$ are 5, 2 and 3).

prime number: A whole number that's evenly divisible only by 1 and itself, such as 2, 3, 5 and 7.

product: The answer of a multiplication problem (for example, in the equation, $4 \times 5 = 20$, the product is 20).

proper fraction: A fraction with a numerator that's smaller than the denominator (such as $\frac{1}{2}$).

proportion: A set of equivalent ratios or fractions (an example of a proportion expressed by ratios is 2 : 3 :: 8 : 12, which is read as '2 is to 3 as 8 is to 12'. The same proportion expressed with fractions is $\frac{2}{3} = \frac{8}{12}$).

quotient: The answer of a division problem (for example, in the equation $20 \div 5 = 4$, the quotient is 4).

ratio: A numerical way to compare items or show a relationship between numbers, with numbers separated by a colon, which represents the words, 'is to' (for example, the ratio 4 : 5 is read as '4 is to 5'; ratios are commonly used to describe the relative proportions of ingredients such as the amount of drug relative to its solution).

reciprocal: An inverted fraction; used when dividing fractions (for example, to divide $\frac{1}{2}$ by $\frac{2}{3}$, multiply $\frac{1}{2}$ by the reciprocal of $\frac{2}{3}$, which is $\frac{3}{2}$; in other words, $\frac{1}{2} \div \frac{2}{3} = \frac{1}{2} \times \frac{3}{2} = \frac{3}{4}$; when a fraction is multiplied by its reciprocal, the

product is 1; for example, the reciprocal of the fraction $\frac{2}{3}$ is $\frac{3}{2}$, and $\frac{2}{3} \times \frac{3}{2} = \frac{6}{6}$ or 1).

rectal route: Drug administration (usually by suppository) through the rectum.

reduce: To simplify a numerical expression by using the lowest possible numbers – or lowest terms – to describe it (for example, the fraction $\frac{15}{45}$ may be reduced to $\frac{1}{3}$).

rounding off: Reducing the number of decimal places used to express a number (for example, a decimal fraction that's expressed in thousandths may be rounded off to the nearest hundredths or tenths; the number 12.827 rounded off to the nearest hundredth is 12.83; the same number rounded off to the nearest tenths is 12.8).

subcutaneous route: Drug administration into the subcutaneous tissue.

topical route: Drug administration through the skin (after absorption through the skin layers, the drug enters circulation), usually in cream, ointment or transdermal patch form.

trade name: The drug's name given by the manufacturer; also called the brand or proprietary name.

transcribe: To transfer information from one type of form to another.

transdermal route: Drug administration in which the drug is absorbed continuously through the skin and enters the systemic system.

unit system: A measurement system that expresses the amount of a drug in units, or International units (IU). Drugs measured in units include insulin, heparin, the topical antibiotic bacitracin, benzylpenicillin and phenoxypenicillin. The hormone calcitonin and the fat-soluble vitamins A, D and E are measured in International Units.

Selected references

Abrams, A.C., Pennington, S.S. and Lamman, C.B. *Clinical Drug Therapy: Rationales for Nursing Practice*, 8th ed. Philadelphia: Lippincott Williams & Wilkins, 2006.

Aschenbrenner, S.D. and Venable, S.J. *Drug Therapy in Nursing*, 2nd ed. Philadelphia: Lippincott Williams & Wilkins, 2007.

Brown, M. and Mulholland, J.L. *Drug Calculations: Process & Problems for Clinical Practice*, 8th ed. St. Louis: Mosby, 2007.

Buchholz, S. *Henke's Med-Math*, 6th ed. Philadelphia: Lippincott Williams & Wilkins, 2008.

Cohen, H. et al. Getting to the root of medication errors: survey results. *Nursing* 33: 36–45, 2003.

Conroy, S. et al. Interventions to reduce dosing errors in children: a systematic review of the literature. *Drug Safety* 30: 1111–25, 2007.

Craig, G.P. *Clinical Calculations Made Easy: Solving Problems Using Dimensional Analysis*, 4th ed. Philadelphia: Lippincott Williams & Wilkins, 2008.

Ford, N.A. et al. Administration of I.V. medications via Soluset. *Pediatric Nursing* 29: 283–6, 319, 2003.

Gray Morris, D.C. *Calculate with Confidence*, 4th ed. St. Louis: Mosby, 2006.

Greenfield, S., Whelan, B. and Cohen, E. Use of dimensional analysis to reduce medication errors. *Journal of Nurse Education* 45: 91–4, 2006.

Greengold, N.L. et al. The impact of dedicated medication nurses on the medication administration error rate: a randomized controlled trial. *Archives of Internal Medicine* 163: 2359–67, 2003.

Griffith, R., and Davies, R. Tablet crushing and the law: the implications for nursing. *Professional Nurse* 19: 41–2, 2003.

Guy, J. et al. Drug errors: what role do nurses and pharmacists have in minimizing the risks? *Journal of Child Health Care* 7: 277–90, 2003.

Karch, A.M. *Focus on Nursing Pharmacology*, 4th ed. Philadelphia: Lippincott Williams & Wilkins, 2007.

Kee, J.L. and Marshall, S.M. *Clinical Calculations: Applications to General and Specialty Areas*, 6th ed. Philadelphia: W.B. Saunders, 2006.

Lehne, R.A. *Pharmacology for Nursing Care*, 6th ed. Philadelphia: W.B. Saunders, 2007.

Macklin, D., Chernecky, C.C. and Infortuna, H. *Math for Clinical Practice*. St. Louis: Mosby, 2005.

Manias, E. et al. Self-administration of medication in hospital: patients' perspectives. *Journal of Advanced Nursing* 46: 194–203, 2004.

Nursing 2008 Drug Handbook, 28th ed. Philadelphia: Lippincott Williams & Wilkins, 2007.

Ogden, S.J. *Calculation of Drug Dosages*, 7th ed. St. Louis: Mosby, 2003.

Pharmacology: A 2-in-1 Reference for Nurses. Philadelphia: Lippincott Williams & Wilkins, 2004.

Roach, S.S. and Ford, S.M. *Introductory Clinical Pharmacology*, 8th ed. Philadelphia: Lippincott Williams & Wilkins, 2007.

Springhouse Nurse's Drug Guide 2005, 6th ed. Philadelphia: Lippincott Williams & Wilkins, 2004.

Straight A's in Nursing Pharmacology, 2nd ed. Philadelphia: Lippincott Williams & Wilkins, 2003.

Wright, K. Barriers to accurate drug calculations. *Nursing Standard* 20: 41–5, 2006.

Yaffe, S.J. and Aranda, J.V. *Neonatal and Pediatric Pharmacology: Therapeutic Principles in Practice*, 3rd ed. Philadelphia: Lippincott Williams & Wilkins, 2004.

Additional resources

British National Formulary, www.bnf.org

National Institute for Health and Clinical Excellence, www.nice.org.uk

Paediatric Drug Information Advisory Line, tel: 0151 252 5837

National Poisons Information Service, tel: 0844 892 0111

Index

A

Abbreviations
dangerous, 138
in metric measurements, 84
in prescriptions, 110,
misinterpreted, and drug errors,
131, 137
a.d., 138
Administration errors. *See* Drug errors.
Administration records,
documentation in, 122–126. *See
also* Documentation.
record-keeping systems for, 119–121
review of, 127
Administration routes. *See specific route.*
Allergies, and drug errors, 133–134
Analgesic, converting dosages of, 163
Andropatch, 175
a.s., 138
a.u., 138

B

Bags, I.V., 92, 115, 216, 225i
Benzyl penicillin, 198
Blood and blood product infusions,
237–238
B.P., 153
Body surface area method, of dosage
calculation, 254
British National Formulary, 115, 137
British Pharmacopeia, 153

C

Calculators, 37, 161, 248
Calories, calculating paediatric fluid
needs based on, 265
Capsule administration, precautions
for, 162
cc, 85

Centi, 89
Centilitres,
converting, to litres, 88–89
Centimetres
converting inches to, 103
cubic, 85
Charting, computer, 120
Charts, equianalgesic, 163
Children. *See* Paediatric.
Climara, 175
Closed-system device, 191
Co-amoxiclav, 153
Codeine, converting dosages of, 163
Combination products, topical and
allergies, 174
Common denominator
finding, 8–15
lowest, 8–10
Common-fraction equations, 50–53
Common fractions,
converting
to decimal fractions, 32
to percentages, 37–38
converting decimal fractions to, 33–34
converting percentages to, 35–37
in dimensional analysis, 70–75
Complex fractions,
dividing, 21, 223,
simplifying, 21
Computer charting, 120
Controlled inventory record, 125
Controlled substance
documenting, 125
Conversion factors,
common, 70
Conversions
between measurement systems,
70–75, 102–104, 169
drug therapy, 317–318
equivalent measure, 102–103
metric, 86–89

Co-trimoxazole, 152
Critical care drugs,
common, 286
flow rates for, 288–293
hypertension and, 293
hypotension and, 294
infusing, 285, 290
review of, 295
Cross product principle, 59i
Cross products, 59
Cubic centimetre, 85

D

D/C, 138
Deca, 85, 87
Deci, 85, 87
Decimal-fraction equations, solving, 54–56
Decimal fractions,
adding and subtracting, 28–29
converting, to common fractions,
33–34
converting mixed numbers to, 32–33
converting percentages to, 35
dividing, 29–30, 31
multiplying, 29
rounding off, 30–32
Decimal numbers, 26
zeroes in, 27
Decimal place, 26, 32, 87
Decimal place finder, in metric
conversions, 87
Decimal points, 26
aligning, 28, 30
and medication errors, 138
in division problems, 29–30, 31
Decimals,
multiplying, 29
review of, 43–44
Denominator,
common. *See* Common denominator.
in dimensional analysis, 69

t refers to a table; i refers to an illustration